Medicine and the American Revolution

Medicine and the American Revolution

How Diseases and Their Treatments Affected the Colonial Army

by

OSCAR REISS, M.D.

McFarland & Company, Inc., Publishers
Jefferson, North Carolina and London

The present work is a reprint of the library bound edition of Medicine and the American Revolution: How Diseases and Their Treatments Affected the Colonial Army, *first published in 1998 by McFarland.*

LIBRARY OF CONGRESS CATALOGUING-IN-PUBLICATION DATA

Reiss, M.D., Oscar, 1925–
    Medicine and the American Revolution : how diseases and their treatments affected the colonial army
        p.   cm.
    Includes bibliographical references and index.

    ISBN 0-7864-2160-6 (softcover : 50# alkaline paper)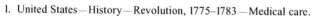

    1. United States—History—Revolution, 1775–1783—Medical care.
    2. Medicine, Military—United States—History—18th century.
    I. Title.
    E283.R45   2005
    973.3'75—dc21   98-20088

British Library cataloguing data are available

On the cover: *background* smallpox (Library of Congress); *foreground* ©2005 ClipArt.com

Manufactured in the United States of America

McFarland & Company, Inc., Publishers
  Box 611, Jefferson, North Carolina 28640
  www.mcfarlandpub.com

This book is dedicated to the people of Bristol, Connecticut. I came among you armed only with my craft. You accepted me as one of your own, and I prospered. In your small-town, New England atmosphere, we raised five children to be law-abiding, productive, contributing members of society. We have left Connecticut because of my failing health but our minds, our hearts, and our roots will always be in Bristol.

Acknowledgments

Most of my information came from the stacks at the University of California, San Diego Medical Library. I want particularly to thank Patricia Kinnison and Diane Eells for breaking the logjam of bureaucracy at the library. With their help and a letter from the Medical Branch of the Library of Congress, I was able to study old articles and manuscripts sent from libraries in other parts of the country. The undergraduate library on the campus afforded me access to the nonmedical literature of the Revolution. (My only complaint is that they have no facilities to make it easy for disabled people to get to the library.) I also received help from the Mira Mesa Branch of the San Diego Library, and particularly John Stevens, librarian. The local library branch can obtain any book in the entire library system within 48 hours. Although I singled out a few librarians who were very helpful to me, I'd like to tip my hat to librarians in general. There must be something in their personality or make-up that prompts them to choose this profession. To paraphrase Will Rogers, "I never met a librarian I didn't like." They have always been cheerful, friendly, and eager to help me.

During my research, I returned to Connecticut several times to visit with old friends. I used the Medical Library at the University of Connecticut in beautiful Farmington on several occasions. While at home, I visited the Historical Museum of Medicine and Dentistry of the Hartford Medical and Dental Society, where Diane Newman, librarian, was most helpful in directing me to exhibits and literature in the shelves.

I want to thank Kim Moore Cavanaugh of Morristown, New Jersey. Kim was a classmate of my wife's at Vassar and is a historian herself. She directed me to Allen Stein, librarian at the Morristown National Park Library, who supplied me with a massive bibliography of material related to the Revolution and, specifically, to the Morristown encampments.

Finally, I must acknowledge my wife, Elinor, for her patience and forbearance. I locked myself in the end bedroom while writing this text with a resultant loss of social engagements. Elinor was careful not to move my papers while trying to clean around me. In addition, I depended on her knowledge of English grammar and her writing ability to edit this text.

Contents

Preface

I started this project with the idea of writing a book on the medical aspects of the American Revolution. My early research soon showed that the "pickings" were limited. The physicians and surgeons involved in the war were too busy, too unimpressed with their activities, or too marginally literate to leave reports of the medical problems related to the fighting. Most modern writers refer to Dr. Thacher's *Military Journal on the Revolution*, but I found it to be more military than medical. The journal left by Isaac Senter on the invasion of Canada through Maine had more medical material. However, the fact that Senter asked the commanding officer, Benedict Arnold, for permission to leave his hospital and lead a company in the assault on Quebec tells us something about his attitude toward medicine. Posterity and Senter himself benefited when Arnold advised him, "Shoemaker, stick to your last,"—my words, not Arnold's. The attack was a fiasco, with many soldiers killed or wounded and many taken as prisoners of war.

Accounts of the war offer at best a bird's eye view of the events. Any reasonable public library has shelves or sections devoted to the Revolution and its participants. I could not hope to compete with the accumulation of knowledge about the events of this era so vital to our history. Rather, I have used the Revolution's battles and progress like the cord used to string pearls, the "pearls" being the illnesses I have associated with the battles and the progression of the war. I hope I have not fallen into the trap of fixing on a particular disease and attempting to prove that it was responsible for the outcome of a war. Medical historians have blamed smallpox for the loss of Canada, syphilis for the end of the Siege of Naples, typhus for the retreat of Napoleon's Grand Army from Russia, and so on. I am aware that illness caused far more casualties than actual fighting in the wars of the past. However, most leaders of mercenary armies did not worry about the individuals in their "pickup" armies. Furthermore, bacteria and viruses did not choose sides. Malaria incapacitated both sides in the battles in the southern states, and typhus was magnanimous in bestowing its favors on all participants. It was true that British troops had greater immunity to smallpox than their antagonists in the American armies, but the replacement for a lost British soldier had to be pulled off the streets of London or another English city, placed on board a leaky wooden ship, exposed to enteric disease, malnutrition, and scurvy, and then deposited on a foreign shore where climatic differences as well as "bugs" foreign to his immune system awaited him. Furthermore, the average British infantryman did not fully understand the reasons for his involvement in the war, or care passionately about its outcome. The Americans, whether Patriot or Tory, were strongly motivated by their cause. The point is that disease, while important, was only one of many factors determining the outcome of a battle or war. I hope my associates in the field of medical history will not accuse me of heresy.

This book does not attempt to provide a general history of the American Revolution. For example, I have not mentioned the war in western New York State in which the Patriots fought Tories, a few British troops, and native tribes. Perhaps it deserves inclusion because of the nature of the wounds produced by the native Americans. More interesting to an internist like myself, however, is the suggestion of an outbreak of ergotism in western New York State because of an infestation of the fungus *Claviceps purpurea* in the grain used to make the bread to supply the Patriots. I saw only one brief reference to this problem, and I could mention it only in passing. I assume it was not as drastic as the outbreaks in Europe described in more recent medicine. Similarly, I have not discussed the westward expeditions by men like George Rogers Clark.

Finally, I want to briefly explain my interest in the Revolution. In college, too many years ago, I took a course in colonial American history. There was no textbook, and we were required to read a book each week on any subject related to the period. This was the start of a lifelong interest in that era. I have always envied those people who could combine their vocations and avocations to produce a full life. This book has been my opportunity.

In closing, I must acknowledge my frequent use of the American Heritage book of *The Revolution* as well as Commager's *Spirit of '76* to refresh my memory about some of the events in our War of Independence.

— 1 —

Army Medicine

Care of the Army in Camp and in Action

Before we plunge into the American Revolution, some general discussion of the care of soldiers in the field and in camp is in order. From early historical times to the present, the treatment of casualties depended on the nature of the army. In the classical city-states of Greece and the armies of Rome, as in our own era, a citizen army was cared for to the best ability of the state. These men represented the wealth of their nation. On the other hand, from the mercenary armies of Carthage to the pillaging rabble of the Middle Ages, soldiers were given short shrift. They took care of their illnesses and injuries as well as they could. The disabled veteran lived or died without assistance from a "grateful" nation.

Aesculapius was a naval surgeon on the Argonautic expedition of Castor and Pollux (1263 B.C.). (His care of his charges, both in the navy and as a civilian doctor, was so good that they made him a god. A doctor cannot do better than that, but some act that way.) His sons, Machaeon and Podalirius, were military surgeons in the expedition against Troy (1192 B.C.). They were not as good as their father, and they remained mortals. Pythagoras, of the theorem, was an army physician who treated King Darius's dislocated ankle and Queen Atossa's breast cancer. Pythagoras was a prisoner of war at the time.[1] Cyrus of Persia (530 B.C.) appointed the best physicians and surgeons to care for his troops. In Alexander's army the wounded were carried on the backs of fellow soldiers. Xenophon publicly scourged a soldier who tried to bury his wounded comrade to get rid of the load. Glaucus, a surgeon, was crucified because he could not save Haephiston; the relationship between Alexander and young Haephiston having been something more than that of comrades-in-arms. Hannibal had doctors to accompany his troops, but they carried off and disposed of the wounded to prevent the rest of the army from observing the pain of war wounds. Doctors accompanied Roman armies and supervised their food, clothing, hygiene, camp location, and exercise. Caesar had any of his troops who were sick or wounded brought back to the valetudinareum, a part of the camp set aside for casualties (i.e., a hospital). There was one surgeon per legion of 7,000 men.[2] Leon VI of Byzantium had surgeons and field hospitals for his troops in the ninth century. One function of his cavalry was to transport the wounded back to the surgeon as soon as possible. The casualty was carried in leather straps on the left side of the horse. In the Byzantine army there was one surgeon for every 250 men as well as six to eight stretcher bearers. The Norman lords had personal armies and hired doctors ("leeches") to care for them. During the crusades, the Knights of St. John of Jerusalem cared for sick pilgrims and crusaders.

In the Middle Ages in England, surgeons and physicians were hired for the duration of the war. They were in the king's retinue and cared for the king and his staff. Casualties were sent to monasteries, local homes, or back to their own home if they were able to travel. Edward I of England set up the first military medical service in his war against Scotland (1298–1300). A surgeon in Edward II's army received four pence per day. One of his duties was to shave the soldiers. The severely wounded were frequently killed by their comrades because they were aware that the surgeon had little to offer them.

The King of England paid army surgeons. In addition, each soldier had some of his pay withheld to add to the surgeon's salary (called stoppages). During the reign of James I of England, the concept of an army medical staff developed. Two physicians were appointed to the forces at six shillings eight pence per day. In addition, two apothecaries received three shillings four pence per day. Every regiment of 1,800 had one surgeon who earned four shillings. He had twelve assistants who received one shilling each. In 1620 a surgeon major to the camp was appointed. Charles II in 1660 developed a standing army and created a need for permanent career army surgeons. They were regimental officers who purchased their positions. Some were combatants as well; that way they could purchase an ensign's commission and then receive two salaries.[3] Supplies were limited, and soldiers paid for medicine. If the soldier became sick, his pay stopped. William III developed the concept of the "marching hospital," one of which accompanied his army in Ireland. Marlborough developed collecting or regimental aid posts to supply first aid. Medical officers of higher rank were needed to staff the medical service of the army. A physician general, surgeon general, and an apothecary general were appointed. In addition, a physician was a member of the staff of the commanding general. In 1756 the English secretary of war established a hospital board for the medical service.

Care of Veterans

The care of casualties after the war was an expression of the level of civilization of the society that sent its sons to war. In 222 B.C., after the defeat of the Spartans at Sellasia, every house in Sparta opened its doors to refresh the wounded and bind their wounds. Ancient Greek cities gave pensions to their disabled soldiers. The citizen army of Republican Rome also cared for its casualties. They carried their wounded with them after a battle and stayed with them until they could move or a safe place could be found for them. In 478 B.C. Fabii distributed the wounded to the patricians to be nursed back to health. Aurelian (270–275 A.D.) proclaimed free medical care for soldiers. The Romans set up colonies for their disabled veterans, where they could hold land without paying taxes. The government supplied seeds, fruit, cattle, and money to run their farms. Byzantium put up asylums for its disabled veterans. The Swiss Confederation antedated the rest of pre–Renaissance Europe in its care for veterans. There were municipal ordinances notifying soldiers of their rights. Swiss archives show that after 1330 payments were made to the wounded and their dependents. The Swiss paid barber-surgeons to take care of the wounded after a battle. Zurich ordered that the wounded were to receive full pay as long as the army was in the field. In 1467 Berne and later Basel sent barbers (surgeons) along with their troops. In 1476 Zurich ordered that living expenses and medical care for veterans were to be paid out of the common purse. The Swiss spent 300 guilders to care for 200 wounded. Zurich also protected the property of children orphaned by war. In 1499 the Bernese voted that all booty captured was to be used to maintain the wounded and care for widows and orphans of the slain. After the battle of Kappel in 1536, Zurich paid 1,358 pounds for the care of the wounded and sent the convalescents to mineral baths. Those wounded who could not be transported were treated locally.

The French soon followed the Swiss in the care of their sons wounded in war. An ambulance hospital (a moving hospital that followed battle lines so that soldiers could be treated as early as possible) was established at the siege of Amiens by Sully, minister to Henry IV in 1597. Henry IV also ordered that the House of Christian Charity in Paris was to be used to care for destitute and disabled soldiers, as well as for widows and orphans of those killed in battle. During the reign of Louis XIV, disabled soldiers received pensions of 30 to 50 livres; officers received 300 to 400 livres. In 1676 Louis XIV used the Hôtel Royal des Invalides for his disabled veterans.

In 1643 the parliament of England ordered the collection of funds for relief of disabled soldiers, widows, and orphans. Charles II had the first peacetime standing army with permanent enlistments. His disabled troops were cared for in a domiciliary. Chelsea Hospital, started in 1681 and completed in 1692, was built to house 500 disabled veterans, and the public had to pay for its upkeep. The Greenwich seaman's hospital in 1695 did the same for seamen. James II in 1685 offered a pension for one year for the loss of an eye or limb if certified by the surgeon general. Frederick the Great of Prussia was most careful with his human resources. He ruled a country with a small population, but he had plans for conquest and expansion. In 1746 he allotted 40,000 thaler for veterans' care (the thaler was a German silver coin, the unit of their currency equal to two shillings, eleven pence). Two years later he founded the Invalid's House for medical pensioners, and he built more garrison hospitals. The emperor also increased the number of surgeons to care for the pensioners.[4]

In early Colonial America, attempts were made to care for soldiers. As early as 1636, Plymouth Colony passed a law to care for its soldiers injured in wars with the Indians. They were supported for life. Virginia and Rhode Island soon followed this lead. The newly formed United States, restricted by a lack of money, also tried to care for its soldiers. In 1776 Congress made provisions for pensions to invalid soldiers and officers. Officers received one-half pay for total disability and proportionate amounts for partial disability. The ranks received about $5 per month. However, poor records were kept, and a lack of funds prevented adequate payment to the 6,000 wounded in the war. Several of the states passed minimal laws to care for their wounded.[5]

Examination of Recruits

The early citizen armies were composed of men who put aside their agricultural tools and took up the tools of war. Any man who could wrest a living from the soil could carry a sword or spear. In the armies of the Middle Ages, anyone who wanted to join did so. As experience developed and a professional cadre replaced the "pickup" army, leaders learned what to look for in a soldier. Regulations for fitness of potential recruits were spelled out. Men from the country were preferred. It was believed that they could bear the vicissitudes of weather, could carry larger burdens, and were more active and sober than their city brothers. Foot soldiers had to be five feet four inches, dragoons or hussars five feet three inches to five feet four inches, grenadiers five feet five inches to five feet six inches (these were eighteenth-century standards). The acceptable age for a recruit was 18 to 25. Men could remain in the army until age 40. After 40, the body was thought to be weighty and stiff. The recruits were examined by a medical officer and a line officer. The potential soldier had to be sound of body and limbs, free of skin ulcers, without venereal disease, rupture, itch, or scrofula. Habitual drunkards or epileptics were rejected. (Doctors were aware of convulsions in habitual drunkards.) Potential recruits sometimes tried to hide medical problems. The medical officer was instructed to examine the movements of the recruit's body and limbs. A compressed (concave) chest was a sign of weakness and poor health, as were a pale face and dull eyes. Medical officers were advised to turn down those with bowed legs, poor respiration, chronic cough, scrofula scars, mutilation of the "noble parts," herniae, obstructions, blindness in one eye, lameness, a hunched back, a disagreeable odor from their bodies, watery eyes, large abdomens or a stutter.[6] Dr. Benjamin Rush, who observed the troops of the nations involved in the Revolution, believed men under 20 caught the greatest number of camp diseases. Southern troops were more sickly than northern or eastern men. Native Americans were more sickly in the army than foreign-born ones. The hardiest soldiers were above age 30. Southern troops became sickly "for lack of salted provisions."[7]

Diet

In Colonial America service in the militia was compulsory. Each colony, at the time of its charter, established a militia unit. Every able-bodied male within certain age limits had to bear arms and train periodically, and he could be mustered into actual military service if necessary. The militiaman reported to his designated station with his own arms, clothes, and provisions. At his station he received his dietary ration uncooked. If duty lasted more than a few days, a commissary was organized to purchase food locally. The diet of the soldier varied with the time of the year, the cost of the food, the value of the currency, and the location of the troops. In the opening days of the Revolution, militia units from Connecticut were the best-fed troops around Boston. The Connecticut Assembly voted daily rations for their militia. Each man received three-quarters of a pound of pork or one pound of beef, one pound of bread or flour, and three pints of beer (or equal amounts of cider). Once a week, he received rice or one pint of Indian meal, six ounces of butter, three pints of peas or beans or other vegetables. Each soldier received a gill (one-quarter pint) of rum on fatigue days. In season he received milk, molasses, vinegar, coffee, chocolate, sugar, and vegetables. Vinegar was to accompany all troops because it was believed to stave off disease in hot weather. It was also mixed with molasses and water to make a "refreshing," summertime drink. This quantity of food was much greater than that of a working man and almost equaled the diet of the rich. The efforts of the other colonies to provision their troops were not as successful. The commissary general of the Connecticut troops, Joseph Trumbull, became commissary general of the entire army after General Washington observed his ability. The Connecticut diet was then made available to all the troops around Boston.[8] It cost the government 11 cents per day per soldier.[9] The diet described provided more than adequate calories, twice as much protein as needed, and an adequate quantity of minerals. However, it was low in vitamins A and C. Spruce beer was included to prevent scurvy. The men joined in groups to cook their rations. The officers formed a regimental mess and frequently employed private caterers or "mess contractors."[10] The enlisted men could supplement their rations by working for civilians around the camp. Many also left camp to go home and work their farms, returning to camp with farm provisions. Water was best obtained from flowing rivers free of impurities. Water from mountains and highlands was considered good if it did not have too many minerals. Lake and pond water was unsafe unless it flowed rapidly and was replenished from springs. Marsh water was very bad. If necessary, unsafe water could be cleaned with two to three grains of alum, which precipitated the impurities. Chalk could also be used for this purpose. "Dirty water" could be cleaned by agitation with the bough of a tree. Then it was filtered through a sponge or sand. It could also be boiled to remove animalcula and then strained through a colander. Sometimes vinegar was helpful. Any water could be used for washing, and the troops received 24 pounds of soft soap or 8 pounds of hard soap per 100 men per week.[11]

Soldiers had to be prevented from buying whiskey: "It cuts the appetite for solid food, affects the venous system and intellect. It obstructs the liver, swells the legs and causes convulsions." New whiskey caused bleeding from the intestines. Cider was good for health when aged and used moderately. If new and used in excess, it caused flatulence, colic, and diarrhea. This could be prevented with additions of a teaspoon of powdered ginger or if a heated iron was plunged into it. Cider boiled with spirits produced "cider-royal," which intoxicated rapidly. Aged beer was safe, but new beer caused flatulence. All alcoholic beverages could lead to indiscriminate commerce with females, which could cause syphilis. This in turn resulted in poor healing of wounds and other diseases. Alcohol was imbibed to excess in all armies. The soldiers received some spirits as part of their rations, but more could be purchased from the sutler. Officers believed alcohol resulted in dereliction of duty, while the surgeons felt it left men vulnerable to sickness.[12]

Feeding an army on the march was a difficult problem. Meat, which was an important staple of the diet, had to be salted for preservation. Salt was obtained largely from Britain. With the outbreak of hostilities, this source was cut off abruptly. Consequently, meat had to be "driven on the hoof" behind the troops and slaughtered locally. The cattle were mostly skin and bones after a march with minimal forage. The men supplemented the meat with flour, which could be added to water and cooked on hot rocks at a fire (fire cakes).[13] Later in the Revolution, talented cooks became company cooks.[14] Purchasing fruits and vegetables from local farms was often difficult. Farmers usually preferred the hard currency of the British to the paper money and promises of the Colonial commissary agents. Frequently, the troops were borderline avitaminotic. In places like Valley Forge and during the first winter at Morristown, New Jersey, scurvy was common. B vitamin deficiencies were not recognized.

Food was seasoned only with salt and vinegar. Meat had to be thoroughly dressed to help digestion. Salt in moderation was believed to help digestion and favor secretions and excretions. Bakers were advised to add rye to wheat to give it an acid taste. Bran was added to slow digestion and decrease hunger. Bread had to be well baked, or it produced acidity and led to flatulence. The soldier's ration was one pound of bread per day. Biscuits could be prepared for future use if bread could not be baked. White bread was believed to be more nourishing, but coarse brown bread helped evacuation. Additives to flour had to be checked, because chalk and plaster of Paris could be slipped in by the seller.

Soldiers required one-half to one and one-half pounds of fresh meat daily. The surgeon's duty included inspection of cattle for disease before slaughter. Cooks were advised that salted beef or pork had to be eaten within one year, or it would lose its value as nourishment. Fat meat was preferred in cold weather. If tainted meat was used, it was boiled with charcoal, ashes, lye, or potash. Vegetables were considered important additions to the diet, particularly in the summer (cabbage, potatoes, onions, turnips, beans, peas, and rice were common staples of the diet). Troops were supposed to have vegetables when they ate salted meat. Vegetables boiled with meat produced an agreeable acidity that prevented scurvy. Rice or barley prepared as flour were considered excellent foods that could be easily preserved and stored. Indian corn was equally nourishing. In besieged forts or hospitals without meat, bones were saved for gelatin, which was made by continued boiling of ligaments, tendons, hooves, and bones. This gelatin, when made into broth with vegetables, made a nutritious substitute for meat. If the army went where fresh fruit was not available, orange and lemon juice were to be evaporated and stored for future use (heating and storing, however, destroyed the vitamin C content).[15]

The food ration was fixed by congressional law (although Congress had no money to pay for it). This included one and a quarter pounds of fresh beef or one pound of salted beef or three quarters of a pound of salt pork, 18 ounces of bread or flour, and one gill of whiskey. For every 100 rations, the soldiers were to receive four pounds of soap, four quarts of vinegar, one and a half pounds of candles, and two quarts of salt.[16] The French army in America received 24 ounces of wheat bread, one pound of meat, and one pint of wine or two of beer. The cavalry received one and one-half times this ration. The feeding of the British army was let out to contractors. Great profits were made and split between the contractors and officers at the expense of the soldiers. Quality and quantity were short. Toward the end of the eighteenth century, medical men were appointed to supervise the food purchased for the English army.[17]

Uniform

The uniform in modern armies served three purposes: to protect the wearer from the elements, to separate him from the enemy, and to be a badge acting as a morale booster for the wearer. Added to that were the buttons and piping that advised a knowledgeable individual that the blue was infantry, the red artillery, and the gold (not yellow) service groups. In other times it had other purposes. Dr. Lind of the British navy advocated uniforms for seamen so the vermin-infested clothes they wore could be burned or discarded. He associated the clothing of the impressed recruits with typhus epidemics on board ship. It was not until 1751 that uniform regulations were established in England.

Edward Cutbush, in a book devoted to the preservation of the health of soldiers and sailors, described the nature of a proper uniform. The soldier was to have a cap of varnished leather, which would be impervious to the rain. It was shaped like a truncated cone eight to nine inches high in the crown and lined with linen. A woolen cap with wings to cover the neck and shoulders was used for bad weather. Iron-bound shoes for longer wear were best. The men wore flannel shirts rather than linen to absorb moisture because perspiration that remained next to the skin was implicated in many illnesses associated with army life. Dr. Rush had recommended that officers wear flannel shirts next to their skin rather than linen to protect them from fevers and disease. The soldiers carried a cloak or coat rather than a blanket, because the former could be used for the latter. The clothes worn by the men had to be examined weekly for cleanliness by the sergeant under the captain's supervision. The camp sutler was not to carry uniforms. This prevented soldiers from trading uniforms for liquor.[18]

The need for different clothes in different weather conditions was not recognized by the Hessian military. Summers in Germany were much cooler than those in America, and the Hessian soldier wore a woolen uniform all year. In addition, he had leggings, a gun, 60 cartridges, rations, and a knapsack. The Battle of Monmouth, New Jersey, was fought in a record-breaking heat wave in June. Fifty-nine Hessians died of heat exhaustion and sunstroke before meeting the Colonials. Dr. John Jones, in his early book on medical care in the army, called for lighter clothes during the excessive heat of colonial summers, recommending a short linen coat or waistcoat with sleeves under a tanned rifle shirt. The linen could be taken off frequently and washed. Jones also called for marches and exercise to be conducted before the heat of the day. Sentry duty was to be shorter in the heat. He urged the soldiers to wear a short flannel waistcoat covered by a warm fur coat for sentry duty in cold weather. Moccasins kept the sentry's feet warmer than leather shoes. When shoes were worn, they had to have thick soles.[19]

Housing

Housing of the army was important to the maintenance of the soldiers' health. Private homes were used if barracks were not available. Barracks were built on high, dry land, distant from noxious effluvia, preferably near a river where the soldier could wash himself and his clothes. Barracks were built a safe distance from the privies, and the currents of air were considered in siting them.[20] According to descriptions of the winter encampment at Jockey Hollow (near Morristown) in 1779–80, ten thousand to twelve thousand men were housed on 2,000 acres. There were 24 huts to each regiment, arranged in rows of 8, and 12 men were housed in each hut. The officers' huts were in front of those of their troops. The officers' quarters were divided into two apartments, and each hut housed three or four officers. The enlisted men's beds were stacked along the walls. The troops' quarters were 14 feet wide, 15 to 16 feet long and were lined up on a company street. However, the officers' huts were larger. Each building had two fireplaces, two chimneys, two windows, and one door. Straw used for bedding was changed every two weeks. Bedding was aired and sunned frequently, and no food or dirty clothes were allowed inside the building, and rooms were kept cool.[21] It was believed that hot rooms caused perspiration, and when men left the warm room for the outdoors, they chilled and became sick. Coming from the cold weather to a hot room led to nosebleed. During encampment, soldiers were forced to wash themselves regularly and were occasionally whipped or drummed out of the service for the enforcement of this regulation.

All authorities agreed that an army on the march was healthier than one in a permanent encampment. The obvious reason was that their waste was left behind, and polluted water would purify itself after the army left. The danger of a move to a new encampment was that the men perspired on the march. They were told never to expose their chest to the air, because this would result in pulmonic and bowel disease. A soldier was prohibited from drinking water when he perspired. If he did and felt bad, he was given whiskey, and the surgeon was called. The choice of an encampment was determined by the surgeon as well as the commander. The surgeon had to hunt out a healthy area. The camp was located away from swamps, because the ground was believed to produce exhalations that were responsible for intermittent and remittent fevers (malaria). Troops were kept on high ground, but not on high ground above swamps, because exhalations moved up. A wooded area was preferred. Camp sites were changed frequently if dysentery developed. Deep pits were dug for privies and were covered daily with fresh earth. When nearly full, they were completely covered with earth and a new site was found.

Pitched tents were aired every other morning. Troops slept on painted cloth (waterproof) to prevent the humidity of the earth from getting through. Men did not eat in tents. Camps were kept away from towns. The surgeon also inspected the civilian inhabitants of the area to decide on the salubrity of the camp site. He looked specifically for big bellies and yellow skin, sure signs that malaria was present. Tents were pitched in the shade of trees in hot climates. Freshly cut tree boughs covered the front of a tent. In an encampment of moderate duration in the Revolution, the shelters were as varied as the uniforms the men wore. They used boards, sailcloth, stones, brush, and turf. Fence rails and straw were liberated from farmers. The floor consisted of packed earth or boards if a sawmill was nearby. Otherwise, logs were laid down. If huts were built, clay, moss, or straw was packed in crevices to keep out the wind and rain.[22]

Training the Military Surgeon: Diseases He Saw

Handbooks for the surgeon were made available to treat the problems developed by the soldiers. One of the earliest was Baron Von Swieten's *Diseases Incident to Armies*, published in 1758. This was actually a primer for anyone who could read if a surgeon was not available. The reader could compare the symptoms of the patient with those described in the book and reach a diagnosis. The therapy for the illness was listed in order by number which corresponded to medications at the back of the book (the ancestor of the old *Merck Manual*). Von Swieten's book was published in England in 1762 and was used by surgeons in the American Revolution; it was republished in Philadelphia in 1776 and in Boston in 1777.[23]

Von Swieten and most other writers were aware of homesickness. They described nostalgia or melancholia when the soldier left his family or his familiar locality, advising that the soldier must be kept busy with exercise, marching, amusement, and diversion when not actually in battle. The individual responsible for the health of his unit also had to supervise the diet. Each soldier needed garden vegetables, fresh fruits (not unripe or "acid") and other fresh greens to prevent and cure scurvy. Pure water was vital to the troops' health. Water could be tested with "oleum tartari per deliquium"—a few drops in water would cause a milky white precipitate if impure. Von Swieten urged that water should be drawn from the middle of a river rather than from near the shore. If the only available water was impure, he advised the addition of six ounces of vinegar to three quarts of water. Another treatment was the use of pieces of root of calamus aromaticus steeped in the water. The camp was to be on dry land with a low water table. It had to be located a distance from a dense forest, because the trees prevented the wind from circulating the air, resulting in damp, close air. If a camp was on damp ground, the straw for bedding was changed more often, and a wax cloth was placed on the ground beneath the straw. Trenches were dug around the tents to drain away rain. Camp sites were changed often, because a large group in one place created unwholesome effluvia from so many bodies and resulted in sickness. Soldiers were forced to wash their hands, faces and feet regularly. If the weather permitted, they bathed in running water. The men were not crowded together, because this prevented free circulation of air.

Von Swieten discussed the illnesses the surgeons confronted. In the early spring they often saw sore throat, cough, pleurisy, pneumonia, and rheumatism. These were believed not to be contagious. Patients were not moved too much, and they were bled before being sent to the hospital. Tertian and quotidian intermittent fevers were seen in the spring; rarely were the quartans seen. All, however, were diseases of the autumn. Coughs were more troublesome than serious, but if neglected they could lead to phthisis. The patient was forbidden wine and salted or acid food. Rice, barley broth, fresh milk, and egg yolk were prescribed. If he developed a fever, he was bled to prevent inflammation. Species of pectoral and cynoglof—perhaps a botanical related to artichoke—were prescribed. The patient was better when his expectoration was thick and easily spit up. A sore throat could be fatal if it impeded breathing. A large bleeding was called for and followed by cupping around and on the nape of the neck. The diet consisted of light broth with rice or barley, and the patient had to gargle with a mixture of flower of elder, red roses, and nitre. The next day, the patient was purged with the remedy known as number six (senna leaves, scurvy grass, agaric, tamarinds, and rhubarb). If his throat went to suppuration and was red and swollen for more than three days, number seven (a species for emollient decoction) was warmed and kept in the victim's mouth. Cataplasm number eight, a poultice made of the residue of the emollient plus linseed meal and linseed oil, was applied to the throat night and day. When an abscess formed, it was drained with a lancet, and then the patient had to gargle with a tea made from red rose, agrimony, and honey (number nine). If the patient could not eat, he received a clyster of twelve ounces of milk and six ounces of barley water every four hours and he had to keep it in as long as possible. Von Swieten also described trench mouth and the stench emanating from the victim's mouth.

Rheumatism was a frequent complaint of soldiers exposed to cold after the body became heated. It also occurred after they wore wet clothes, and during cold nights which followed warm days. The disease started with shivering, heat, thirst, uneasiness, and fever. After two days there was pain in the joints, which moved from one to the next. Joints were red and swollen. The tendons were involved with severe pain. Fever dropped in a few days, but the pain persisted. If the disease passed inward and affected the lungs and brain, it became serious. The disease was seldom fatal, but if not treated, an incurable stiffness of the joints remained for life. The disease was treated first with the removal of 10 ounces of blood from the arm on the afflicted side. After this treatment, the painful area was wrapped in flannel soaked in one of Von Swieten's numbered remedies (warm fomentation 12). A light diet and dosing with other remedies followed, along with further bleeding if the pain persisted.

It is hard to differentiate here between acute rheumatic fever and rheumatoid arthritis. Young people crowded together certainly can develop rheumatic fever after a strep infection as was demonstrated in the training camps of World War II. The movement from joint to joint is usual in rheumatic fever.

However, the persistence of pain and stiffness once the attack subsides sounds more like rheumatoid arthritis.

Jaundice was another problem faced by the surgeon. Von Swieten talked of jaundice after a prolonged fever (typhoid?) or an autumnal fever (malaria). Other common illnesses were dropsy and pneumonia. It is interesting to note that although most soldiers were discharged from the military after a bout with pneumonia, those in the calvary remained in service because horseback riding was good therapy for the lungs.

Dysentery was seen in the late summer and autumn. There was flux, griping and painful straining at stool. The stool may have been bloody. It was caused by the heat and fatigue of war, which turned the bile acrid; by exposure of the heated body to cold air; by sleeping in wet clothes; by drinking stagnant or marsh water; or by eating tainted meat or musty bread. This disease spread through the army. The healthy soldiers were affected by putrid exhalation of fecal matter of the sick if they used the same privies. (The privies of the sick were to be kept separate, deep, and repeatedly covered with a layer of dirt during the day.) The camp site had to be changed frequently. Von Swieten recommended a number of remedies including ipecachuana and crude opium, the latter for its constipating powers.

Von Swieten's monograph should really be considered as a general textbook of internal medicine. Despite its name, it was actually a book that any doctor, civilian or army, could keep and refer to as needed for the treatment of illnesses he might see during his career.

Illness always accompanied an army, and before World War I it was responsible for the majority of casualties suffered in wartime. Plague destroyed Xerxes' invasion army in Greece. Not being partial, it probably also caused Athens' downfall in the Peloponnesian War as well as the cessation of the siege of Syracuse by the Carthaginians. Although they were on God's side, the Crusaders were struck down by the plague as well as by smallpox and scurvy. The plague, widely known as the Black Death, had gradually subsided after a destructive epidemic outbreak in Europe, and did not affect armies very much after that. However, there were many other diseases waiting in the wings to take center stage. While probably none were as destructive as plague, their persistence over the centuries as armies grew larger, nevertheless led to great numbers of casualties. Smallpox was destructive to the Saracens before Mecca and recurred whenever the number of nonimmunes proliferated, even until our American Revolution. Typhus was easily on a par with smallpox if not of greater destructiveness. Charles V's army, the army of Maximillian II of Germany, the Austrian army at Prague, and Napoleon's Grand Army in Russia were all destroyed by typhus.[24] Dysentery never caused the mortality rates of the other three, but it broke the army's morale and its will to fight. Imagine an army on the march or actively engaged in battle with the men suffering tenesmus that required them to stop every few minutes to evacuate or made them feel like they had to. It weakened the army and made the more serious diseases mentioned far more lethal. Malaria was in the same category as dysentery. Influenza by itself was not destructive of life, but it could put an army out of commission for weeks or months at a time. The English army in New York during the Revolution had this problem. On occasion, the flu was the forerunner of pneumonia (usually staphylococcus), which was fatal before antibiotics (as in our expeditionary force in World War I). In the Revolutionary War, the doctors saw fevers predominantly. These were thought of as the disease rather than as a symptom of many diseases. The fevers were associated with diarrhea, dysentery, pneumonia, pleurisy, jaundice, rheumatism, venereal disease, smallpox, jail or hospital fever (typhus) as well as a widespread "itch." Dr. Tilton remarked that illness caused ten to twenty times the casualties of arms and, on a percentage basis, more physicians died in the Revolution than did line officers.[25]

A breakdown in sanitary regulations was always followed by an outbreak of dysentery. A patient could still move around camp with little or no fever, but his skin was dry and dusky. Men would "melt away from running off at the bowels." Dysentery was treated with a blood letting followed by a vomit. Then the bowels were kept open (as if they needed to be) with small amounts of calomel and repeated doses of epsom salts. Medication was continued until the griping abated. Treatment was continued with astringents and anodynes, but opium and ipecac were useless. The only real cure came if the soldier was furloughed away from camp. He was sent "to the country" and kept on a milk diet. Dr. Craik, who became George Washington's family physician, tried tincture of Huxham and tincture of Japonicum, two tablespoons twice a day. This palliated the suffering but did not cure the disease. All attempts to "direct the current of humors from the bowels failed."[26]

The "itch" or scabies was a debilitating problem. The skin was covered with vesicles, which broke open when scratched. These became secondarily infected by staphylococcus. First the victims were treated by fumigation of their clothes with brimstone, then they were purged every eight days. Flower of sulphur and "Ethiop's mineral" were also applied daily. At night sulphur in hog's lard was smeared on the sores. When the surgeon ran out of sulphur, the men could go to the artillery section to get the sulphur, which was then mixed with tallow and applied to the skin. Instead of a purge, they often took liquor liberally.

Dr. Tilton developed "putrid fever" while he was a physician at the Princeton Hospital.[27] This may have been typhus, but typhoid fever is a more likely diagnosis. He did not describe the petechial hemorrhages characteristic of typhus. The doctor complained of listlessness for a few days, followed by a severe headache associated with a synochus type of fever. (Synochus meant continuous or persistent. In the eighteenth century it was considered a type rather than a form of fever.) After the early symptoms, his pulse became weak, and his tongue was dry. He then showed nerve disorders and delirium. Tilton did not mention being bled, which would have been done if the pulse had been bounding. In signs of inflammation mercury was given. If the pulse dropped, the tongue became dry, and the patient became delirious, he received bark as well as wine, volatile salts, and blisters. If the victim survived, a crust formed on his tongue, which peeled off and left a tender surface. The skin peeled as well, and his hair fell out.

Smallpox was a constant threat as long as nonimmunes entered the army. With the occupation of Boston in 1776, inoculation of the nonimmunes was started, and the procedure was continued throughout the war. Mortality from inoculation was kept to a minimum, probably because the men were young and healthy. Also, the various techniques of "preparation" were discontinued, because these frequently weakened the inoculee. A single dose of calomel and jalap or extract of the inner bark of the buttermilk tree was given before the onset of symptoms. If the patient developed smallpox the natural way and was seen by doctors, he was bled heavily and given mercury for inflammation.[28] Pneumonia and pleurisy were winter diseases and were also treated with bleeding and mercury. Bark was used as a tonic if the pulse grew weak.

Preventive Medicine in Armies

Anyone in the business of medicine will agree that the prevention of disease is better than the treatment of disease. To my mind, the concept of immunization and the discovery of the relationship of dietary deficiencies and disease far surpassed the discoveries of antibiotics and other advances in modern medicine. Similarly, the prevention of disease in the military was far more successful in keeping down casualty rates than was treatment. Physicians and line officers alike called for preventive techniques to keep their armies strong and functional.

As far back as Biblical times, Moses led his nation (his army) for 40 years and maintained a level of health unequaled by armies until the present day. The Mosaic code divided animals into clean and unclean. Leviticus proscribed carnivores as food because they carried diseases (parasites). Pigs ate garbage and offal, and the Hebrews, like the ancient Egyptians, considered pigs unfit as food. Animals with cloven hooves who chewed their cud were considered clean, while those walking on paws and those eating carrion were unclean. Animals that died naturally also were considered unclean, as were those mangled by other animals. Blood was unclean because it decomposed rapidly in the heat and caused disease. Fish without scales or fins were unsafe, because several scaleless fish were known to be poisonous, and shellfish carried diseases. Moses also recognized the need for pure water, and stipulated the use of earthenware vessels to carry water. If they came into contact with unclean things, they were broken and discarded. If someone died in a tent where there were uncovered containers, the contents were discarded because of the danger of flies, which flew from the dead body to the food in the container. The need for pure air guided the location of a camp. Moses tried to place his camp on a hillside to get better circulation of breezes—of course, it was easier to defend as well. He insisted that the camp remain clean because "God walks among you."

According to Deuteronomy, body wastes were kept outside of camp. Every man was to have a digging object to dig a hole for body waste. This was then covered after use. This was certainly more sanitary and less ill-smelling than the privies for a camp that were covered with a layer of dirt once a day. Leviticus urged washing of body and clothes in water. In Psalm 26 and in Job, the need to wash one's hands is mentioned frequently and urged particularly before meals to prevent reinfection with enteric diseases.

All army commanders had problems with venereal disease. In their war against the Moabites, the Israelite soldiers were intimate with the enemy women, and they brought an infection back to the tribes that resulted in the death of 24,000 Israelites. (Gonorrhea would not have had this effect, but syphilis could.) Moses learned from experience, and when his troops conquered Midian, he ordered all non-virgins to be executed to prevent a recurrence of the epidemic.

Moses also kept his people's dwellings safe from disease. Dwellings with discolorations from fungus or lichen due to overcrowding and humidity were treated. If this did not clear up the problem, the house was destroyed. The fear of communicable disease in camp kept lepers away from the community and in isolation. Those suspected of leprosy were separated and examined by priests who also served as doctors back then. Those who recovered from leprosy had all their body hair shaved off, and they and their clothing were thoroughly washed before they were allowed to return to the camp. There were probably few spontaneous cures of leprosy, so those readmitted to camp probably had suffered from another skin disease that had healed. People exposed to the dead had to stay out of camp for seven days, obviously considered an incubation period. Any communicable disease in the community was announced to the community by the blowing of the shofar or ram's horn.[29]

Sir John Pringle of Britain is credited with being the father of modern preventive medicine and hygiene as it relates to the health care in armies. Born in 1707, Sir John was the son of a baronet of England. He attended the University of St. Andrews and at age 20 went to Edinburgh to study medicine. This was followed by a period of training under Boerhaave at Leyden. The young Sir John practiced medicine in Edinburgh until he was appointed physician to the British army in 1742.[30] Early in his career he worked to develop the concept of a military hospital that came to be a neutral oasis in war. At the

Battle of Dettingen (War of the Austrian Succession), he and his French counterparts succeeded in creating a special place for hospitals in war. Their commanders, the Earl of Stair and the Duc de Noailles, agreed with this concept. With this agreement in place, the sick and wounded would not have to be removed hurriedly at the approach of enemy forces, which increased mortality among the casualties. In addition, those serving in a hospital would not become prisoners of war. Instead, they would be returned to their army along with the casualties as soon as possible. Furthermore, surgeons could cross lines to care for their wounded. The sick and wounded enemy soldiers were to receive the same care, medicine, and food as the victor's casualties.[31] This agreement existed through the French and Indian War. However, with the outbreak of the Revolution, it was abrogated by the British, because the Americans were considered rebellious Englishmen. Richard Huddleston, a British surgeon, was captured by American forces during the invasion of Canada. With reference to this agreement, he petitioned the American Congress for his freedom. Congress sent him to General Carleton, British governor of Canada, on his parole, to see if he would accept the release of all physicians and surgeons as per this agreement. Carleton refused. However, during the war, physicians could pass through enemy lines with a flag of truce to care for their wounded. Later in the war, the British finally accepted the concept developed 40 years earlier.[32]

In 1752, Pringle, through astute observation, discovered that hospital fever and jail fever were the same illness, namely typhus. He saw this connection when British deserters in jail developed spotted fever, and patients in a hospital near the detention compound developed the identical disease. To prevent the spread of jail fever, he suggested that no prisoner should be allowed to carry out his clothing upon his release. Instead, the clothing was to be burned, and the recent inmate was given new clothes at public expense. Pringle also called for the destruction of all clothes of executed prisoners. In addition, when prisoners were brought to court, they were to be washed and given special clothes to be worn for this appearance. The court uniform had to be washed frequently. (This probably derived from the experience of the "Black Assizes" to be described later.)

In 1752, Dr. Pringle published *Observations on the Diseases of the Army*, based on his experiences during the War of the Austrian Succession when he was in Flanders with the British army (1740) and he saw the British army almost destroyed by illness. Pringle believed the chief cause of death in the army was the hospital. To prevent cross infection caused by crowding, Sir John Pringle urged good ventilation and adequate space between patients, weather-appropriate clothing, and cleanliness of body and uniform. He described the need for proper disposal of waste in addition to well chosen campsites and latrines. Recognizing the relationship between impure drinking water and disease, he urged careful supervision of the selection of water supplies and urged line officers not to quarter their troops in barns, churches, and houses previously used as hospitals.

Dr. Pringle believed that animalcula were the cause of the spread of dysentery among soldiers and that scabies was due to insects in pustules on the victims, as had been described earlier by Leeuwenhoek. Pringle recommended treating scabies with sulfur ointment applied externally. Sir John recognized that lowered resistance of soldiers made them more susceptible to illness and that therefore undue fatigue and exposure to extremes of the weather should be avoided. He preceded Dr. Lister by a century when he described and used the term "antisepsis" when calling for the treatment of stool from a dysentery patient with strong acids.[33] Pringle's beliefs and ideas probably played an important part in the medical care the army received in our Revolution. Many of the young American medical students, who were to become leaders of the American medical department, studied in Britain, learning there about Pringle and his concepts of hygiene. However, like their British counterparts, Americans often failed to follow his commonsense advice.[34]

Dr. Richard Brocklesby, another physician stationed in Flanders, wrote a monograph, *Observations of Military Hospitals*, in 1764. He was surgeon general of the British armies after Pringle's tenure. Dr. Brocklesby urged the line officer to accept responsibility for the health of his troops. He believed strict discipline among soldiers was required to maintain their physical well-being. Like Pringle, he opposed large general hospitals and preferred small regimental hospitals to care for sick troops, pointing out that infection could be kept to a minimum if the sick and wounded were scattered in small lots. It is probably from Dr. Brocklesby's work, among others, that Dr. Tilton derived his concept of the "Tilton Hospital" in his regulations for field hospitals to follow the troops.[35] Surgeon general Donald Monro (or Munro) described the need to maintain cleanliness to keep the army healthy, referring frequently to the Mosaic code. Dr. Monro was particularly interested in clean water for the troops and discussed additives to develop purity. Wine, vinegar, and cream of tartar may have made it appear and taste better, but his idea of boiling it was more effective.[36]

On this side of the ocean, Dr. Benjamin Rush wrote directions for preserving the health of soldiers in 1777. He felt it was the line officer's duty as well as the medical officer's responsibility to care for the health of the troops. They had to enforce sanitary regulations. Rush believed the surgeon general of the army should be near the commanding general. The surgeon must express an opinion on orders for marching, camping, eating, and even fighting. Rush opposed "spirits" for the army, referring frequently to the Roman army and its ration of vinegar rather than alcohol, which he believed helped in its victories. Rush counseled against crowding and sleeping in wet clothes, urged that camps be kept clean of all animal waste and filth, recommended the avoidance of undue fatigue, and insisted on a "complete bath" twice a week, weather permitting. Dr. Rush wanted soldiers to change underclothing frequently and to wash their eating utensils after each use.[37]

Dr. John Jones was primarily a surgeon, and his description of the care of battlefield injuries will be discussed later. However, his innate wisdom and common sense came through in his monograph, *Medicine in Armies*. The appendix of the book was a discourse on hygiene. A layman today might think this material is pretty basic, as indeed it is, but the work was completed over two centuries ago when the germ theory of disease did not exist, and most American soldiers were individualists who had grown up in places where there was room to "spread out." Dr. Jones urged that uniforms appropriate to the weather be supplied. Exercise should be performed only when the weather permitted. He discussed sleeping accommodations for the troops. If in a tent, trenches were to be dug around it to carry off rain; tents were to have extra blankets; tent and bedding were to be aired frequently; some waterproof material was to be placed on the earth floor of the tent. If the men were in barracks, they had to have enough fuel to keep them warm and dry. The troops had to have mattresses filled with straw which were changed regularly, sunned as often as possible, and filled with corn husks if clean straw was not available. The men were allowed to build fires behind camp to dry their clothing. Campsites were to be changed frequently. According to Dr. Jones, this protected the camp from the effects of putrid air from marshes and stagnant water. Like all medical officers, Jones was aware that a moving army was healthier than a stationary one. Deep privies were to be dug where the wind would carry the putrid effluvia away from camp, and Jones also urged strict punishment of the soldier who did not use the privy to "ease himself."

The doctor knew that a large group of men packed together was a forerunner of dysentery. When it broke out, he advised the use of even deeper privies and that fresh dirt be shovelled in every night. The victims of the disease were not to be packed into general hospitals. It was safer to keep them in camp. If the numbers increased, the excess could go to a regimental hospital, which was housed in a large, airy structure, such as a church or a barn, rather than in close private dwellings. Dr. Jones urged space between patients in the hospital and, if possible, the ceiling of a room was removed to make the room and garret one large, airy place. Doors and windows of a hospital were to be kept open. The hospital room had to be kept clean, and all patients' discharges and dressings removed immediately. Vinegar was to be sprinkled around the room frequently. Dr. Jones felt that soldiers should eat in mess groups so that food was properly prepared and nourishing. Pork could be used in camp, although it was forbidden in some installations. He believed that suet was more nourishing than lean meat. According to him, on long marches, suet and fat pork were thus preferable to lean meat. Jones believed alcohol was necessary to counteract extremes of weather. Rum mixed with vinegar was good in the heat to prevent corruption of the humors. He felt that both fatigue and indolence were bad for the soldier, but indolence was worse. The men were exercised frequently for short periods. Armed drills, digging trenches, cleaning clothes, and competitive sports were good to keep the men busy. Officers participated in these activities, but they should not push the troops to fatigue.[38]

Doctor James Tilton served throughout the Revolution. In 1803 he published *Economical Observations on Military Hospitals*, based on his personal observations.[39] His administrative skills were recognized when he was appointed director general of the medical department in the War of 1812. Dr. Tilton was obviously aware of the "indiscretions" during Shippen's administration, and he called for the separation of a doctor's duties from those of purveyors and commissaries to prevent questions of ethical misconduct.

Tilton described the "swallowing up" of half the army by the hospitals in 1777–78. Like his predecessors in England, he related this misfortune to putting all the sick and wounded into a large general hospital. He urged that casualties be retained at a regimental hospital under the care of a competent regimental surgeon chosen after a thorough evaluation by a board of physicians and surgeons. Between the regimental and the general hospital, Tilton called for a "Flying Hospital." This was a temporary hospital while the army was in the field. It would be a branch of a general hospital and controlled by its senior physician. Only soldiers with serious wounds and chronic illnesses were to be sent to the general hospital. The doctor urged proper payment to keep competent physicians in the service.

Dr. Tilton believed there should be a medical board for each army consisting of a chief surgeon, two or more hospital surgeons, and a line officer who served as president. The board was to meet once a month, appoint regimental and hospital mates and examine regimental and hospital surgeons, delineate the duties of the regimental and general hospitals, and supervise the purveyor to prevent extravagance. The board was directly responsible to the army's commander. Tilton's table of organization called for a regiment to have one surgeon and one mate, raised to two mates in war. There was one hospital surgeon per division. Tilton did not believe in the separation of duties for the surgeon and the physician as practiced in the British army and wanted the hospital surgeon to control his hospital and to be able to order necessary provisions and equipment. The army had a physician-in-chief with two mates whom he appointed and one purveyor and assistant. The office of the physician-in-chief was near the army commander's for easy consultation. In addition to the physician-in-chief, there was an apothecary-in-chief to prepare and deliver all medicines and dressings to the hospital upon receipt of written orders. Surgical instruments were delivered to the surgeon who paid for them and was reimbursed by the purveyor. The general staff had one surgeon at headquarters whose responsibility was the health of that group. The physician-in-chief established the necessary hospitals, and in emergencies he was empowered to place hospital surgeons in the field. The physician inspected all hospitals in his area. The regimental surgeon was responsible to the physician-in-chief; the mate was responsible only to his surgeon. The purveyor received money from the treasury to pay salaries and expenses. He purchased the necessary medications and utensils and reported to the board monthly to show his expenditures and stock. The purveyor appointed the steward who purchased vegetables, straw, and similar supplies for the hospital. The steward appointed the matron and nurses. If the army was split and a medical section left the main group, it developed its own chain of command similar to that of the main group, but in miniature.

The hospital had to avoid infection to function. Wooden buildings with wooden floors were not recommended as hospitals because they retained infection. Wooden hospitals in winter resulted in the penning up of foul air that "becomes exalted to such a poisonous malignancy as to make all approach to them hazardous." Tents were best for summer hospitals and were safest if they were erected on an earthen floor. For winter use, the "Tilton Hospitals" developed during the Morristown encampment were best. These were built on earthen floors. The building itself was of rough logs chinked with clay. New patients were washed and given a new set of hospital clothes upon admittance. The patients were instructed to wash their hands and face daily with vinegar. Clothing was changed frequently. Excrement was removed from the ward daily. The sick were separated from the wounded and the convalescents from the sick. Hospital diets required substantial amounts of milk and fresh vegetables. The regimental hospital treated acute illnesses; patients with chronic illnesses and wounds went to the general hospital. This concept was also propounded by Frederick the Great. Tilton repeatedly urged that casualties be kept out of crowded hospitals and concluded his chapter on hospitals with a panacea for all contagious diseases and all fevers where there was an inflammatory diathesis, namely, calomel two drams, opium one dram, tartar emetic 15 grains, and syrup to make 60 pills. This worked in inflammation of the lungs and liver and might work in inflammation of the stomach and bowels, and it definitely helped colic.

Tilton also advocated strict discipline by the line officers to enforce cleanliness. Military activities in camp were conducted in the cool of the morning. The men were exercised and marched to keep them occupied. They had to have clean clothes and bedding and were forced to bathe their entire body in warm weather. Trenches were dug around tents to keep them dry. Bedding was aired regularly. Privies were dug on the north and east sides outside of camp, or outhouses were built over running streams. (I saw this in France in World War II. Children swam in these streams close to the effluent of the outhouses. This was done in Thailand as well. The village people washed themselves and their clothing in the same stream.) Summer uniforms were made of cotton, winter uniforms of wool. Soldiers ate in messes, each of which had an old veteran to teach recruits how to use food and avoid spoilage. Each mess received fresh vegetables and well-baked bread. The soldiers were advised to rub their skin daily with a blanket, because the friction kept their skin healthy and prevented colds and pneumonia as well as consumption. Cold baths in the heat were also good for the skin. Dr. Tilton believed it was the duty of the line officer to maintain hygiene, particularly when the soldiers were removed to a different environment. Their ignorance of local conditions could subject them to numerous diseases. In addition, troops required exercise, games, amusement, and short marches for morale. Tilton was ahead of his time when he talked of the need to maintain a soldier's self-esteem, urging officers to refrain from striking their men.

In the present era, we expect the trained physician to promulgate orders to maintain the health of the fighting services. However, two or more centuries ago laymen, through observation and experience, were frequently as important as the surgeon in promoting the health of the men under their command. Frederick II, King of Prussia, paid intense attention to the health of his troops. He insisted on strict examinations for his army physicians and surgeons. The king did not commit his army to battle until he had installed field medical stations connected to permanent installations behind the lines. Frederick used hospital boats, and he tried to make dressing stations artillery proof. He had his surgeons look after enemy casualties only after all of his own were cared for. The king read medical books and believed strongly in purging. He had his army purged on days when he felt it to be necessary. Frederick ordered those ill with dysentery to be treated with emetics. On marches the men were not allowed to drink water from suspicious sources.[40]

In Belgium, Prince De D'Ligne supervised the entire medical care of his troops despite his lack of formal training. To my mind, he showed great common sense that more than made up for the lack of medical education. According to the prince, soldiers became sick due to poorly cooked food, too much water in the food, bad fruit, too much farina, muddy water, and drinking water when the soldier was overheated on a march. Other causes were brandy, overheated rooms, rotten straw, filth in camps, foul air, tight clothing, buttoned garters, small uniforms that stopped circulation, collars, garters, too long a period spent under arms, exercise during hot days, straps that crossed the chest, and a heavy knapsack that cramped the stomach. He wanted his men to march and eat at proper hours. They were forced to bathe regularly. He felt that surgeons who bled and purged and experimented with casualties and contractors who cheated should all be hanged. The diet of the sick included wine, veal, milk, broth, and chicken. Garlic, water, bread soaked in butter, and vinegar were good for men on the march. No oil or coal was stored in soldiers' rooms. No woolen clothes were worn because they absorbed sweat and stank. The troops needed fresh air and ventilation, and candles were extinguished because they used the air. The prince ordered urine troughs built that entered covered receptacles in order to keep the odor down. The prince felt tin-covered copper vessels were dangerous, but iron and tin plates could be used in the field. Earthenware was used in garrison. He did not allow the use of stagnant water or rain water. The men drank from rivers or springs. If water was taken from pools, it was filtered. The primary drink of soldiers was beer. They were not permitted to buy wine because what they usually received was not really wine. If men were imprisoned, they were not to be kept in dark, unsanitary places. They could be fed on bread and water. Whipping with switches was permitted because this increased circulation. No sticks or clubs were used. Soldiers were not whipped on the back or buttocks, because this prevented them from marching. Men were not to march in close order because this prevented circulation of air. Officers had to realize that soldiers were children and treat them as such. If troops were camped in damp soil, trenches were dug around tents. He advised that they build and keep a sand filter in the regimental wagon. Damp bread was not eaten. Instead, it was saved and toasted. New latrines were dug every eight days. He urged his surgeons not to cure disease, but to prevent it. The soldier was kept fit and his legs dry. Worn clothing was not left lying around. Officers were ordered not to humiliate and torment the men. Officers who annoyed men were mentally deranged. Gaiety was good for soldiers.

Concerning the medical service the prince insisted that too much surgical lint prevented wounds from uniting. A good surgeon major was one with sense enough to know he knew nothing; he was experienced and liked by soldiers and could skillfully treat ruptures. He rarely had more than 10 of his men in the hospital at one time. In the hospital, expenses were kept down in order to have money for necessities, but two patients were never kept in one bed. Patients were not to see a man dying of the same disease they had. The prince recognized that the transport of wounded was done poorly as they were piled in wagons and left there too long. However, he offered no suggestions for improvement.

Barracks were to be built instead of housing men in peasant huts. Barracks had trophies, good architecture, and swinging beds supported by slats. Each man had his own mattress. No fire was permitted in a room where men slept. Sixty beds in a large bright room was considered the optimum. The barracks had two other large rooms, heated moderately in winter, for the men's assembly. In the middle there was a general kitchen. Windows were kept open when possible. Soldiers never slept in a room with food fumes. After meals in the assembly room, all pots were brought to the kitchen. The assembly rooms were also for the men's entertainment and for exercise in bad weather. There was a small attic or garret for women and children as well as storerooms. Floors were laid three feet above ground level. Windows were five feet above the ground. Barracks were placed in the middle of a large field and not surrounded by a wall. Instead, he recommended a low hedge. The field was used for exercise and sports. The men had to have clothing with finery because this gave rise to vanity and vanity gave rise to esprit.[41]

Like the Belgian prince, George Washington was a layman well versed in the hygienic needs of an army. In the collected writings of the general there are many references to military health precautions, cleanliness, and policing of camps, huts, and quarters. He discussed food, diet, rations, and proper dressing of provisions. Washington also wanted proper clothing for his troops. He was a strong advocate of inoculation for smallpox, therapy for the itch, and many other medical matters. In his earliest general orders after he took command of the army around Boston, he ordered his line officers to make certain their men were kept clean. They were to visit the men in their quarters every day and to enforce cleanliness as essential to their health and to the service. The officer must be certain his men had clean straw upon which to sleep, and they were to report if this was lacking. The officer had men dig "necessaries" (latrines) of adequate number and depth. The men were instructed to cover them with a fresh layer of earth daily to prevent their becoming offensive and unhealthy. Officers and men who followed the general's instructions were singled out for commendation. Sanitary orders were repeatedly issued, and officers who did not follow instructions were punished. The general also demanded that animal remains were to be burned outside the camp's perimeter.

When Washington reached Cambridge, he ordered a chain of command set up for the care of casualties. The General Order of July 7, 1775, required a sick or wounded soldier to be treated at a regimental hospital. If he could not receive adequate care, the patient was sent to a camp hospital with his name and company on the transfer order. If the camp hospital was full, he was moved further back to the general hospital at Watertown with a similar certificate. The General Order of July 14, 1775, related health to cleanliness. Streets of the camp and the barracks were to be swept daily. All filth around the barracks was removed. Company commanders inspected the kitchen daily to see that food was dressed properly and was prepared in a wholesome manner. Washington also recognized the need for a medical establishment to care for casualties. He sent a letter to the president of Congress in which he described such a creation. Congress was of a similar mind and had already developed the hospital (medical) department. Of course, as with many laymen and doctors of those days, many of Washington's directions were based on medical misconceptions. In the General Order of August 28, 1775, he associated bloody flux (dysentery) with new cider. If it was brought into camp, the barrels were destroyed.[42]

Washington's greatest contribution to preventive medicine and hygiene was his call for the inoculation of non-immune soldiers and recruits. Smallpox broke out in Boston during the British occupation of 1775–76. After the British evacuation, Washington allowed only those troops into Boston who had immunity to the disease. He then had Dr. Morgan institute inoculation of all non-immune soldiers left in the Boston area, while he took his army to New

York to try to defend that city. After his victories at Trenton and Princeton, he pulled his army north to Morristown, New Jersey, for winter encampment. With the consent of Congress, he instituted an army-wide inoculation program. The men at Morristown were isolated into an inoculation hospital for treatment. In addition, hospitals were set up in Virginia and Maryland to immunize all new recruits who joined the army from the South. As late as 1781, while encamped at the Highlands in New York (near West Point), an immunization program was carried out. It was due to these programs that the debacles of Canada and New York State in 1776 were never repeated.[43]

Next to Washington, the layman most responsible for the maintenance of the soldier's health was Baron Von Steuben. The Baron had been an aide to Frederick II of Prussia who, as we have seen, was a strict disciplinarian in the matters of his soldiers' health care. Von Steuben learned his lessons well to the benefit of the American army. Like many European soldiers who were "out of work" in the interlude between wars, Von Steuben presented himself to Ben Franklin and Silas Deane in Paris to obtain employment. He admitted to a minor rank in the Prussian army, captain, unlike so many other European "generals." Franklin was aware of his ability and raised his rank to lieutenant general, so he would be more acceptable to Congress. The Baron was sent to America in time to join Washington's forces at Valley Forge on February 23, 1778. Von Steuben received the rank of major general and was appointed inspector general of the army. The new general was the author of *Regulations for the Order and Discipline of Troops of the United States Army*. This was adopted by Congress on March 29, 1779, and became a manual for the army. The regulations covered drill, served as a manual of arms as well as a code of health regulations. Von Steuben ordered all line officers to maintain sanitation in camp and on marches. The Baron believed the commandant's first and greatest responsibility was the health of his troops. The commander was to supervise his junior officers to see that they enforced personal hygiene among their men. A captain was required to send men with infectious disorders out of the company area to a hospital or other place to prevent the spread of infection to the rest of the company. All officers and non-coms were responsible for the men's cleanliness as well as that of the camp. Latrines were to be dug 300 feet away from tent lines. The quartermaster was responsible for digging and covering latrines. Latrines were to be used no longer than four days before they were covered over completely. In summer, they were used for shorter periods. Von Steuben not only promulgated these regulations, but he enforced them personally.

The line officer also concerned himself with the comfort of his sick men. Each regiment had two or three tents set aside to house the sick who could not or need not be sent to a general hospital. Each company had two sacks to fill with straw for their sick. These sacks were supplied by the regimental clothier to the captain. When the patient died or returned to duty, his straw was burned, and the bedding was washed and aired before its next use. At roll call, corporals reported the sick of their squad to the sergeant who reported to the first sergeant. The first sergeant wrote up his report for delivery to the regimental surgeon, who examined the sick to decide who would go to a regimental or general hospital. The regimental commander examined the sick to help weed out malingerers. The regimental surgeon reported the number of sick to the surgeon of the army. Between these two members of the medical service was the brigade surgeon who supervised the activities of the regimental surgeon. Once a week the regimental surgeon reported the list of sick to the regimental commander along with the nature of the disorder and whether the patient required hospitalization. The arms and supplies of the sick soldier were locked in the regimental arms chest. The surgeon decided when the soldier was ready to return to duty. The surgeon remained with his regiment on marches to care for any emergency. One non-com per regiment helped the sick and lame who were unable to keep up with the regiment. Empty wagons were to follow the march to carry the arms and knapsacks of the infirm.

Von Steuben was also responsible for the regulation, first approved by Congress but later withdrawn, to fine officers and men who caught venereal disease. Overall, Von Steuben's contribution to the Revolution was to create a healthy, disciplined army that left Valley Forge with high morale. They marched into Philadelphia after the British left, and they showed their mettle at Monmouth, New Jersey. If it was not for the failure of Lieutenant General Charles Lee (another European "general"), they would have administered an overwhelming defeat to the British Army.[44]

Surgical Treatment of Casualties

Illness was responsible for at least nine times the casualties as those produced by actual combat. However, the care of wounds was certainly the prime reason for army surgeons. To my mind, Ambroise Paré (1510–1590) should be considered the father of military surgery. He was observant and did not follow the dogma prescribed by his predecessors or contemporaries. Paré came to Paris in 1532 to be apprenticed to a barber-surgeon. At that time, there were three classes of healers. The highest were the physicians (Faculté de Médecine). They controlled all who practiced healing. Below them were the surgeons (Confrérie de St. Côme), the surgeons of the long robe. The lowest were the barber-surgeons who performed venesection, cups, and leeches and they did some minor surgery and dressed wounds. Surgeons of the long robe did not do surgery. To treat surgical conditions they used plasters, ointments, and cautery. They also treated wounds and abscesses. In addition to these groups were the wanderers, the empirical physicians. They cut for stones and operated for hernias and cataracts. They were not authorized to practice, but they were tolerated.

A separate grouping were the bonesetters who kept their secrets in the family. At the very bottom were the midwives.

Paré became house surgeon at the Hôtel Dieu where he remained for three or four years. He left in 1536 to become a surgeon in the French army in the invasion of Italy against the German Emperor Charles V. He still had not passed the examination given by the barber-surgeons guild. Early in his army career, Paré learned that burning oil was not as good for gunshot wounds as was generally believed. It was used to prevent "poisoning by the gunpowder." He ran out of oil during the bloody capture of the Castle of Villaine, and so instead of oil, he applied a digestive of egg yolk, oil of roses, and turpentine. The following morning, the soldiers treated with his concoction were much better than the "oiled group." He returned to Paris in 1539 and passed the examination in 1541 to become a master barber-surgeon. In 1542 and again in 1543 he went with the army. In 1545 Paré wrote his book on the treatment of wounds caused by an arquebus, an early musket. The young surgeon returned to practice in Paris and also worked as prosector while Dr. Sylvius lectured on anatomy. He dissected many bodies and wrote a book on human anatomy, in which he discussed obstetrics and podalic version for breech presentations.

At the Siege of Danvilliers, he amputated the leg of an officer and used arterial ligatures instead of a hot iron to control the bleeding. The officer was soon able to use a wooden leg. In 1554 Paré became a member of the College de St. Côme. The doctor then left for the Siege of Rouen. He gave up dressing wounds with the "oil of puppies" and used Egyptiasum made of honey and alum. Paré followed his Rouen adventure in 1564 with his book on surgery. In 1559 he retired from army work and returned to Paris. In 1568 the surgeon wrote a medical text on plague, smallpox, and measles. He wrote another book on surgery in which he discussed the manual induction of labor. In 1575 Paré produced the work that became the first true surgical treatise. In it he ridiculed some of the bizarre therapies of his day. The author attacked the use of unicorn horn as a universal antidote, because he knew it did not exist. He denied the benefit of "mummy," a medication in vogue in Europe supposedly taken from Egyptian mummies. In his *Apology and Treatise*, he described several interesting surgical procedures. For migraine and "fluxions of the eyes," Paré cut the artery behind the ear. The author described an incision in the chest to treat empyema. He described a plastic reconstruction technique for large breasts where he made a cruciate incision, removed some fat, and resewed it. The surgeon described paracentesis for ascites. His treatment for sciatic pain was to damage the nerve by burning the back of the hip. He included a treatment used by Hippocrates for a displaced vertebra. The patient was tied straight to a ladder. The ladder was raised to the top of a house and dropped like a dead weight. This bit of therapeutic wisdom was illustrated in texts of the period.

Paré apparently was also strongly interested in psychotherapy in connection with surgery. He was called to see the Marquis D'Auret, who had been shot near the knee seven months earlier with an arquebus, resulting in a fracture, followed by an abscess, fever, and loss of body strength and mass. He performed an incision and drainage and removed the bone splinters. The surgeon next applied friction to all parts of the body with linen. (This technique of friction was advocated in the Revolution, but flannel was used instead of linen.) Paré also applied various fomentations around the thigh. The patient was served good food and kept in a clean bed with fresh linens. He had flowers brought to sweeten the smell. Paré created an artificial rainfall when he poured water from a high place into a cauldron to lull his patient to sleep. The surgeon also ordered that violins be played in the room, and he employed a jester to make the patient merry. (He antedated Norman Cousins in the therapy of rheumatoid spondylitis by 400 years.) After six weeks, his patient had gained weight and could walk around on crutches.[45]

Two hundred years passed between the writings of Ambroise Paré and the American Revolution. In that interlude weapons of destruction improved, and the wounds they caused required considerable improvement in treatment. The standard American infantry man of the eighteenth century carried a musket, bayonet, tomahawk, and a long knife. The rifle was given to sharpshooters and specialized companies. The officers and non-coms wore a straight sword and one or more pistols. Artillery was available in the form of mortars and howitzers to shoot above and beyond obstacles in an arc, as well as the basic cannon that shot straight ahead. Artillery could be armed with grape shot against personnel or with round shot to batter down obstacles. Burns were a fairly common injury to those manning these instruments of destruction. This occurred from flashback of the black powder in the firing pan of the musket or the touch hole of the artillery piece. Burns of over twenty percent of the body were fatal. Wounds from muskets, rifles, and grape shot as well as overwhelming destruction of tissue by a cannon ball were suffered by the infantry. The musket had a non-rifled smooth bore, which hurled a jagged ball of soft lead at low velocity. It flattened on contact and created a large wound, forcing in bits of skin and clothing, tearing the flesh savagely, and splintering bone. Bayonet and sword points were fairly sharp and caused penetrating wounds free of foreign material. The sides of swords were duller and were used for slashing, resulting in massive tearing and contusion of flesh. Bayonets and swords were used in close combat. When the thorax and abdomen were penetrated, the wounds were fatal.[46]

The American military surgeon had some experience in the treatment of wounds because he lived in an agricultural society. The repair of gunshot wounds from hunting, as well as broken bones and lacerations in falls or from instruments used in farming were a part of his daily activities. However, the military surgeon required preparation for the destruction he would face. The monograph produced by Dr. John Jones answered this need. Dr. Jones believed the surgeon should be ambidextrous with firm steady hands, clear vision, calm mind; he must be intrepid, humane, passionate, and he must avoid any cruelty to his patients. Dr. Jones described wounds as a separation of vessels of various kinds. He believed a wound was mortal if it was inflicted in "those parts whose cohesion was inseparable from life." Any wound that destroyed a reflux of blood to the heart or expulsion of the blood from the heart was mortal. Limb arterial bleeding could be controlled with tourniquets and ligatures, but many wounds could cause death if not treated rapidly. He referred specifically to the need to trepan the skull when there was bleeding under it. Those soldiers with wounds associated with great loss of blood could be lost due to improper therapy. These patients needed nourishing broths. They were not to be given spiritous liquors, which were stimulants or dilators of the blood vessels and caused more hemorrhaging. He used bark because he felt it had vasoconstrictive properties. Dr. Jones described wounds as incised, contused, lacerated, and punctured. He described how wounds progressed with time. On the fourth day pus was seen. This material separated the lacerated vessels and extravasated fluid from the sound parts, which grew up fresh. This was laudable pus and a good sign. After pus formation, the redness, heat, pain, and retraction of the lips of the wound diminished. These symptoms were due to an obstruction of circulation as a result of the contraction of the orifices of wounded vessels. These effects were removed by laudable suppuration. Pus started the stage of digestion. The wound then filled with new flesh, and the margins united. It dried and was covered with a cicatrix produced by the body. The surgeon was admonished not to use balsams and balms. Rather, he should let nature do its healing. The best treatment was the application of dry, soft lint. It stopped hemorrhage with less injury than styptic medicines and was the best digestive as well. Lint was soft and could still compress "sprouting fungus" or granulations. When a wound degenerated and lost its proper florid appearance, it was called an ulcer.

Incised wounds healed by first intention. The lips were brought together and sutured or bandaged to keep them together. Linen or thin strips of leather were used as suture material. Plasters could be used as well. In oblique incised wounds, the patient required interrupted sutures. Initially the wound was cleaned out, the lips were brought together, and a needle dipped in oil was used as the suturing agent. The surgeon started the suture a distance away from the wound equal to the depth of the wound and brought the needle out on the opposite side, the same distance from the wound. The lips were brought together without puckering, and a double knot was used in the suture material. As many sutures as necessary to keep the lips together were advised. Adhesive was applied over sutures. The sutures were removed on the second or third day. (This advice is still good except for the oil, and nowadays we keep sutures in longer.) Punctured wounds that did not penetrate a body cavity required no special therapy unless deep and winding. They responded to dilatation of the external orifice to permit discharge of fluids.

Concerning lacerated wounds, Dr. Jones admonished surgeons to save as much skin as possible. If there was a bad laceration, enough skin was to be removed so that it resembled a simple incised wound. In severe contused wounds, suppuration followed. The surgeon had to cut an opening for drainage. Warm fomentations were applied. Also, the patient was bled, purged, and placed on a reduced diet. When tendons were divided, the ends were brought together. Jones then described a procedure for joining a torn Achilles tendon. Wounds of the thorax and abdomen, the head, cerebellum, medulla, and receptaculum chyli were considered fatal.

Despite Dr. Jones's words, occasionally soldiers with wounds of the thorax survived.[47] Dr. James Thacher's military journal described a soldier who was shot through the lung and then attended by Dr. Eustis, who dilated the wound and advised that the patient be "bled to near death." The soldier survived.[48] Dr. Eustis was an apprentice of Dr. Joseph Warren of Boston who was killed at Bunker Hill. The preceptor turned his practice over to his student when he became a general in the Massachusetts army. Dr. Eustis did not remain a civilian very long. He became a regimental surgeon in an artillery regiment. He learned so much about artillery that he was offered a lieutenant colonel's commission in the artillery. He refused, despite the fact that a surgeon at this time had no rank in the army. Dr. Eustis was later transferred to the Robinson House at West Point where he cared for a hysterical Mrs. Arnold after her husband's treason.

Wounds of lungs, liver, intestine, kidneys, pancreas, gallbladder, large vessels, spleen, mesentery, bladder, and stomach were hazardous but not necessarily fatal. In wounds of the abdomen, the surgeon introduced a probe with lint on the tip. He then removed it to check for gut contents—probably by smell. If gut contents were present, the patient died (peritonitis). Occasionally, the surgeon tried to look for the intestinal perforation. He then exteriorized the area or sutured the wounded gut. The gut was then attached to the body wall. If the intestines protruded through the abdominal wall, they were immediately pushed back with two forefingers. If this was not possible, the abdominal wound was increased in size. Mortified omentum was cut away. In penetrations of the thorax, air passed through the wound in respiration, and the patient expectorated frothy blood. If the soldier suffered a wound from a bayonet or sword, the external orifice was enlarged to allow blood to discharge. Heavy hemorrhage was restrained by heavy venesections. After venesections, the patient received frequent doses of nitre and barley water, and he was placed at complete rest. In non-penetrating wounds of the abdomen and chest, bleeding and antiphlogistic (anti-inflammatory) therapy were provided. To determine which organ was injured in penetrating injuries, examination of the evacuations was required. This determined prognosis rather than therapy.

In simple fractures, limbs had to be relaxed. The limb was placed in the best position to relax the muscles and bring the ends into apposition. This was followed by medications applied to keep the skin lax, moist, and perspirable as well as to decrease inflammation. Gentle compression was applied to restrain the bones. This was done with a cerate (a stiff ointment) prepared from a solution of litharge in vinegar to which soap, oil, and wax were added until the mixture had a consistency allowing it to be spread without injury to the part. An eighteen-tailed bandage was applied over it, so the fractured part could be seen easily without disturbing the limb. Then splints of wood or pasteboard lined with linen and flannel were applied. These splints were an adaptation of an invention by Mr. Sharp of England.

In compound fractures, Mr. Potts called for amputation, but Mr. Gooch was conservative. (These were authorities to whom Dr. Jones referred. Note the designation Mr., which meant they were surgeons.) If the patient was in a hospital with noxious air, amputation was preferable. In the country, the patient was treated conservatively. If the fracture involved joints, Jones amputated immediately.

If there was great destruction of tissue, a mild digestive was applied, and the limb was enveloped in a relaxing cataplasm and fomentation. Purges and gentle bleeding were used, and pain was relieved.

Abscesses formed from extravasation and splinters. Foreign bodies were extracted, and the lesions were opened. After inflammation, the patient was supported with a nourishing diet and bark. If no healing occurred, and the patient continued feverish, he needed amputation, but first a consultation should be obtained.

For gunshot wounds, Dr. Jones admonished the surgeon to remove the shot if possible and to stop hemorrhage by tie or with styptic. The openings were dilated for extravasation, and a light dressing was applied. This was followed with a bleed and gentle purge, clysters, an easy perspiration, and a light diet. If there was a need to amputate, it was done immediately.

In superficial burns, spirit of wine was used. In deeper burns, linseed oil and a cerate of oil, wax and spermaceti was applied. If a patient was burned down to the muscles, he was bled early, purged and given clysters. Then, the surgeon applied an emollient poultice, anodynes and fomentations until the part sloughed. Then a digestive was applied. He used a soothing ointment of leaves of the thorn apple. The juice was made by boiling, then absorbed by hog's lard with wax added for consistency. This could be applied until scarring developed. The fungus was treated with escharotics (Roman vitriol or lunar caustic). This burn could need therapy for a year. Lint or rags dipped in strong tea and wrapped around a burned area with a compression bandage was a later useful discovery. (The tea supplied tannic acid which was used in the treatment of burns into the twentieth century.)[49]

Amputation of a limb and trepanning the skull were the most serious operations performed by the military surgeon as well as his civilian counterpart. Amputation of an extremity was rare before gunpowder and it was first reported in 1338. Hippocrates amputated a limb because of vascular occlusion. (Did patients live long enough for arteriosclerosis to decrease circulation or produce emboli?) He advised an incision through devitalized tissue to decrease hemorrhage. Hippocrates's aphorism of therapy was the following: "Those diseases that medicine did not cure, iron cures. Those which iron did not cure, fire cures. Those which fire cannot cure are to be reckoned incurable." Hot oil, hot cautery, or boiling water were used to stop hemorrhage.[50] These methods were later replaced by Paré's ligature. Cautery was used to prevent suppuration and encourage healing despite the concept of "laudable pus." Cautery was considered anti-putrefactive. Paré used cautery for gangrenous wounds. The hot iron was advised by Hippocrates for debridement. Because the surgeon frequently had no assistant to help in surgery, cautery worked better than ligature. In 1718, Pettit invented the compressive tourniquet, which provided hemostasis, so the ligature came back into use. In compound fractures with protruding bones, Hippocrates tried turpentine ointment. With protrusion, he tried to slip bones back. If unable, he cut off the protruding ends. If a compound fracture was associated with fever, Paré advised amputation. After amputation through devitalized tissue, the wound was left to heal by granulation. Contraction of the soft tissue after healing left bone exposed, which had to be sawed off. If amputation was performed through viable tissue, this required closure, so the bone was cut proximal to the amputation site, and the tissue was drawn over the edge. The edges were sutured or taped. A flap over the amputation was first developed by Yonge. The wound was left partially open for drainage.[51]

The "Gold Standard" of the period under discussion relating to amputation was a treatise by Baron Larrey of France, *Les Memoires de Chirurgie Militaire* (1812). James Mann examined Larrey's work but developed a more conservative approach. Larrey's axioms included the following: When a limb was carried away by a ball, prompt amputation was necessary. When a ball struck a limb and bones were fractured with the soft parts severely contused, extensively torn and broken up, amputate immediately. If a large portion of soft parts was taken away along with the principal vessels and the bone was fractured, prompt amputation was required. When a ball struck the thick part of the limb, broke bone, cut and tore muscles and nerves, and left the main artery intact, Larrey advised amputation. Mann felt watchful waiting was indicated, because he had saved some limbs with conservatism. If a spent ball struck and did not break the skin, but underlying tissues were badly shattered, amputation depended on the site and the amount of trauma. The area was incised for investigation, and the hematoma was relieved. If a missile fractured bones around a joint, particularly the knee or ankle, with laceration of the ligaments, Larrey urged amputation, but Mann waited. If part of a bone was denuded, but not fractured by a missile passing through, Larrey amputated,

but Mann treated it conservatively. If a joint was cut in two by a saber or bayonet, Larrey amputated to prevent fatal infection, but Mann waited. In a compound fracture with persistent drainage of pus, Larrey amputated. Mann urged
patient observation to get the sufferer in better shape for amputation. This
resulted in a lower mortality. The surgeon who performed the amputation was
taught to show no emotion in the face of the screams of his patient. However,
he had to be fast in order to end the procedure as soon as possible.[52] An above-
the-knee amputation was performed in thirty seconds, a below-the-knee one
took slightly longer. The surgeon's assistants had to be strong muscled and
strong willed. They had to hold the patient, as well as the limb that was being
severed. After surgery, the patient was given a sweat-producing anodyne to
relieve pain and cause diaphoresis. The stump was then covered with a knit-
ted woolen cap.[53] The need to amputate early served two purposes for the military surgeon. First, the shock of the wound affected the patient's mental status
so amputation, if done immediately, was performed with less pain. Second, a
severely contused limb usually became gangrenous. This weakened the patient's
general health and increased the mortality when the operation was performed.
As the Revolution progressed, the conservative approach became the norm of
therapy, and many limbs were saved that would have been sacrificed earlier.
Occasionally, amputations were not performed when the patient refused the
procedure. One such patient was Benedict Arnold after his leg was injured at
Saratoga.[54]

Trepanation of the skull was a technique carried out as early as the Stone
Age in order to let the evil spirits out. There is evidence of regrowth in the
skulls, which suggested that the patient survived for some period after the
procedure. Hippocrates promulgated rules for trepanning in trauma. He advised
the procedure in contusions whether or not the bone was laid bare and when
there was an indentation of the skull with or without a fracture. Galen developed a guard on the trepanning tool to prevent entrance into the dura. In the
twelfth century, the Bamberg text on surgery in Salerno also described this
treatment for compound fractures of the skull. Paré operated on skulls injured
through trauma. He removed osteolytic portions of the cranium and incised the
dura to relieve pus and blood. Dr. Percival Pott of England urged trepanning
to remove pus and blood under the skull. Dr. John Jones in America also
described the operation. He performed the operation for delirium in a
patient 80 days after a head injury. The patient probably had a subdural hematoma.[55] The operation was done occasionally during the Revolution for head
injuries. The following incident was related by Dr. Drowne, an army surgeon
from Providence, Rhode Island. In General Sullivan's expedition in Rhode
Island, a soldier received a severe skull injury. Most doctors who saw the
patient felt the case was hopeless. Dr. Drowne trepanned his skull and removed
a piece of bone from the brain. At that point, the wounded man shouted out

the balance of a command he had started in the field. Dr. Drowne hammered a Spanish silver quarter to fit the space and replaced the missing piece of skull with it. The man lived for more than thirty years after the incident. The piece of bone is still in the Drowne family's possession.[56]

Blade and bullet wounds of the face, neck, and extremities required most of the battlefield surgeon's attention. He tried to arrest hemorrhage, clean the wound, and remove any foreign bodies. He could restrain hemorrhage by pressure bandages, tourniquet, or ligature. New surgeons had to be taught the proper application of a tourniquet to stop the flow of blood from any artery until it could be otherwise secured. Care had to be taken against its application in such a manner that it would interfere with circulation, increase inflammation, and "excite a fever." If it was applied too loosely, it would slip and cause a fresh loss of blood. It had to be fortified with a ligature of thread.[57] Once bleeding was controlled, the surgeon had to clean the wound and probe for foreign material. Before the search, the surgeon usually gave his patient a grain of opium or a good swallow of alcohol. He opened wounds with his scalpel and made additional incisions in the belief that healing was speeded by changing the shape of the wound. When he located a ball, he removed it with a spoon or his fingers. If a ball was too deep, forceps could be used. If the surgeon extracted a piece of metal, he showed it to the wounded soldier (if he was still conscious) to improve his morale. (Today, after gallbladder surgery, the surgeon leaves the stones at the patient's bedside table in a hospital cup so that the patient can see them and show them to visitors.) If the metal was too deep, it was left inside to "extricate itself."[58] The wound was then cleansed with dry lint or lint soaked in oil. Then it was packed with fresh lint soaked in wine, brandy, or vinegar and bandaged.

The use of alcohol in the treatment was serendipitous. Dr. Charles Gilman of New Jersey accidentally discovered the disinfectant properties of alcohol. He was wounded in the hand at the Battle of Harlem Heights, and it continued to drain pus. The good doctor was a tippler, and once during a drinking session he accidentally spilled rum on his injured hand. When the surgeon removed the dressing two days later, there was no more odor, and the wound was clean. Thereafter all wounds were soaked in rum before they were covered.[59] (We know that 70 percent alcohol is required for antisepsis. The distillation of a rum with that much alcohol is unlikely, but it made a good story.) If the surgeon did not have lint, he stuffed the wound with grass, moss, leaves, rags, or even a piece of a tattered flag. In the second stage of treatment on the fourth day, infection usually followed with suppuration and a free discharge of pus. This was encouraged in the belief that the evacuation would dislodge any foreign body. It also separated the lacerated vessels and tissues from sound parts and allowed the regrowth of normal tissue. "Laudable pus" was believed to be part of the healing process, and surgeons would leave lint or a piece of sponge in the site in the belief that inflammation would promote the healing process. Later, in the third stage, the wound was washed with a digestive (a substance used to draw pus) and covered with a milk and bread poultice with oil to maintain the moisture. The surgeon felt the patient should be kept cool during the prolonged period of granulation. The cooling process was accomplished with a light diet without heated foods. Cooling medications were also prescribed.

After removing foreign material, the surgeon set any incidental fractures and splinted them to prevent displacement in the future. He could then turn his attention to the patients' less serious injuries, including sprains, dislocations, simple fractures, and burns limited to a small area. Frequently, his mate could handle these problems while the surgeon was taking care of the serious injuries. Surgery was carried out on tables, doors, or planks across barrels. The table, instruments, and doctor's coat were covered with blood or secretions from previous operations. Frequently there was little heat or light. A simple wash basin was all that was available to rinse the instruments, sponges, and the surgeon's hands. The surgeon used one instrument to probe dozens of wounds. The same filthy sponge "cleaned" wounds. If a rag was not available, the surgeon wiped his hands on his bloody coat. Gangrene was a frequent accompaniment to surgery.[60]

Early Treatment to Save Lives

The understanding of the urgency of getting the casualty to a military surgeon promptly evolved with time, as did the care the surgeon gave. In earlier mercenary armies, the wounded lay on a field among the dead until they died or their mates put them out of their misery. If the field belonged to the opposing army, they were killed and looted by the victors. With the growth of national armies, attempts were made to get the wounded to a surgeon as soon as possible. In 1487 Queen Isabella of Spain introduced bedded wagons to carry the wounded to hospital tents in safe areas. Her grandson, Charles V, placed surgeons in the rear of his armies, with heavy wagons (fourgons) that could be pulled by horses to the battlefield. It sometimes took twenty-four to thirty-six hours to reach the site of carnage.

During the Revolution, neither the British nor the American army had a routine for removing the wounded. A casualty might be carried in a wheelbarrow, ox cart, a sailcloth held by four men, or in blankets or clothing over two shafts. In 1777 Congress gave the quartermaster general responsibility to provide litters in wagons to remove the wounded. It appeared on paper but went no further.[61] There was no safe way to move casualties over any distance. Before Britain agreed to give Americans legitimate enemy status and respect their sick as a special group, casualties had to be transported with the army in retreat to avoid capture. In the withdrawal from New Jersey to eastern

Pennsylvania ahead of the advancing British, many casualties from New Jersey hospitals died of pneumonia due to exposure in the open wagons.[62]

Wounded soldiers were first transported to the regimental hospital facility. In a permanent encampment, this might be a house, barn, or church near the camp. During actual combat, this might be an area behind the lines protected by a small hill or other elevation to protect it from direct fire. The regimental hospital was manned by a surgeon and one or two mates. The surgeon in combat gave first aid and treated life threatening wounds before the patient was transported further. In periods between battles, the regimental surgeon handled the illnesses and injuries of camp life.[63]

During the encirclement of Boston, most of the regimental medical chests were filled with material that the surgeons brought from their own offices. After some time, these had to be supplemented. The Continental Congress in Philadelphia gave the contract to Christopher and Charles Marshall, the main pharmacy in that city. They supplied 20 chests used by seven states. Even the largest pharmacy in Philadelphia, the most populous city on the eastern seaboard, could not keep up with the increased demand. The colonies had imported their pharmaceuticals from the mother country since their beginnings, but shipments were abruptly cut off with the onset of hostilities. However, certain items were required in most chests. Peruvian or Jesuit's bark was used for all fevers, although it was effective only in the treatment of malaria. This was in short supply until privateers' prize ships made up the deficit. The chests also contained opium in the form of gum opium, opium tincture, and paregoric elixir. Purges, the "chicken soup" of eighteenth-century physicians, were also needed. These included jalap, rhubarb, senna, aloe, and castor oil. Cathartics, the baby brother of purges, in the form of Epsom and Glauber's salts, were also required. To help the purging, emetics were needed. These were ipecac and tartar emetic (antimony and potassium tartrate). To add to the victim's misery, blisters were used to remove the noxious humors. Cantharides or Spanish fly was the item of choice. This was ground and applied, then covered with a plaster. Other items included camphor for fevers and venereal disease. Nitre (potassium nitrate) was used for fevers. Mercurials in the form of corrosive sublimate, red mercuric oxide, calomel, and mercurial ointment were used to treat wounds and venereal disease. They also acted as purges. Sulfur in hog's lard and other soothing ointments was required for skin conditions. The surgeons also needed mortars and pestles to grind medication, glass vials, lint, bandages, splints, probes, bullet extractors, amputation saws with extra blades, several Pettit tourniquets, trepanning instruments, and lancets.[64]

Types of Army Hospitals

The benefit of the regimental hospital was that the men knew the surgeon from previous exposure during training. They were usually from the same area, and they were more comfortable in his hands. Furthermore, there were not many patients in the regimental hospitals, so crowding and cross infection rarely occurred. By and large, the officers and men preferred treatment in their regimental installations. During the early years of the Revolution, the regimental surgeons were of poor quality and were not above illicit activities to increase their income. They would give furloughs and medical discharges for a price. The surgeons demanded more stores and equipment than needed to sell later. Medical men who had the backing of their colonel resented control by the directors of the hospital department. George Washington, early in the war, referred to them as rascals. However, too often they were the "stepchildren" of the medical department. The surgeon frequently had little or nothing available to treat casualties. On occasion, their colonels were forced to write to the State Committees of Safety to obtain medical equipment. Many colonels refused to allow their casualties to go to the general hospitals, some even going to the general hospital to take their men out and deposit them in farm houses for better care.[65]

Sir John Pringle developed the concept of the flying hospital during the War of the Austrian Succession. As its name implied, it was a movable hospital (later called a field hospital) that could follow the lines of battle and provide more definitive care for casualties before they were moved to the rear or sent back to the battle line.[66] The French adopted this concept and improved upon it. They placed their "ambulant hospitals" about 1,200 yards behind the front lines, usually behind the artillery. These were staffed by very competent surgeons who did major surgery. When they finished, the patient was moved back to a larger hospital in a nearby city. During the Revolution, the American flying hospital was in size between the regimental and the general hospital. Because of its smaller size with less mixture of medical and surgical casualties, the mortality was lower. The hospital at Valley Forge was considered a flying hospital. It was like a regimental facility but larger and consisted of several brigade hospital huts under the control of the physician and surgeon general of the army, Dr. Cochran at the time. Patients here were made ready to return to duty or were prepared to move to a general hospital. There were two hospital huts per brigade located 100 to 300 yards behind the brigade. The hut was fifteen feet wide by twenty-five feet long by nine feet high. They were covered with boards or shingles, but cracks were left open for ventilation. There were windows at each side and a chimney at one end.[67]

Washington quartered his army around Morristown in the winter of 1779–80. It was here that Dr. Tilton developed the Tilton Hospital or "Indian Hut." Like all medical observers, he knew that the increased mortality in the larger hospital was due to crowding and unsanitary, poorly ventilated rooms. The Tilton Hospital was based on a plan developed by Marshal Saxe, a German in the French army. Tilton believed that the entry of air through crevices between timbers slowed the spread of typhus. It was at Jockey Hollow near Morristown that he tested his ideas by having a one-story log cabin built to house 28 patients in three separate sections. It had a central ward of seventy-eight square feet for 12 patients and two side wards of fifty square feet each with eight patients. The structure had one entrance to each ward. There were no windows and the floor was packed earth to neutralize infection. Each ward had a fireplace with a four-inch hole in the roof. The smoke of the fireplace passed through the room before it found its way through the hole. The men were placed with the heads of their beds to the wall and their feet toward the fire. From Tilton's sketches, it is apparent that the building supplied a small, amply ventilated open hospital in which patients could be separated depending upon the nature of their disease. Noting the effects of isolation, Tilton remarked on the importance of separating those with fever and fluxes from the wounded and those with minor problems. The smoke from the fire circulated above the beds of the patients. He believed this acted as a form of disinfectant, because there was no spread of contagious disease in the hospital. The facility was the most practical achievement of the medical service that year. The winter of 1779–80 at Morristown was the coldest winter of the century. Food was limited and men were weak from exposure. However, the sick rate was very low. About three to five percent of the army of 11,500 spent time in the hospitals.[68]

The general hospital was a fixed or stationary one. This was always well behind the lines of battle and well behind the huts in an encampment. The general hospital could be in a church, a barn, a large private home, or the barracks-like home of religious orders in eastern Pennsylvania. When the general hospital served one purpose, e.g., as a smallpox facility or an inoculation hospital, it served its purpose well. The patients in an inoculation hospital were mildly ill and all had the same problem. There was little other infection if the men were examined before admission. After all the scabs fell off, the inoculees were discharged back to duty, and a new group was admitted. However, the general hospital came up short when it acted as a receiving facility for all sick and wounded. Regimental and flying hospitals would send their convalescents back when their census climbed, but the general hospital had no place to send excess numbers. Patients piled in and were mixed together. Surgical patients were next to typhus and flux inmates. Convalescents shared the same ward. General hospitals treated patients for all kinds of diseases, from fevers, dysentery, diarrhea, rheumatism, and venereal disease to small pox, jaundice, rash, itch, measles, mumps and scurvy. Fevers were inflammatory, intermittent, bilious, putrid, nervous and hectic. Bilious intermittent was probably dengue (also called break bone and scarlatina rheumatica). Additional problems included scarlet fever, throat distempers (malignant quinsies, putrid or malignant sore throat and cynanche trachealis) and nostalgia (homesickness). The results of packing infectious diseases together was a mortality rate that astonished the attending physicians.[69] The physicians, nurses, and orderlies were caught in the web of infection and frequently paid with their lives. The general hospitals of the American army were "sinks of human life." "They robbed the country of more citizens than the sword," according to Rush.[70] Another surgeon, Francis Allison, described the hospital in Bethlehem in these words: "While I am writing these few lines there are several brave fellows expiring within 50 yards of me from being confined in a hospital whose air has been rendered putrid by the sick and wounded being crowded together."[71] If the soldier survived his treatment at the hospital, he might be ready to return to duty. Others required more convalescence or permanent care.

The concept of a small convalescent hospital was pioneered by Connecticut in 1776. There citizen soldiers received care in a familiar atmosphere. While some were able to return to duty from these institutions, others joined the "Corps of Invalids" developed by the Continental Congress to use disabled soldiers for garrison duty, so that the able bodied could report for active duty.[72]

The need for a permanent hospital to care for disabled servicemen arose with the development of national armies of citizen soldiers. The first military hospital in Great Britain was at Portchester Castle in 1563. In 1600 Dublin was the site of the second such hospital. In 1644 and 1648 two military hospitals were set up in London (the Savoy and the Elizabeth House) each with fifty beds. Others were started in Edinburgh. All of these hospitals were closed at the start of the Restoration because of the expense, and the patients were referred to their home counties for care. In 1680 and 1681 Charles II opened two new hospitals. All army officers and men contributed to their upkeep. The French, like their neighbors across the channel, had veterans' hospitals throughout the country. Louis XIV is supposed to have built 85 such hospitals.[73] The American Congress, at Washington's insistence, authorized the first new permanent hospital at Yellow Springs, Pennsylvania. This was ten miles from Valley Forge and was started as a camp hospital for Valley Forge. The Yellow Springs area was an old established health resort with medicinal springs and baths. The building at Yellow Springs was three stories high. During the Revolution, 1,300 men were patients there until the winter of 1781. The hospital also had a large apothecary installation for the manufacture of drugs for regimental chests.[74]

Army Physicians and Surgeons

The physicians and surgeons manning the American hospitals were predominantly apprentice-trained. Of the 1,200 men who served as physicians, about one hundred had earned medical degrees either from European schools or from the infant American schools. The length of apprenticeship varied greatly. The usual duration was seven years, but as little as one year could suffice. This was the case for Ebenezer David, a Seventh Day Baptist preacher who enlisted after Lexington and Concord as chaplain to Rhode Island regiments.

After a short time, he resigned and apprenticed to a physician in Rhode Island. After one year of apprenticeship, he became a surgeon's mate at the Lancaster hospital that served Valley Forge. Unfortunately, he developed typhus and died in March 1778.[75] The better-trained physicians usually were promoted to the top of the service and ended up in administrative capacities. The poorly trained ones were regimental surgeons' mates, hospital mates, and hospital surgeons.[76] Many reputable physicians did not join the army because the pay was bad— if they were paid at all, and it was in paper money. They had no rank and they did not receive the benefits given to line officers until the end of the war, when they were awarded bonuses for service.[77]

The surgeons of the three European armies that participated in the American Revolutionary War had similar early histories, but that changed with time. The earliest surgeons were the progeny of the "bath men" who worked in the bath houses of the Middle Ages. They shaved and cut hair. They then learned cupping, and they dressed wounds and bled patients. The barbers developed and separated from the bath men. They did similar work, but they called themselves "wound surgeons." There were physicians present, but their training consisted of reading the medical literature. The physician decided on a course of therapy, and the bath man or surgeon did the technical work. The barber-surgeons, to keep their reputations intact and separate themselves from the itinerant tooth-pullers, stone-cutters, and cataract-couchers, formed guilds, and developed examinations and regulations for their members. These men became the military surgeons. Early in their history they volunteered their services in return for booty from their patients. They often fought as soldiers during engagements. Later, barber-surgeons were hired by army commanders to treat the wounded. They ranked below fifers and drummers. They reduced fractures, probed for bullets, cauterized bleeding wounds, and amputated. In time, physicians were hired by monarchs and nobles to supervise these technicians. The surgeon gradually received better training and higher rank. He also received special instruction specific to the military.[78]

The almost constant warfare in Europe in the seventeenth and eighteenth centuries required standing armies with surgeons to care for them. As the armies grew in size, so too did the medical services. The British medical service was administered by a surgeon general, a physician general, and an inspector general. The physician general placed physicians in general hospitals as well as on the staffs of field commanders. The surgeon general appointed staff surgeons and apothecaries for the general hospital, but the regimental commanders appointed their own regimental surgeons and mates. The inspector general inspected medical installations. Each field army of 20,000 had an inspector general. He had four assistants, one for each of the four divisions. The surgeon general supervised the purveyor who had commissary duties and purchased straw, linen, bedding, and provisions for the sick. The three leaders of the medical service were usually well known London practitioners, but they were civilians without military experience. However, in the War of the Austrian Succession, the concept of military surgeons and physicians developed. The army physician had to be a graduate of a medical school but held no rank. The army surgeon was a technician usually with enough money to buy a commission, which sold for 500 to 600 pounds. He was listed below the youngest ensign.[79]

During the American Revolution, the British flying hospital ceased to exist. Its duties were taken over by the general hospital, which had developed a "staff" that could follow an army and set up satellites removed from the larger group. These satellites existed for the duration of a campaign and then closed. Their occupants were then sent to a larger base hospital. The general hospital had about 400 beds and serviced 20,000 to 30,000 troops. Its complement included a director, a purveyor, a physician with two mates, a surgeon with one mate, an apothecary and mate, a steward, three ward masters, two dispensers, a seamstress, and five laundresses as well as bathers, cooks, servants, and laborers. Physicians and surgeons treated the patients. The physicians were still prestigious and received one pound per day. Staff surgeons were still craftsmen and received a half pound per day, as did the apothecary. Mates of physicians and surgeons received five shillings per day. The senior staff of the hospital was of high quality and did not purchase their positions. This was attested to by the observations of Jonathan Potts, who watched them work on their men in hospitals in Albany after the Battle of Saratoga. The lower ranks in the hospital generally came from regimental hospitals. Women, usually wives or widows of soldiers, were hired as servants and nurses for the hospitals in the British army and were paid six pence per day. Laundresses received one shilling, cooks one shilling eight pence, and matrons two shillings and six pence per day. Soldier's wives picked up very little experience as nurses, because they were rotated out of their position every six weeks. As a rule, they did not want the jobs, and occasionally they had to be supplemented by misfits from among the infantry regiments. They served meals and reported to their superior, the matron. They made sure the patients took their medicine and cleaned them and the wards. They had to keep their own clothing clean and dress properly. They could be court-martialed for infractions of the rules. In a large hospital, a nurse and orderly cared for twelve patients. Some nurses were permitted to change dressings.

Generally, regimental medical and surgical officers were of poor quality. They received a formal commission from the king. The surgeon's mate was a warrant officer who took over the surgeon's duties as needed, and assisted him in surgery. The mate was poorly trained and may have been a line warrant officer before becoming an assistant. Mates were chosen by the colonel, and they paid for the position. A regimental surgeon received four shillings per day, mates received three shillings six pence per day. The surgeon also received approximately one penny per week of each man's pay, which amounted to about eighty pounds per year. This was called stoppage and was used to buy supplies. The surgeon kept what he did not spend. The regimental surgeon also received fifty pounds per year to rent a hospital and pay for its fuel and some salaries. In wartime, he cared for 700 to 1,000 men. He did first aid and shipped the patient back to the general hospital satellite. If the distance was great, as many as one-third of the patients died on the way.[80]

The choice of surgeons and mates changed after the War of the Austrian Succession (1740–48). The Company of Surgeons of London obtained the right and monopoly to choose these officers. This monopoly persisted until 1780 when the Company of Surgeons of Edinburgh was permitted to give a warrant to a surgeon's mate.[81] The surgeon was an officer, but the lowest ranking one. He could be flogged before the troops, on the colonel's order, for infractions observed by his superior officer.[82] The theater commander was generally in charge of all medical services, but he usually delegated these duties to a medical director. The secretary of war was in total command, but he consulted with the physician general, the surgeon general, and the inspector general. These three were the true controllers of the medical service. One of their major functions was to keep the cost of services down and thus, as a war approached its conclusion, they discharged most medical officers. At the start of hostilities, they had to start from square one. This resulted in increased mortality among casualties until the new surgeons learned their trade.[83]

The allies of the British in America, the Hessians, had a more primitive organization. Like their British associates, they were observed in action at the American hospital in Albany. Potts felt they were unskilled, unsympathetic to their charges, and generally unable to perform the major operations needed to repair the wounds of war.[84] The British hired 17,000 Germans to help fight the war in America. The mercenaries came from several principalities, but since Frederick II, landgrave of Hesse-Kassel, supplied the largest number, all Germans were called Hessians. The landgraves had been in the business of selling soldiers for 140 years.[85] They supplied two corps, each with its own hospital complement that included four physicians (three of whom were graduate medical doctors), two surgeons general, eight surgeons, an apothecary, two purveyors, three clerks, four commissaries, and two cooks. In the field they placed forty-five regimental surgeons, most of them "self-taught." Below the regimental surgeons were company surgeons. Below the company surgeons were squadron surgeons. The German surgeon was held in low esteem even by his own army. He was still the barber, and one of his duties was to shave the officers and bleed them when necessary. A bleed was a commonplace treatment for a myriad of symptoms, much as we nowadays take two aspirins for relief of all kinds of symptoms. Officers paid for their own medical needs. After the war, more than half of the German surgeons stayed in Canada, with or without permission, rather than return to Germany.[86]

The French have a long history of trying to supply the best medical care for their armies. In 1718 France opened schools of military and naval medicine and established the first set of medical regulations. The English followed this example in 1762. In 1766 the first medical journal devoted to military medicine was introduced. The Academie Royale de Chirurgerie was founded in 1731. Its members were predominantly military surgeons, and they developed the mobile hospital to follow the troops. These were well equipped with competent surgeons who had their own means of transportation and thus did not have to request wagons from field commanders. The supplies for the medical service were sent for bids by private contractors, and this naturally resulted in abuses. These contractors received a specific sum per patient, and they supplied food, medicine, and bed linen. Food was sent in carts that were then used to evacuate casualties to larger hospitals. In the eighteenth century, the king hired and paid monks to attend at hospitals and supply spiritual care. After the war, disabled veterans were cared for in military hospitals.[87]

The French expeditionary force in America comprised about 5,000 men. They were cared for by more than 50 physicians, surgeons, pharmacists, and ward masters as well as 44 surgical and apothecary apprentices plus 100 infirmary attendants. Count D'Estaing set up hospitals at the sites of debarkation of the troops—Newport, Boston, Savannah, and Williamsburg. The chief medical officer, 39-year-old Jean Francois Coste, established general hospitals at the State House in Newport, at Brown University in Providence, and at Popnowquash Point. Those of his troops who became sick with scurvy and dysentery during the trip from France were treated on land. On the trip across the Atlantic, Coste authored a pharmacopoeia that was published in Newport in July 1780. It consisted of 16 pages and presented 79 formulas. When Dr. Coste was at Yorktown, he established a general hospital at William and Mary College. American casualties at Yorktown were placed in the French hospital after the American one had burned down. Dr. Tilton was in charge of these casualties, and he was able to observe the poor sanitation of the French. As he described it, they had one "common toilet" for the three-story hospital. It was a chute in the shape of a half hexagon of boards that passed from the roof to a pit in the earth. Doors from each floor opened into the chute and all filth and excrement was thrown down. This stank up the entire hospital. Tilton also noticed that French surgeons did not use bark for fevers. They used little or no "chemicals," and most did not use opium. Their pharmacopoeia consisted of decoctions, potions, and watery drinks.[88]

Nurses and Apothecaries

There are two paramedical groups that should be mentioned; the nurses and the pharmacists. As described earlier, the nurses in British hospitals were "servants" and often the wives of soldiers. They laundered, emptied slop pails, scrubbed the floors, provided cooked meals, and washed dishes. In the American army, they fared little better.[89] Major General Schuyler, on July 13, 1776, requested one woman from each company of the Pennsylvania regiments to be sent to the general hospital at Fort George to receive the customary provisions from the medical director of the Northern Department, Dr. Stringer. Their ability and training were of no consequence. Some women worked as private contractors. Esther Burke is mentioned in a record of the Committee of Safety of New York on November 29, 1776. She was paid five pounds ten shillings for ten weeks of nursing care. Sarah Burke was a nurse in a military hospital between 1777 and 1779. In 1776 Dr. Shippen offered to raise the nurses' salaries from three shillings nine pence to ten shillings to induce them to work in the general hospital at Perth Amboy. In the reorganization of the medical department in April 1777, nurses' salaries were raised from two dollars to eight dollars per month. In 1778 Washington suggested that women should be enlisted at the same salary as soldiers to replace men in noncombatant roles and thus to free more men for active service. One hundred and sixty years later, during World War II, that suggestion was put into practice.[90]

In England the apothecary became the general practitioner to the poor, and his social and economic position was equal to that of the surgeon. Similarly, in Philadelphia, medical director Shippen's father started out as an apothecary and became a well respected member of the medical fraternity of that city. Generally in America, the physician or surgeon was his own druggist. He compounded the medications he prescribed, which represented a major source of his income, and he sold many "patent medicines" as did other shopkeepers. There were specific pharmacies in the colonies as well that made up and shipped medicine chests to plantations and ships. The pharmacy also sold the usual therapeutics such as antimony, mercury, and sulfur as well as folk remedies such as viper's fat, and the usual British patent medicines. It was only in the American Revolution that the pharmacists' specialty became distinct from that of his medical associates. Early in the war, Dr. Craigie was made apothecary general by Congress, which also appointed apothecaries to work in general hospitals. Approximately two hundred apothecaries served in the Revolution on the patriot side. The hospital apothecary received, prepared, and delivered medications to the hospital. Before the war, most remedies were imported from Britain. With the outbreak of hostilities, drugs were obtained from British ships taken as prizes as well as smuggled from France and Holland. The difficulty with obtaining drugs from these foreign suppliers was the lack of hard currency needed for their purchase. The regimental medical chests always lacked items the surgeons needed. A pharmaceutical industry had to develop to "take up the slack." A manufacturing laboratory was started at Carlisle, Pennsylvania, and another at the hospital at Yellow Springs. Early in the war, deficits in medical chests were sizeable, but by 1778 most needed medications were available. Many of these were shipped from Marseilles. Bark, which was wastefully used for all fevers, was in short supply until privateers and the French brought enough so that Carlisle had 6,000 pounds by 1778. The various forms of opium were available, as were ipecac and tartar emetic and jalap, rhubarb, senna, aloe, castor oil, Epsom, and Glauber salts, all of them used as purges. Cantharides sold for twenty pounds per pound, but at least available. Camphor and nitre were also available as was mercury for wounds and syphilis. Surgical supplies, however, were scarce. Glass vials were blown in South Jersey and were in adequate supply. If medication was not available, substitutes were suggested. In July 1778, Dr. Brown, physician general of the middle medical department after Rush resigned, brought out the 32-page Lititz pharmacopoeia in Latin. (His assignment was the general hospital at Lititz.) The booklet was designed to assist surgeons and mates who had little training. It standardized material for regimental chests. The monograph discussed the simplest, cheapest, most available drugs, particularly botanicals indigenous to the region. It suggested substitutes for materials in short supply such as linseed oil for olive oil, cider and vinegar for wine, molasses for sugar, and crude ammonia for volatile salts.[91]

The Revolution and Its Consequences

There are no accurate mortality statistics for the early wars. The failure of a son or husband to come home from a battle was a significant statistic only for the family involved. During the Revolution, educated guesses on mortality were available. The mortality from sickness in the American army was at least nine times as high as that from combat, although some say it may have been as high as nineteen times as great. The predominant fatal illnesses were smallpox, typhus, and pneumonia. In addition, there were diseases not fatal in themselves but weakening the afflicted soldiers so that other diseases became fatal. Among them were malaria, dysentery, influenza, scurvy, malnutrition, and exposure to the elements. The American troops usually came from isolated communities and lacked antibodies to the diseases to which they were newly exposed. In addition, many of them signed up only for short periods and were not professional soldiers as were the British and Hessians. About 250,000 Americans served during the entire Revolution as regulars or militia. At no time were there more than 50,000 men under arms. Their mortality rate was about twelve to twenty percent per year. The mortality figures decreased as the Americans became more seasoned veterans and recovered from the diseases to which they were exposed early in the war. After 1777 mortality decreased considerably. Prior to 1778 the debacle in Canada and upstate New York, the destruction in the hospitals of New Jersey and Pennsylvania, and the loss of more than two thousand men at Valley Forge can be compared to the winter of 1779–80 when

Washington was quartered at Morristown. Supplies were limited because of a lack of finances, which was exacerbated by the indifference of Congress and uncoordinated procurement. However, only eighty-six men died. Sickness rates at Morristown ran well below nine to eleven percent of the army of 11,361 men and officers. British losses in battle were eighteen per thousand per year. Illness cost the army about a hundred men per thousand per year. The Hessians suffered similar losses. Overall, approximately 25,000 Americans died in service in the Revolution. The deaths on British prison ships (about 8,500, perhaps many more) almost equaled the numbers of those who died in the hospitals (about 10,000). Battle casualties were about 6,500. The total mortality represented approximately seven-tenths to nine-tenths of one percent of the population,[92] and was second only to that during the Civil War where 1.6 percent of the population died. Dr. Rush had his own set of statistics; their validity is open to question, however, because he had a political axe to grind. He believed two percent died in battle. If hospitalized, this went to twenty-five percent. If the casualties were transported from one hospital to another, the mortality was fifty percent.

One positive effect of the war was that with the sudden cut-off of drugs and surgical instruments from England, the colonists had to develop their own pharmaceutical industry. The Lititz pharmacopoeia described medications that could be substituted for those imported from the motherland. Separation also prevented the import of nostrums and that of medications that were useless as well as dangerous. Within the next century, American drug companies were producing medications to rival any that could be imported.

Surgeons in the Revolutionary army had to treat men from all over the country as well as from Europe. They saw and treated illnesses they would not have seen in their own communities. They also learned surgical techniques from foreign surgeons. One important benefit in surgery was conservatism in amputation, the number of which dropped dramatically toward the end of the war. Surgical aphorisms that had previously been accepted uncritically were questioned, and this was of benefit to the patient and his limbs. The mortality of an amputation at mid-thigh level was close to fifty percent. The interested surgeon could learn anatomy from autopsies performed on unclaimed bodies, both American and British. Dr. John Warren of Boston was notable for taking advantage of this opportunity. He lectured to army and lay surgeons on the basis of experience gained in his military hospital. This same Dr. Warren later became a professor of surgery and one of the founders of Harvard Medical School. Lectures to army surgeons were also given in Philadelphia. George Washington encouraged his surgeons at the Morristown encampment to attend these lectures when they were off duty.

The benefits of a formal medical education became obvious. Surgeons with a better education passed the entrance examination more easily and advanced more rapidly. Those with a poorer education were relegated to

"Staten Island." Thacher explained in his *History of the American Revolution* how he started as a hospital surgeon. He was examined by Dr. John Morgan, the new director general. Thacher was removed from the hospital in Cambridge and made a regimental surgeon's mate. He served for the duration of the war, gaining experience, before he returned to his former position. The benefits of a "formal medical education" resulted in an increased demand for schools after the war. A plethora of schools opened, unhappily with little capacity or ability to teach fledgling doctors. Taking a page from the army, which required prospective surgeons to pass examinations, states began to examine prospective medical practitioners. In addition, states started to license doctors in order to cut down on quackery. Well-trained men formed medical societies for the diffusion of knowledge and to control their numbers. Medical monographs written before and during the war, such as those by John Jones and Benjamin Rush, gave rise to the development of medical journals for the dissemination of knowledge. The first medical journal published in the new United States was the *Medical Repository* in New York City in 1797.[93]

Probably the greatest medical benefit to come out of the war was the advance of smallpox inoculation. After 1777 the disease never affected the army again as it did in the retreat from Canada. The safety of the procedure had been demonstrated beyond a doubt. Overall, mortality from inoculation was less than one percent. The army experience disposed of the need to "prepare the inoculee." During the preceding decades, patients were prepared for the "operation," sometimes for weeks, at great expense. This expense made the procedure unaffordable for the poor. Of course, the inoculees were isolated until the scabs fell off. This was an expense that could not be dispensed with. Inoculation became commonplace, and physicians planned to do the procedure even without the presence of an epidemic. Earlier, the procedure had largely been used to stop an epidemic. The benefits of inoculation lasted less than two decades after the war. Dr. Jenner, a country doctor in England, wrote of his experience with cowpox vaccination. It required many years before physicians gave up inoculation for vaccination. In 1830 the British parliament finally outlawed the use of inoculation.

Along with the credits, we should examine the debits. King's College closed for the duration of the war. Enrollment at the Philadelphia College dropped. The Philadelphia school became enmeshed in political squabbles resulting in two competing schools that were finally united near the end of the century. The worst result was the fallen stature of the physician in the lay public's eyes. The prewar physician was not at the highest level of social acceptance—the minister and the lawyer were usually a few rungs above him—and the American physician of the eighteenth century frequently had to have another means of livelihood. Some were farmers, others owned or worked in bars, and many left the profession to take political jobs.

The number of physicians who put away their medical tools to take line officers' positions indicates their attitude toward the profession. During the war, the medical profession sank to further depths. The first medical director, Church, was a convicted spy. The second medical director, Morgan, could not work with his subordinates and was relieved of duty. The third was even worse; Dr. Shippen speculated in medical stores for his own benefit, failed to visit hospitals and give them the benefit of his training, and he frequently kept a large coterie of medical personnel around him to treat few casualties. Shippen was eventually court-martialed. Although exonerated, he was censured. Added to these problems were the violent disputes among the leaders of the medical service which found their way into the lay press. Dr. Rush repeatedly attacked Dr. Shippen in the *Pennsylvania Packet*. The same Dr. Rush was involved tangentially in the Conway Cabal that attempted to replace General Washington with General Gates after the latter's success in northern New York. In terms of mortality, however, the army hospitals received well-deserved abuse. The "decimation of regiments and the swallowing of armies" became common knowledge among the people. There were other infractions of duty among the medical officers. After the American army left Boston to prepare for the invasion of New York, Dr. Warren was told to close down his hospital. He refused. The existence of a superfluous hospital added to the burden of the limited medical budget. Dr. Philip Turner attempted to have a hospital erected in New London at government expense for his personal use and profit. Isaac Foster stockpiled medicine in New England for his own use. These activities led Dr. Barnabas Burney to say, "The dirtiest, basest actions are everyday depreciating the profession till the very appellation of doctor has become a butt of satire and contempt."[94]

— 2 —
Leaders of the
Medical Department

The Medical Department started with a catch-as-catch-can system of local physicians to care for the wounded of Lexington and Concord. This was followed by a system developed by the Massachusetts Provincial Congress, which was taken over and expanded by the Continental Congress. It went through growing pains, in-fighting between regimental surgeons and the central authority, intrigues, recriminations, and courts-martial, only to end completely broken up and discarded on the junk heap in 1783. What of the men who led (or perhaps were dragged by) the medical department in the Revolutionary years?

Benjamin Church

Benjamin Church was the first to accept the title of director general, and he lasted three months. Dr. Church was born in Newport, Rhode Island, on August 24, 1734, but his family moved to Boston in his youth. He attended Boston Latin School and then Harvard. (This path to Harvard has been trod by the boys of Boston to this day.) He graduated in 1754. Church trained for the medical profession and completed his studies at the London Medical College Hospital. While in London, he married an English woman and brought her home to Boston. The doctor was a skilled practitioner who earned a reasonable sum for a physician of his time in a city in the midst of a long recession. Dr. Church was an accomplished writer and could express himself in poetry and prose, and he was a contributor to *The Times*, a Whig newspaper of the period. Church was active in the patriot cause and came to the attention of leading Whigs, such as the Adamses, John Hancock, and Dr. Joseph Warren. In 1770 Church belonged to a committee sent to Governor Hutchinson to protest the Boston Massacre. In 1774 he was elected a delegate to the Massachusetts Provincial Congress that legislated for the colony in Cambridge and Concord while the Governor remained in Boston. The division in the government developed after Parliament passed the Port Bill that imposed restrictions on Massachusetts following the Boston Tea Party. Members of the Provincial Congress formed a Committee of Safety that acted as the executive branch of the government, similar to the English system. Church was a member of that committee, and he enjoyed a position of trust and responsibility just below that occupied by Warren, Hancock, and Sam Adams.[1] With the outbreak of hostilities and the need for regimental surgeons, Church was appointed a member of the committee to examine potential surgeons. Church was then appointed director of the newly created hospital department of Massachusetts, which was later taken over by Congress. Dr. Joseph Warren had been the first choice, but he preferred a fighting appointment and was made a general of the Massachusetts army. Warren fought as a rifleman on Bunker Hill and was shot through the head and killed. He was buried in a mass grave by the British after their pyrrhic victory. Six months later, after the British departure, the grave was opened, and Warren's remains were recognized by several silver teeth that Paul Revere had constructed for him.

When the Continental Congress took over the Medical Department on July 27, 1775, Church was appointed director and chief physician.[2] Immediately upon assuming his position, he had the same complaint as all directors after him. There was never enough medicine and equipment, and the regimental surgeons could not be managed. He felt that the regimental surgeons from the other colonies were poorly trained, and they demanded complete independence from his control. He had had a hand in choosing Massachusetts surgeons, so he felt they were adequate. Only Massachusetts surgeons considered him their superior officer.

Church early recognized the shortcomings of the regimental hospital. He felt it was expensive to run individual hospitals and wasteful of limited supplies. He wanted regimental hospitals closed and all patients sent to general hospitals. The problems reached Washington's headquarters, and Washington ordered an inquiry carried out at each brigade to solve the problem between Church and the surgeons. Apparently little came of it. Church submitted his resignation on September 20 because of ill health and weakness, but it was not accepted by Washington.[3]

Church was later found to be in correspondence with the enemy and was court-martialed, with Washington presiding over the court. Church was found guilty, but the new Articles of War listed no punishment for treason, and so he was turned over to Congress for trial and punishment. The Provincial Congress of Massachusetts tried him, found him guilty, and removed him from membership in that body. He was then tried by the Continental Congress, found guilty, and dismissed from his office as director general. He was immediately sent to jail in Norwich, Connecticut, where he was not permitted to have pen and ink or to talk to anyone unless a magistrate or sheriff was present. Church became sick with asthma from his underground confinement, and he was allowed out of jail, under guard, by order of Governor Trumbull of Connecticut, and returned to Boston. A condition of his parole was that he was not to communicate with the enemy or leave the province. Church would have been allowed freedom to move about on parole, but his life was in peril from the Massachusetts mob. The government tried to exchange him for Dr. McHenry, an American surgeon who had been captured in the Canadian invasion, but the mob refused to allow this. The prominent prisoner remained in jail in Boston for several months and was then exiled to the West Indies. The ship foundered on the trip down, and he was apparently lost at sea.

History was not able to judge Church until General Gage's letters were opened to public scrutiny. First, Church had been in need of money. He had built a rather elegant house in Boston that was beyond the means of even a successful practitioner. The physician also took a mistress who must have been a drain on family finances. Second, Church had been educated in London. Though we know nothing of his experiences in England, we can perhaps interpolate from Shippen's experience. Shippen enjoyed his life as a student in England. The rigid class system in England, particularly in the cities, must have created a massive chasm between the haves and the have-nots. To live with and be entertained by the haves gave one a positive view of society, if he did not look around too carefully. In addition, Church had taken an English wife.

There is evidence that Church was in the pay of Governor Hutchinson and General Gage before the outbreak of hostilities. Before Concord and Lexington, General Gage, his troops, and Governor Hutchinson sat in Boston. The Provincial Congress sat in Cambridge and Concord. Congress collected taxes, trained militia, and passed laws. They were felt by General Gage to be in open rebellion. He knew of all of their activities from a paid informer who was high in the echelon of leaders in the state. Gage sent out his troops to capture stores in Concord, prompting Paul Revere's famous ride to warn the inhabitants of Concord. In Lexington, Sam Adams and John Hancock were notified of their impending capture. Revere was captured in Lincoln, but Dr. Samuel Prescott carried the message to Concord. General Gage received letters (two written in French) from paid informers who described where the stores of powder were hidden. A sudden move to capture the powder would have left the colony defenseless and prevented other New England colonies from supporting beleaguered Massachusetts. Gage knew exactly what homes and other hiding places had the powder, muskets, and cannon, but he told Lieutenant Colonel Smith not to harm the inhabitants or their property. The troops were simply to destroy the ordnance. After Lexington and Concord, Gage was hemmed into Boston. He received news from a spy that rebels would fortify Bunker Hill and the Hills of Dorchester. This caused the Battle of Bunker Hill, which was actually fought on Breed's Hill.

On May 16, 1775, the Massachusetts Provincial Congress sent a letter to the Continental Congress to ask advice about how to rule the province in view of the absence of the governor and council who, naturally, were loyal to the king. They also asked Congress to take control of the army forming around Boston. This letter was sent to Philadelphia with Church. Church sent a letter to General Gage in which he described his vexation at having to go, which would make it impossible for him to communicate further with the general.[4]

While Church was in the midst of his problems with the regimental surgeons, General Washington ordered an investigation as described. His bookkeeper at the time reported that Church suddenly had hundreds of new British guineas, which could not be accounted for.[5]

Church's downfall came as a result of an intercepted note to the British forces in Boston. Prior to the actual outbreak of hostilities, British soldiers and Tories occupied Boston; the Patriots occupied the rest of Massachusetts. Civilians could pass between the strongholds. Once bullets were exchanged, the causeway from Boston to the mainland was closed. (Boston was like the head of a lollipop stuck into the harbor with the handle attached to the mainland.) On his trip back from Philadelphia, after he had delivered the note to Congress, Church "met" a woman who carried a note to him from his Tory brother-in-law in Boston. The note told him to come to Boston and receive a pardon for his revolutionary activities before the situation worsened. What was more significant was how this messenger was able to get from Boston to Cambridge. Church learned that one could travel to Newport, Rhode Island, and contact Captain Wallace of the *Rose,* which would convey him to Boston.[6] At his trial, the medical director claimed this had given him an idea to send the wrong information into Boston in code, via this route, to mislead the British high command. Church wrote such a note in which he described the great spirit of the Patriots, and the feeling of unity between Massachusetts and the other colonies. He also said that they had a large supply of ordnance, and he described the high morale of the soldiers. The note was addressed to Major Carne and was given to Church's mistress to deliver. She approached Mr. Wormwood in Newport, Rhode Island, and asked his help to get to Captain Wallace or to Mr. Dudley or Mr. Rome. Wormwood, a Patriot, took the letter, and with a friend, one Mr. Maxwell, opened the letter. He could not read it, because it was in cipher. They gave the letter to Henry Ward who was secretary to the Whig government in Providence. The letter then was sent to General Greene and from him to Washington in September, two months after it had been written. Church's mistress was arrested, and she named Church as the author. The code was deciphered by the Reverend Samuel West. The letter described American forces around Boston. Church was taken into custody and admitted it was his letter, but he claimed his purpose was to fool the enemy. Washington ordered Church's home to be searched for any incriminating evidence, but nothing was found. However, it is known that a confidant of Church had rummaged through his papers before Washington's messenger arrived. The three trials and convictions followed rapidly, and Church was replaced by John Morgan as director general.[7]

Thus, the first blemish on the record of the Medical Department occurred. This one was certainly the most serious, but it was followed by stains that left Congress and the people with a "bad taste in their mouths" for the medical service.

John Morgan

Dr. John Morgan was chosen by Congress to replace Dr. Church. He was the best trained academically and the most qualified physician for the position, at least on paper. He had spent his life in pursuit of a medical education. He then trained others and tried to raise the level of American medicine to a higher plane. He was the acknowledged leader of Philadelphia medicine and therefore of American medicine. Unfortunately, his successes were not equal to his abilities, perhaps due to a personality problem.

John Morgan was born in Philadelphia in 1735 of Quaker parentage. His family had come to Philadelphia from Wales. He was the son of a successful merchant. Morgan matriculated at Nottingham Academy under the Reverend Samuel Finley of Maryland.[8] In 1750 he was apprenticed to Dr. John Redman who had recently returned from an extensive period of study in Europe. During this apprenticeship, which lasted until 1756,[9] Morgan attended the College of Philadelphia and graduated in 1757. After college and apprenticeship, Morgan took the position of apothecary to the new Pennsylvania Hospital. This position gave him excellent training, because he filled the prescriptions of the eminent physicians of Philadelphia who were working at the hospital. During the French and Indian War, he enlisted with a militia detachment to join an English army expedition to Fort Duquesne. He was a regimental surgeon as well as a line officer in the unit.[10] The regimental surgeon had very low rank in the English army, and this was particularly true for anyone from the provinces in that position. Provincial surgeons took no exams but were simply appointed, and their pay scale was below that of chaplain. In a provincial regiment, the surgeon was quartered with the colonel. He traveled to different posts of the regiment where sickness was reported. The isolated detachments had "first aid stations" under the care of whomever was literate and could understand a book of symptoms and therapies. Morgan observed the work of the English surgeons during the war, and he found them to be well qualified for their tasks. Ever ready to learn, Morgan gathered considerable experience from this "hitch," which he was able to use in this position as director general.[11]

After completing his service in the French and Indian War, Morgan sailed for Europe to complete his education and studied there for five years. In London he studied at the private academy of the Doctors Hunter, where he learned specimen preparation by injection and corrosion.[12] This technique was an important skill that would open doors to him when he went to Paris. While in

London, Dr. Morgan was taken under the wing of Dr. Fothergill, an eminent Quaker physician, who mapped out his plan of study.

Morgan and Shippen, both from Philadelphia, discussed the development of a medical school in Philadelphia with Fothergill. According to their plan, Shippen, who returned to Philadelphia first in 1762, would approach the trustees of the College of Philadelphia to sponsor a medical school. Despite his academic background and excellent family connections, his idea was turned down, and he opened his private academy of surgical anatomy and midwifery.[13] Meanwhile, Morgan continued his training. He walked the wards in London, then moved to Edinburgh for theoretical studies for his medical degree. He matriculated in the fall of 1761 and found Edinburgh to be a community about the size of Philadelphia. At this time, the university taught theory with little or no practical hands-on instruction. Morgan graduated with honors on July 18, 1763. His graduate thesis was entitled "The Secretion of Pus by the Blood Vessels in Certain Inflammatory Conditions." He believed pus was a product of the blood vessels rather than of the tissues, the concept held at the time. The possibility of pus being derived from a component of blood was not advanced.

After graduation, he sailed to France and studied surgery under Jean Joseph Sue, chief surgeon at La Charité. Morgan's demonstration of the technique of specimen preparation, learned at the Hunter School, won him membership into the French Royal Academy of Surgery in 1764. He received this honor after he begged Dr. Sue to sponsor him. Morgan did not give credit to the Hunters for his dissertation. The young American was also elected to the Royal Society of Edinburgh and received various other honors and honorable memberships. Morgan then visited Italy where he met Morgagni (who wondered about the similarity of their names) and was made a member of the Society of Belles-Lettres of Rome.[14] Morgagni gave Morgan a personal copy of his book, *De Sedibus*. Several decades earlier Morgagni had developed morbid anatomy, the study of the body after death, to correlate symptoms and findings in the tissues. His work was to start a revolution in medical thinking and help discard the medical theories of the period. Morgan then went to Switzerland where he met Voltaire.

In 1765 he returned to America, married Mary Hopkinson, and set up a practice of medicine in Philadelphia. The young physician discussed his plans for a medical school with the trustees of the College of Philadelphia. Morgan had a letter from Penn, the proprietor of the colony, who supported the school plan. This carried great weight with the trustees. His idea was to practice medicine only. Morgan did not want to do any surgery or apothecary work at the beginning. He brought with him from England Mr. David Leighton, a surgeon and apothecary, to carry out this aspect of practice. That he remained true to this belief is seen in his medical relationship with Thomas Jefferson, who was referred to him for smallpox inoculation, a practice that was illegal in Virginia.

He turned this eminent Virginian over to Dr. Shippen, Jr., because inoculation was a surgical procedure. It was later in his career that the needs of a family forced him to do "general practice."

At commencement exercises of the College of Philadelphia in 1765, Morgan gave his "Discourse Upon the Institution of Medical Schools in America." He deplored the concept of a trained physician forced to perform surgery as well as prescribe, prepare, and sell drugs to the patient. He felt the physician should be paid only for his visit. Morgan wanted a trained physician to have enough time to study the patient and his illness without concern about the other aspects of care. Most other physicians carried out all the other practices he deprecated. He further alienated the prestigious physicians in his audience by indicting American medical education. Morgan wanted physicians to receive a medical degree from a recognized institution rather than simply completing an apprenticeship, which was how most in his audience had become practitioners. Morgan demanded excellence of himself and others and would not settle for less.[15] In his battles later in life Morgan had few allies.

The only early physician in Philadelphia to practice medicine similar to Morgan's concepts was an eccentric, Dr. Abraham Chovet, who arrived in 1774. Chovet had been a physician in London. One of his adventures included a visit to a condemned highwayman in a London jail. For a large sum of money, he promised to return this person to life after he was hanged the next day. At the time, hanging caused death by strangulation. A rope was placed around the prisoner's neck and was pulled tight when his support was kicked away. The knot did not snap down and break his neck which caused destruction of the medulla with its control of respiration and heart action. Rather, the victim struggled for as long as forty minutes before he was declared dead. Chovet did a tracheostomy on the highwayman and inserted a silver tube to keep it open. This was covered by the man's clothing. After the hanging, the body was cut down and brought to Chovet's rooms where he worked to revive the prisoner. The victim was indeed alive and might have survived. Chovet, however, performed the panacea of the period, and he bled the patient to death. This incident may have been responsible for Chovet's early move from London to the British West Indies. He remained there until a slave insurrection frightened him enough to leave. The doctor made his way to Philadelphia where he practiced only internal medicine and gave lectures in anatomy. During the Revolutionary War, when the British occupied Philadelphia, he was an outspoken Whig. When the Americans occupied the city, he was a vociferous Tory. However, he was able to avoid imprisonment under either occupation.[16]

The Medical School of the College of Philadelphia opened on November 18, 1765, and Morgan was named professor of theory and practice of physic at the advanced age of 29. Morgan wanted the new students to complete an apprenticeship with a recognized physician before matriculation. He believed they could pick up the rudiments of medicine and pharmacy before classes started. He also wanted them adept in Latin, math, natural sciences, and a modern language. Students attended lectures in anatomy, botany, the effects of drugs, theory and practice of medicine, and chemistry. After they attended rounds at the Pennsylvania Hospital for one year, and completed the lectures at the school, the students were required to complete three years of practice and submit a creditable thesis before being eligible for a bachelor of medicine degree.

Morgan recommended that William Shippen, Jr., be given the post of professor of surgery. Shippen sent in his application and was accepted. In 1768 Dr. Adam Kuhn became professor of materia medica and botany. In 1769 Dr. Rush became professor of chemistry. This completed the medical school faculty. At the school, Dr. Morgan would lecture three times a week for three or four months. The tuition for this course was four pistoles (three pounds eight shillings), plus a one dollar fee to help build a medical library. Morgan's lectures were basically Cullen's lectures that Morgan had copied while a student at Edinburgh. Morgan taught his students the benefits of fresh air and diet as well as the benefits of the "baths," particularly the one at Yellow Springs in Chester County, later to be the site of the first permanent army general hospital. He advised his students that nature was the physician, and the physician was the assistant. The doctor should "embrace her indications to strengthen her when weak, to correct her when too violent, and show her the most salutary way." This had been Hippocrates's dictum 2,000 years earlier. Among Morgan's first class of students was Benjamin Rush.[17] Morgan next founded the medical society. He wanted this society to emulate the Royal College of Physicians of London and of Edinburgh. Morgan hoped it would grow and become intercolonial in scope. It was also to be a licensing body and have authority in all of British America. The Shippens were not consulted at its inception and did not join. The society did not receive a charter from the colonial government and soon lost its identity.[18]

In October 1775 Morgan was appointed director general and physician of the hospital to replace Church. One disaster after another one befell him during his 15 months as director. He inherited all of the problems related to lack of organization and supplies that Church had had. He also had problems with the regimental surgeons who felt themselves vindicated and in a stronger position in view of Church's treason. Morgan demanded excellence from his surgeons, and this ran counter to the general incompetence, political appointments, and medical hacks friendly with their colonels. Morgan felt he could not delegate any of his work, in part this was because of his distrust for the surgeons, in part because he believed he could do the work better than anyone else (an attitude not unknown among modern physicians). Congress, in its wisdom or lack thereof, did not explicitly instruct Morgan as to the full extent of his duties and responsibilities, and Morgan believed his responsibilities ended at the hospital and not in the regimental establishment. His trials and tribulations with Stringer, Shippen, and the regimental surgeons were insurmountable. Finally, on January 9, 1777, he was summarily discharged from his office.[19]

A man with Morgan's personality could not take this dismissal without a fight. He spent the next two and a half years bombarding Congress, the newspapers, and the pamphlet printers with thousands of words depicting his side of the controversy and his demands for vindication. Morgan presented his letters of support from General Washington, General Greene, and officers of the hospital—namely, John Warren, William Eustis, Philip Turner, and Isaac Ledyard. These letters certified Morgan's excellence in his care for casualties and illness, stating that the mortality among troops in Canada and New Jersey was not his fault because these areas had been taken out of his control by acts of Congress. Morgan's health and his medical practice suffered from this profusion of bile. He felt, and probably rightly so, that Shippen was responsible for his downfall. He turned all of his investigative power on the new director. In this act of vengeance he was joined by Dr. Rush. Morgan remained in Philadelphia during the British occupation and planned to go to the West Indies to start life again. However, after the British left Philadelphia, he decided to stay and keep up his fight.

In 1777 Morgan had a pamphlet published in Philadelphia, *A Vindication of His Public Character in the Station of Director General of the Military Hospital and Physician in Chief of the American Army 1776.*[20] Morgan believed his problem was caused by his control of the stores that had been sent to the general hospital under his care, and he feared they would be dissipated by the regimental surgeons. He also tried to prevent the abuses by those surgeons who tried to raise their positions despite obvious incompetence. Morgan complained that Congress dismissed him without a hearing to defend himself, and appealed to the commander-in-chief. Morgan received no reply for three months, and he composed the tract to vindicate himself. He wanted to set the true facts before Congress so the congressmen could judge him properly. He also wished to present his case to the public. Morgan claimed he could have resigned at the first sign of trouble, but had felt it his duty to his country to stay and try to supervise the medical service. Morgan was accused of confiscation of hospital stores in Boston and of withholding medicine and stores from the regimental surgeons. He had ample proof that he carried out orders from Congress and Washington. Morgan described his personal sacrifices in the job. He had no trial and did not know his accusers' identities—this was a violation of his civil liberties.

Morgan's position as director general had been undercut by Congress when he was reduced to director and restricted to the east side of the Hudson River. The director of the flying camp, Shippen, was made senior to him (in his eyes), and he sent his reports to Congress rather than to Morgan. Shippen set up a hospital west of the Hudson River in New Jersey and received a great amount of hospital stores and almost half of Morgan's surgeons and mates. Morgan had massive duties and responsibilities he tried to carry out. He felt Shippen was undermining him to get his position. Shippen received help and assistance because he had the right connections. Morgan's powers of control of the service were limited, but he was responsible for all the problems and shortcomings of the medical department. In his pamphlet, Morgan included a letter to Washington explaining the deficiencies of the medical service and how he tried to correct them. Among those deficiencies were poor regimental surgeons who did not follow orders and a lack of equipment. Morgan described how he cared for the sick around Boston and eventually discharged all the sick after the army left for New York. The doctor told of his efforts to collect and ship medical stores to New York and how he practiced economy with his limited stores.

In his last act as director—despite his poor treatment and because he still felt responsible for the medical service—the teacher in Morgan prompted him to leave instructions concerning the material a regimental surgeon and mate should have available in the event of action. To support one thousand men in battle, they needed one set of amputating instruments consisting of a large knife, a saw with two blades, a catine (also called catling, a sharp pointed knife sharpened on both sides), at least 300 bandages and rollers, one or two dozen sets of splints, a dozen common tourniquets, six pairs of old sheets or their equivalent in rags for compresses, two or three pounds of lint, a dozen crooked needles, a screw tourniquet, a case of six incision knives, a set of pocket instruments, four bullet forceps, artery forceps, two dozen straight needles, a paper of pins, a case of lancets, three ounces of thread for ligatures, one or two pieces of inch-wide tape, sixteen-inch or eighteen-inch square saddler's leather, and a piece of saddler's inch-wide girting. Bandages, tourniquets, and splints should be made by the surgeon. Six pounds of fine toweling and six ounces of sponge were also needed.

Finally, on June 13, 1779, Congress vindicated Morgan of charges of misconduct and inefficiency. Three days later, Morgan again took up the fight against Shippen with accusations of malpractice and misconduct. After Shippen's court-martial and eventual resignation from his position, Morgan could rest. By this time, however, he was broken in health but not completely in spirit. He took up his duties at the Pennsylvania Hospital. Morgan resigned from that august body over a dispute with "The Overseers of the Poor," who ran the almshouse, related to the care of patients with syphilis. Syphilitic patients at the almshouse were turned over to the doctors of the Pennsylvania Hospital for mercury therapy. He submitted a bill for 70 shillings for each of two patients. They paid only part of this amount. After this, he "gave up on life," and in a letter to his brother, he "looked to a better world with God" and died October 15, 1781, at the age of 53.[21]

What can one say about Morgan? He was a hard-working doctor with an unbending personality. He put his duties to his patients above other considerations. Morgan had no administrative skills, and he could not get along with people who disagreed with what he felt was right and proper. As a doctor, however, he displayed real insight and great commitment to his profession.

William Shippen, Jr.

William Shippen, Jr., became the third director general of the strife-ridden, disorganized, Medical Department on April 11, 1777. He was promoted from his position of medical director of the flying hospital and director of hospitals west of the Hudson. His plan (and Cochran's) for the reorganization of the Medical Department was submitted on February 14, 1777, and it was revised and accepted by Congress on March 24, 1777. At the time, he seemed a good choice.[22] He was from the right stratum of Philadelphia society, well-trained with a medical degree from Edinburgh, a professor of anatomy and midwifery at the Medical College of Philadelphia, and well-placed with Congress with two brothers-in-law in that body. Shippen was handsome, polished, affable, and with enough private wealth to keep him above the needs of "peculation." He took over a department that had functioned poorly, was "full of rascals" (Washington's term for the regimental surgeon), lacked money to operate, and had lost the respect of the officers and men of the line.[23] Unhappily, Shippen did not have the ability or desire to work at his job.

By colonial standards, Shippen had been born into a rich family in 1736. The Shippen family had its roots in Yorkshire, England. His forebear, Edward Shippen, studied at Oxford for a time, left England in 1668, and settled in Boston where he became a merchant. Edward married a Quaker woman, Elizabeth Lybrand, and converted to the Quaker belief. Boston, early in its existence, was a strict Puritan town. It granted religious freedom only to Puritans. With the growth of a merchant class, society became more cosmopolitan, and religious toleration was granted to most Protestant sects, except for the Quakers. During the period of his residence, four Quakers were hanged, and Edward Shippen was whipped twice in public for his beliefs in "the Truth." Despite this, Shippen became reasonably wealthy, but to save his skin, literally, he planned to move to the new Quaker community of Philadelphia. He was widowed and then married a second Quaker lady, Rebecca Richardson, a widow living in New York. He moved his business to Philadelphia, a bustling town of 4,000 souls, in 1690. He was again widowed and, perhaps to forget his grief or to advance his business turned to politics. He was elected to the Provincial Assembly, and in 1695 he became speaker of that body. He was then appointed to the Governor's Council. Edward also became the first mayor of Philadelphia. Perhaps he forgot his grief through the efforts of Esther Jaines, a young woman of Philadelphia. At age 67, he married her, but her "apron rose too fast" after they exchanged marriage vows (a colonial expression for premature pregnancy). Shippen was sorely castigated by the Society of Friends, but he was gradually accepted back into the fold. He died in 1712, leaving a substantial sum to his beneficiaries.

The family grew and spread throughout Pennsylvania, New Jersey, and Maryland. In 1735 William Shippen II, our William's father, converted to Presbyterianism and married Susannah Harrison. He was a merchant and apothecary. As was common in England, a wise apothecary who questioned his customers about their symptoms and compounded the medicine prescribed by the physicians of the community could develop an excellent grasp of medical practice. Shippen did and became a physician. He also apprenticed under John Kearsley. He was accepted by patients and his contemporaries in the business and was called "doctor" without a formal education. He was so well thought of that he was elected to the staff of the Pennsylvania Hospital, the only one with his medical background or lack thereof.[24]

His son, William Shippen, Jr. (1736–1808), grew up in the "old, top stratum of Philadelphia society." He attended Samuel Finley's Boarding School and the Nottingham Academy as did Morgan. Shippen then attended the College of New Jersey at Princeton and lived with its president, Aaron Burr. After having graduated as valedictorian, Shippen returned to Philadelphia and was apprenticed to his father for four years. In 1758 he went to England to complete his education. He married Alice Lee of Virginia in 1762, a union that proved excellent for his future. While in England, he developed some royalist tastes and enjoyed the lifestyle of the upper class.[25] He did, however, spend his time wisely. He moved into the Hunter house and school in October 1759 and studied anatomy under John and William Hunter as well as under Hewson. He trained in obstetrics under McKenzie, who had studied under Smellie. From the diary Shippen kept during his stay in Europe, we know that in addition to his social activities, he attended hospital rounds, watched surgery, sat with doctors, saw and prescribed for patients, and attended lectures on various subjects and diseases. Shippen also made a complete study of the way English hospitals operated and left notes about his observations. For example, at St. Thomas Hospital, every Thursday was admitting day, and outpatients were seen by the senior physician on Thursday mornings. Tuesdays all hospital patients were seen and treated, and Saturdays physicians and surgeons made rounds together. Wednesdays male outpatients were seen by junior physicians, and Fridays women and children were seen. Major surgery was performed as needed, but Mondays were reserved for minor surgery. By arrangement, surgeons made rounds at St. Thomas on Tuesdays, Thursdays, and Saturdays. At Guys Hospital, they made rounds on Mondays, Wednesdays, and Fridays. Nursing was done by women of the servant class who were completely untrained. Three senior physicians and three senior surgeons divided responsibilities for the patients. Each senior surgeon had one or more apprentices bound to him for seven years by the Surgeon's Hall of London. Below apprentices in importance were surgeon's dressers. They carried dressings, performed minor surgery, and cared for accident cases. Pupils were spectators. This group was composed of apprentices or those who had completed apprenticeship. They had to present a certificate from their preceptor before being allowed into the hospital. Surgeons took three to four pupils at a time for a fee. Although bound to one surgeon, the students could follow all surgeons at the hospital. A St. Thomas pupil could attend operations but could not practice at Guys and vice versa. For extra fees, students could attend lectures in chemistry, anatomy, surgery, and medicine — in other words, an early medical school.

Shippen also left a record of the program of instruction at the Hunter private school. The students dissected until 5:00 P.M. Then Hunter lectured daily from 5:00 to 7:30 P.M. His lectures were attended by laymen as well as professionals. Hunter obtained bodies of criminals and paupers, and each student had a body to work on. Students learned dissection, surgery, and injection to make specimens. The injection technique Morgan used so successfully to further his position in Paris had originally been developed by Swammerdam and Ruysch in Holland at the end of the seventeenth century. This technique was improved upon by the Hunters.

After his stay in London, Shippen planned to go to Leyden and France for his theoretical studies, but the Seven Years War intervened. He was advised about the excellent level of teaching in Edinburgh. In September 1761, after one year of study at Edinburgh, he received his degree from that university. His thesis for graduation was "De Placentae Cum Utero Noxii," discussing the development and circulation of the placenta. He demonstrated that the maternal and fetal circulations were separate. Shippen spent a total of four years in the British Isles. He was able to spend one season in Paris before returning to Philadelphia in 1762 to start a private practice. On November 26, 1762, the young physician started anatomy lectures with material sent by Dr. Fothergill, a Quaker "internist" in London, who befriended American students in England. That good doctor sent seven cases of anatomical drawings, a skeleton, a fetus, and castings in plaster of Paris to the Pennsylvania Hospital to be used for teaching anatomy. He also suggested that they be used to help start a medical school in Philadelphia. It was at this time that Shippen presented his plan for a medical school, but the trustees were not ready for the idea. Perhaps the required finances were not available, or perhaps Shippen was not as forceful as Morgan was three years later. In place of the medical school, Shippen started a private school of anatomy similar to that of the Hunters.[26] In fact, his lectures consisted basically of the notes he took while he studied with them. He had not performed any original investigations. Shippen's lectures included anatomy, histology, pathology, and physiology of the organ systems. He also discussed therapeutics. His lectures were open to men interested in the practice of medicine, and those just interested in the human body. The tuition was five pistoles, another five if the student wished to watch and learn the injection preparation technique and dissection. In 1763 Shippen started a course of studies at the hospital. He gave lectures twice a month to all interested gentlemen. The fee was one dollar to be used for the hospital library.[27] Shippen's home and school suffered the same problem of anatomists before and after him. Mobs attacked his home, his carriage, and his person. He had to assure the population that his cadavers were executed criminals and suicides. He took out an ad in the *Pennsylvania Gazette* to explain that bodies were from Potter's field, not from churchyards. The readers apparently were willing to accept this explanation as he had little trouble thereafter.

In January 1765 Shippen advertised a course in midwifery for men and women. He gave twenty lectures. Pupils were to attend two courses and Shippen housed poor pregnant women for demonstrations. With the start of the medical school, Shippen was a natural choice for anatomy and midwifery. Morgan recommended him for this position, and he became the second professor at the school in September 1765. He was to give sixty lectures on anatomy, surgery, bandaging, and midwifery for a tuition of six pistoles.[28]

With the approach of war, the Shippen family took sides, as did many families in the colonies. Shippen's father was strongly pro–Patriot. While he abhorred the actions of radicals like Sam Adams and John Hancock, he eventually accepted the Declaration of Independence. Despite his age, William II went to the hospitals at Bethlehem, Allentown, and Easton to treat the sick and wounded. William , Jr., was a Patriot but not as strong in his beliefs as his father.

William Shippen, Jr.'s, advance in the medical department was described in the previous section. On April 11, 1777, he became director general. He inherited all of his predecessor's problems, but he was not the worker that Morgan was. Under Shippen medical costs skyrocketed, in both real and inflated currency. During his tenure, Shippen did not treat any casualties, and he was lax in his visits and supervision of the hospitals under his care. As in Morgan's case, Congress undercut Shippen's authority. Shippen dispatched physicians, surgeons, and mates to the hospital in Virginia. The director, Rickman, objected to Congress that Shippen was usurping his authority, and Congress sided with Rickman. Shippen was continually sniped at by Rush and Morgan with charges of misconduct, malpractice, and trading in hospital stores. Rush started his attacks in earnest in October 1777 when he corresponded with members of Congress. Rush also attacked Shippen in a letter to Washington. Of course, he himself did not stand in Washington's good graces at this time, because of his involvement in the Conway Cabal. The commander-in-chief, always a gentleman, referred the letter to Congress. A commission of Congress sided with Shippen, and Rush felt he had to resign from his position in the middle department of the medical service. Rush continued his attacks as a civilian. He used the terrible mortality rates in the hospitals of eastern Pennsylvania in his attacks on Shippen. His use of hyperbole could bring his points to the attention of the public. Rush suggested a plan to defeat General Howe. If the Colonials could retreat through any town in Lancaster County with a general hospital, and get Howe to follow with his army, within six weeks not one British soldier would be alive or fit for duty. Rush accused Shippen of trading in hospital supplies for his own benefit. In February 1778 Shippen was relieved of the duty of purchasing supplies for the hospital. He prepared a budget of $1 million for the Northern Hospital in 1779. This was cut in half by Congress. His physicians and staff were accused of eating food and drinking wine meant for patients.

On June 15, 1779, after Morgan's vindication, he formally accused Shippen of malpractice and misconduct. Copies of the accusations were also sent to Washington and Shippen. Washington felt the charges were unsupported and refused a court-martial. Also, Washington was planning a serious military campaign and thus could not afford to have his medical service in disarray. Morgan urged Congress to recommend to the states that all people called to testify in a court-martial be made available, whether in service or a civilian— only New Jersey complied. Congress further directed that prosecutor and accused must be present when a deposition was taken. If he kept himself unavailable, Shippen could put this off indefinitely. Congress countered his action by a declaration that testimony could be taken by a justice of the peace if the prosecutor and the accused were made aware of the time and place. Morgan proceeded to get depositions despite Shippen's refusal to be present. Finally, on January 5, 1780, Shippen was served with papers and placed under arrest. The court-martial was set for March 14, 1780, and General Edward Hand, a physician and a cousin of Shippen's, was the presiding judge. The court denied Morgan's depositions because he had not been appointed prosecutor. Rush testified against Shippen, as did several other army surgeons. The court recessed on April 5, and Morgan was appointed deputy judge advocate to get more depositions that would be accepted by the court. Shippen now accompanied him. The sheriff of Ephrata, probably an ally of Shippen, arrested Morgan on slander charges and kept him in jail with a $10,000 bond. He planned to hold Morgan while Shippen was free to obtain depositions in his favor. Morgan's friends raised the bail, and he was able to get out and accompany his adversary. The court met on May 15, and Morgan presented his depositions. The charges against Shippen included: (1) fraud as a result of the sale of hospital stores as his own property, and his use of government wagons to transport them; (2) speculation in and sale of hospital stores as well as peculation and adulteration of hospital wine; (3) failure to keep accounts of expenditures and neglect to pay proper bills; (4) neglect of hospital duties, and his dispatch of false reports to Congress on the state of the sick in the hospital; (5) infamous practices to try to vilify superior officers in order to supplant them. This last charge was a balm for Morgan's self-image. Shippen presented letters from Washington and Benedict Arnold (at that time still an American hero) as well as testimony from Dr. Bodo Otto. He was acquitted by one vote, that of his relative. However, he was castigated by the court for his private accumulation of funds from improper trade of hospital wine and sugar and for his negligence in the care of soldiers. His behavior was described as reprehensible. The report of the court was sent to Washington who sent it to Congress. Congress was outraged with the result of the trial and was particularly disgusted with Shippen. His brothers-in-law in Congress worked hard to restrain Congress. Congress refused to confirm or sanction the acquittal, and Shippen was temporarily dismissed from the service.

The Medical Department was reorganized on October 16, 1780, and Shippen was reappointed as director as a face-saving device. Morgan then went public. He wrote articles in the *Pennsylvania Packet*. The first was accompanied by the depositions he had obtained for the court. Shippen countered with his own material. Rush joined the fray in print with testimony from Patrick Garvey that Shippen tried to bribe him to change the books. Garvey, however, was not the best witness—he was in jail for trading with the enemy. Shippen finally resigned on January 3, 1781. Morgan published a handbill about his resignation, but in the end the reputations of all three and that of the medical service were tarnished. The documents of Shippen's court-martial were lost, but the court-martial served a purpose. It led to the reorganization of the department, and the appointment of a physician who was honest, capable, and experienced.[29]

Shippen's troubles were not over with his resignation. Rush and Morgan continued to attack him in civilian life. They urged the board of trustees of the Medical School not to reappoint him. As a result of the revocation of the charter of the College of Philadelphia and the formation of the new University of Pennsylvania, there were two medical schools with two faculties. Shippen was on both until they joined on September 30, 1791. Morgan was too worn out to return to his position, and he retired.

Shippen returned to his high position in society. His home became the meeting place of artists, politicians, and visiting dignitaries. However, his private life collapsed. His daughter, Anne, fell in love with Louis Otto, a young French legatee in Philadelphia, but Shippen married her off to Colonel Henry Beekman Livingston. She left him in one year and returned home. She and her mother lapsed into "melancholia." His son, Thomas Lee Shippen, trained as a lawyer in England and returned home to practice. He developed consumption and was treated by Adam Kuhn, a professor at the medical school. He showed no improvement, and Benjamin Rush was called in. As usual, he turned to the lancet and bled Thomas 25 times, but could not save him. Thomas Shippen died in 1798 at the age of 33, and Shippen retired from practice. In 1801 his wife and father died. In 1808 Shippen died under Rush's care. The final diagnosis was anthrax.[30]

Shippen was a good-looking and polished member of Philadelphia society. He was bright and well trained. Unlike Morgan, he was friendly, talkative, and able to get along with people. He was ready to delegate duties rather than burden himself with minute details. In this he resembled politicians of today. But one of the basic requirements of an internist is to keep up with advances in medical science. When he stops reading, his ability deteriorates. Shippen, like some physicians today, was hampered too much by his diffusion of interests to be relied upon as a doctor.

John Cochran

Cochran was the last of the directors general of the medical service. He took over from a prior, scandal-ridden administration. The new director was the first of the four who did not have a formal education and an M.D. degree. His administration was reasonable, and he stayed on until the end of the war and watched the complete dismemberment of the medical service. Cochran did not interfere in problems that were not of his concern or responsibility, but he stood firm where he felt he or his charges were being placed at a disadvantage. He did not involve himself in the Morgan-Rush-Shippen controversy. During those terrible three years he did what was expected of him.

John Cochran was born in 1730 and came of sturdy Scotch-Irish stock, the second most important group in American society and public affairs at that time. Cochran's antecedents started in Scotland. During the reigns of Mary Queen of Scots and James VI, his family migrated to Northern Ireland with the encouragement of the English government. Their descendants are the present inhabitants of the six northern counties who have retained their Presbyterian beliefs. They prospered after the civil war of 1641 and developed industry and agriculture in Ireland. Meanwhile, the English were developing a mercantile class with political strength, and they wished to retain all means of wealth production in England. They passed restrictive legislation against Scotch industry, raised farm rates, and attacked their Presbyterianism. Many people in Scotland migrated to America; others supported Bonnie Prince Charlie's attempt to take the crown. Both groups hated the English. Cochran's family, like many others, headed for Pennsylvania for the excellent farming land. There John Cochran was apprenticed to Dr. Robert Thompson of Lancaster. With the start of the French and Indian War, he enlisted as a surgeon's mate in an English regiment. Cochran stayed in service from 1755 to 1760. There he gained excellent experience in surgery from the British surgeons.

After the service he married into the Schuyler family of upstate New York. This was a rich, politically strong family in New York colonial politics. Philip Schuyler, his brother-in-law, became one of the first major generals to be appointed by Congress at the outbreak of hostilities. John Cochran opened a practice in Albany and remained there for two years. Perhaps he found his wife's attachment to her family too onerous, or perhaps his new family was too overwhelming; in any case, the young doctor moved to New Brunswick in East Jersey. The east side of the Delaware River along with New Amsterdam had been settled by the Dutch. When Holland ceded the land to the British, it was given to the Duke of York. He gave what is the present New Jersey to two of his followers, Carteret and Berkley. This led to the early division of present-day New Jersey. In 1761 Cochran helped form the Medical Society of East Jersey to enlarge the stock of knowledge and experience in medicine for all practitioners. He drew up a petition to the legislature for the right to examine and license all who wished to practice in East Jersey. This was approved in 1772. In 1771 he decided to specialize in smallpox inoculation, and he opened a small private hospital to carry out this work. At the time, New York and Virginia prohibited smallpox inoculation, and Cochran advertised in the newspapers of the four neighboring colonies. He was successful and earned a good reputation in this field. He continued his practice at the outbreak of hostilities and did not become actively involved in the war until Washington's army made its retreat through New Jersey. At this point, he joined the army as a volunteer in December 1776.[31] Cochran helped evacuate casualties to Bethlehem, Pennsylvania. William Shippen recommended him as medical officer for Washington's headquarters. It was at this time that Cochran and Shippen worked out the first major reorganization of the medical service. It was "Shippen's Plan" and was accepted by Congress on April 1, 1777, with Shippen promoted to director general.

Cochran was with Washington when he crossed the Delaware in December 1776, and he saw action at both battles of Trenton. The first was on Christmas Day 1776, the second on January 3, 1777, where Washington was hemmed in on the Assumpink River by a larger force under Cornwallis. Washington sneaked around Cornwallis at night, and by morning his army was outside Princeton. After a successful engagement, his victorious army marched into Princeton. The army then moved to Morristown and arrived there February 12, 1777. Smallpox became a serious problem among civilians and soldiers around Morristown in the early spring of 1777. Washington felt his army should be inoculated, and this was to be performed under Cochran's supervision in view of his expertise. Congress also ordered the inoculation of all troops who came from the south. They were housed in Virginia for the procedure. Cochran's plan for preparation called for a vegetable diet, no salt, no spices, and no antimony. Calomel and nitre powder were given every other day for five or six doses. A cathartic was given one week after inoculation and when pocks were expected. The patient was kept cool and advised to avoid violent exercise. Cochran ordered that huts be kept clean. There were to be only single bunks in the hut with a lot of straw for the mattress. Shippen, at Washington's orders, set up smallpox hospitals at Newton, Bucks County, and in New Jersey.

After the promotion of Shippen to director general, Cochran became physician and surgeon general of the middle department and director of the flying hospital. He treated casualties at the battles of Brandywine and Germantown and accompanied the troops to Valley Forge. He set up an inoculation hospital there and opened the hospital at Yellow Springs ten miles away. After the encampment and the Battle of Monmouth, he was on the field actively involved in the treatment of casualties. Washington recognized his ability and sent him to become the private physician to Lafayette who was suffering with pneumonia.[32] Cochran remained with the army when it wintered at Middlebrook, New Jersey, in 1778–79 and in Morristown 1779–80. The army must have been housed and dressed well during that bitter winter, because there were no major reports of frostbite that year. The winter at Valley Forge was milder overall, yet there were many cases of frostbite requiring amputation. Cochran was faced with the depletion of his medical supplies at Morristown. He had 600 sick who were languishing because of the deficiency. Fortunately, he was wise in the ways of the congressional government at the time and handled his problems quietly with a modicum of success. The alternative option was to refer the problem to the commander-in-chief, who would refer it to Congress, who would refer it to the medical committee of the Congress, who would discuss it for awhile, and then nothing more would be heard about it.[33]

Even while occupied with his military duties, Cochran found time to draw up plans for the reorganization of the Medical Department. They were submitted and accepted by Congress in October 1780. After Shippen's forced resignation, Cochran was made director general and remained at this post until the Medical Department was dissolved. Cochran faced the same problems as all his predecessors. There was no money from Congress to purchase supplies. His subordinates refused to obey orders. His letters (1781–82) tell of a problem with the purveyor for the Eastern Department in Connecticut who refused to give up supplies purchased with public money. Cochran did not describe how the problem was resolved, but it was settled. He had to superintend the closure of hospitals that served no purpose when hostilities subsided. The director was plagued with the problem of good doctors resigning from the service to go home and care for their families because they had not been paid for two years. There were problems of men anxious for promotions who did not deserve them. He was plagued with surgeon's mates who sought elevation to surgeon's rank. As in all dealings with physicians in the past and present, he had to handle different personalities who saw their worth differently from the director.

As the war drew to a close, the board of war (heir to the medical committee of Congress) ordered hospitals in New England to close. The inmates had to be removed and boarded at private homes or transported to other general hospitals many miles away. How the private home owners were paid was anybody's guess. The director also had to retire the "paramedics" (stewards, matrons, nurses, etc.). Cochran was constantly short of funds and ran the service on credit and promises to pay. He wrote Robert Morris, financial dictator of the government, for funds, but none were available. Cochran had to sell his own property to keep his family fed during those lean years.[34]

Cochran was a gentleman in every respect, but he could be stern when necessary to protect himself and his assistants. In a letter to Timothy Pickering, the quartermaster general, dated November 4, 1782, he attacked Pickering for poor quarters supplied for winter camp at Newburgh (1782–83). He ended the letter with an offer to give Pickering any satisfaction he wished. His offer was not taken up by that gentleman. Cochran left the service after the war and died in 1807.

Overall, he was probably the best man who occupied this position even though he had neither a formal medical degree nor a great reputation among the physicians of the country. He was never guilty of the slightest bit of improper behavior or dishonesty. He did the best he could with what was available to him. He obviously had developed surgical skill while he observed the British, and he was willing to use it to treat casualties on the field. He seemed to be a good organizer and administrator, and he might have prevented the destruction of the army in the hospitals of Pennsylvania and New Jersey.

Benjamin Rush

Dr. Benjamin Rush was not one of the directors general of the Medical Department. However, his activities during the war as politician, writer, and physician demand some attention. He and Morgan were instrumental in bringing Shippen down. Rush was physician and senior surgeon of the middle department until his resignation. More important was the swath he carved through American medicine before, during, and after the Revolution. That he had time for his massive writings on a multitude of problems, teaching chores, private patients, and politics is beyond my comprehension. He was described as the American Hippocrates, and his influence persisted long after his death. It was only with the beginnings of statistical review that his bleeding theories finally were discarded.

Rush's great-grandfather was one of Cromwell's officers in the civil war. His ancestor, a Quaker, migrated to Philadelphia in 1683 for religious freedom. Rush's father, an Episcopalian, died at age 39, leaving six children for his widow to support. She opened a grocery and liquor store to feed her family. Benjamin was sent to the Reverend Dr. Finley's Nottingham Academy because Finley was his uncle. At the age of 15, he went to New Jersey College at Princeton in 1759. An entrance exam placed him in his junior year immediately, and in one year he graduated with a bachelor's degree. Rush was prepared to study law, generally more highly esteemed in society than medicine, but Finley urged him to go into medicine. Rush was apprenticed to Dr. John Redman of Philadelphia from February 1761 to July 1766. He started as Redman's apothecary while the preceptor saw patients. Then he accompanied Dr. Redman on his visits to patients at home, office, and hospital. Redman was on staff at the Pennsylvania Hospital, so Rush could attend and observe the other doctors there as well. He also attended the private anatomy lessons of Dr. Shippen in 1762 and the latter's college classes in 1765 as well as Morgan's classes on materia medica that same year. In August 1766 he went to Scotland. On board ship he met Jonathan Potts, who was also going to Europe for a medical education but returned prematurely and completed his education in Philadelphia. The professors at Edinburgh at the time were Monro, Cullen, Black, Gregory, and Hope. Lectures included anatomy, chemistry, institutes of medicine, and natural philosophy as well as practice in the infirmary. In the summer, Rush studied Latin, French, Italian, and math. The second winter Rush studied the practice of physic and materia medica. He received his medical degree in June 1768. His thesis was on the digestion of food in the stomach. The summer after graduation, he took further courses in the practice of physic. In September of that year, the doctor went to London and studied under Dr. William Hunter and Mr. Hewson, a surgeon. He walked the wards of Middlesex and St. Thomas Hospitals with Dr. Huck. While in London he also met Sir John Pringle, the eminent army medical physician. He also met Dr. Fothergill and Ben Franklin. Rush briefly visited Paris but felt it had nothing to teach him. His funds were probably too limited for Paris or any prolonged stay on the continent. On May 26, 1769, he left England, arriving in New York on July 14, and then traveled by stagecoach to Philadelphia.

Rush was aware that his opportunities there were limited. In order to establish a "good business," a physician needed the patronage of a great man, powerful family connections, and the influence of a religious sect or a political party. He had none of these. He started practice by working with the poor. Immediately after his arrival home, Rush introduced Sutton's technique of inoculation for smallpox. He was appointed Professor of Chemistry at the College of Philadelphia one month after his return from England. Like the other professors at the school, he lectured on the notes he had taken at Edinburgh. Rush's lectures were essentially Black's lectures, and Rush charged six pounds for his course, which started on August 1, 1769.

At the time, physicians in Philadelphia adhered to Boerhaave's theories of the humors, while Rush was a follower of Cullen and his theories of the nervous system. One year after his return, Rush published many articles on his theories of medicine. The first was a paper on hives (a term for cynanche trachealis—more of this later). What he described in this paper was probably croup. Rush believed it was due to spasm of the windpipe without mucous or a membrane. He followed this with articles on exercise, alcohol, and slavery, opposing the latter two.[35] In 1773–74 Dr. Rush earned from his practice, apothecary sales, and lectures 463 pounds in cash and 829 pounds on the books. In 1775 his income was a substantial 900 pounds Pennsylvania currency.[36] Rush began to lose faith in Cullen's theories and so turned to Brown before developing his own theories of the cause of all disease. Rush lost many referrals, because the physicians of Philadelphia started to accept Cullen's theories, which Rush had introduced earlier. He also lost a considerable amount of money because he was an outspoken Whig, and most of the wealthy people of the city were Tories. The physician continued to write extensively and urged that many useless drugs be discarded from the materia medica. He urged proper diet and drinks to treat disease. Rush opposed dissertations and prescriptions in Latin because they increased the suspicions of the lay public against doctors, making people feel the latter were trying to keep their knowledge a secret.[37]

The extent and range of Rush's activities are amazing even more than 200 years later. He lectured at the medical school, took care of an active practice, wrote articles on medicine and allied social problems, and still had time for the politics of the day.

Rush was chairman of the group in Pennsylvania that called for independence on June 24, 1776. He was elected to the Continental Congress in time to sign the Declaration of Independence in August 1776. The new congressman became head of the committee to procure provisions for the Northern Army as well as of the committee to obtain medicine for the survivors of the Canadian invasion. Rush became chairman of the medical committee of Congress,[38] and he was a member of the committee for prisoners of war. While still a member of Congress, Rush joined the Pennsylvania militia to defend the state. The congressman visited the site of the Second Battle of Trenton, and he treated casualties on both sides. During this experience, he worked with Dr. Cochran. It was during this battle that Washington and his army slipped around the British and attacked Princeton. The casualties were left in the doctor's care. After their treatment, the casualties were placed on wagons and the physicians set out in search of the army. They learned of Washington's victory at Princeton and repaired to that site to care for the casualties of that engagement.[39] Rush then returned to Congress to take up his duties. He must have been impressed with Cochran's abilities, because he wrote a letter to Richard Henry Lee in Congress to support the appointment of Cochran as director general after Shippens' discharge.

Rush spent only a short time in Congress. On February 22, 1777, he was turned out by the Pennsylvania Assembly because he opposed the new constitution and government of Pennsylvania as developed by the Pennsylvania Convention.[40] During his stint in Congress, Rush was surgeon to the Pennsylvania navy, whose duty it was to keep the Delaware River open,[41] a mission that was not successful. After he had left Congress, Rush was appointed physician and surgeon general of the middle department. During this period, he treated casualties of the Battle of Brandywine. Under a flag of truce, he worked at the British Army Hospital and was impressed with the good food and fresh vegetables the patients there received as well as with the orderliness and cleanliness of the hospital. (Working there took a great deal of personal courage. As a signer of the Declaration of Independence, Rush had committed high treason against the king.) Rush's position as physician and surgeon ended nine months later when he resigned on January 30, 1778, prompted by his acerbic pen and his support for the wrong side in the Morgan-Shippen controversy.[42]

While still in the service, he tried to have the Medical Department changed to resemble the British system. He urged that a purveyor be appointed separate from the director general. This was not accepted until a later reorganization. Rush also urged that line officers and guards surround the hospital perimeter. He asked for a military inspector to examine the hospitals and report on their deficiencies. Rush believed that the director general had too much power in the American system compared to the British arrangement, where his duties were in the hands of three men, each independent of the others. His suggestions reveal his suspicions of Shippen as director general. Rush expressed his thoughts on this aspect of the service in a letter to Washington, who in turn sent it to Congress. Both he and the director general appeared before a committee of Congress. Rush made his charges against Shippen, which were rejected, and resigned his position in the service on January 30, 1778. Shippen, of course, had too much power in Congress, and Rush had burned his bridges with the Conway Cabal.

Rush was probably tangentially involved in the Conway Cabal. Conway was one of the many lower officers who had seen service with the British army. Like others, he had come to the colonies and offered his services to "help" the colonies and to receive a general's commission in return. Conway felt Washington stood in the way of his promotion. He formed a group to oust Washington and put Gates in his place. The group included General Gates, General Charles Lee of Monmouth infamy, Thomas Miflin, the quartermaster general, as well as other officers and members of Congress. They claimed Washington was incompetent, and his appointments were not based on merit. In November 1777 the board of war was reorganized with Gates as president. This made him Washington's superior, and Congress appointed Conway as inspector general with the rank of major general. A letter written by Conway to Gates and critical of Washington fell into Washington's hands and reached the public. This was a breach of etiquette and weakened the cause. Conway was forced out of the army. Rush was involved because he denounced Washington anonymously for inefficiency.[43] He wrote to John Adams to compare Washington's poorly organized army and his great losses to Gates's victorious army at Saratoga. In January 1778 Rush wrote an anonymous letter to Patrick Henry in which he praised the armies in the northern and southern sectors and criticized Washington's army in the middle sector. Henry sent the letter to Washington who recognized the handwriting. Consequently, Rush lost any support he ever had from Washington.

This anonymous letter writing by Rush was most unusual behavior for him. In all of his other arguments with the professors at the medical school, with Shippen as director general, and with the physicians of Philadelphia in the yellow fever epidemic of 1793, he always stood up to his accusers and backed his arguments without ever hiding behind anonymity. Rush was never actually proven to be a member of the conspiracy. At best, he was tactless, brusque, and indiscreet. A postscript to the Conway Cabal was the court-martial of Charles Henry Lee for his failure to attack the British rear at the Battle of Monmouth.[44]

Rush also attacked Shippen in his correspondence with John Adams on October 31, 1777. He urged that the director general furnish physicians and surgeons with medicine, stores and accommodations. The requisitions for the material were to be in writing by the doctor so they could be used as a voucher by the director general for expenditures. Rush also requested that accounts of the director general for medicine and stores be certified as true by the physician and surgeon general before they were passed. In addition, accounts of the sick and wounded were to be delivered to the medical committee of Congress by the physician and surgeon general. The accounts from the various doctors would be a check on the expenditures of the director general. Basically, Rush accused Shippen of graft and claimed he tampered with the census of the sick and wounded in his reports to Congress. Adams took no action and Rush appealed to Congressman Duer who similarly did not want to become involved. Rush then approached Shippen directly about the poor care, lack of supplies, and overcrowding. Shippen replied that he was the only judge of hospital affairs and that Rush's job was to treat the casualties sent to him. Rush sent a letter to Shippen on February 1, 1778, claiming he had no personal animosity toward him but was only acting to help the patients in the hospital. A week later, Rush wrote a letter to Adams to describe all the evils committed by Shippen. These included the use of hospital resources, utilization of hospital horses to transport his personal supply of wine for speculation, and his use of false statistics about the number of men who died in the hospitals. Two weeks after that, he wrote a letter to Daniel Roberdeau and again repeated all of his charges against Shippen. Rush was pleased that his suggestions about reorganization of military hospitals were accepted, but had he known this earlier, he would not have resigned his position in the Medical Department. In his letters, he claimed his attacks against Shippen and the service were not an attempt to replace Shippen but, rather, for the good of the army. To show his good purposes, he resigned in order to take himself out of the running if Shippen was discharged.[45]

When Rush left the service, he openly joined Morgan in his attacks on Shippen. On February 25, 1778, Rush wrote Washington a letter in which he accused Shippen of malpractice.[46] Naturally, the letter was sent to Congress. Rush refused to appear before a committee of Congress after its receipt of his letter. He felt Shippen should be court-martialed on the basis of the evidence he presented. When no action was taken, Rush dropped the affair and returned to the distribution of free medical advice.

He had printed, at his own expense, a pamphlet addressed to the line and medical officers of the army with directions on how to keep their men healthy. Rush proposed that men wash their hands and face daily and their whole body two or three times a week. They were to shave three times a week. Soldiers were to keep their hair "thin" and cut close to the neck. This prevented perspiration from becoming putrid, which led to disease. When on garrison duty, they could powder their hair with flour. A hunting or rifle shirt worn over a flannel shirt was the best protection, but these had to be changed regularly. A linen shirt became impregnated with sweat. This plus rain produced miasmata, which caused fevers. Shoes were to be made of thick strong leather with wax seams to keep them waterproof. The troops were to sleep in tents on dry land, with access to winds and away from marshes, and they were to avoid excesses of heat and smoke. He believed fire with smoke, burning sulphur or gunpowder, preserved the purity of the air. Bedding was stored above ground level with bed straw changed frequently. The bedding was exposed to the sun daily. Privies were to be dug deep and placed downwind from the camp, and the excrement covered daily with a goodly amount of earth. Food should be predominantly vegetables and fresh fruits. Troops were to cut down on meat consumption. No damaged flour was to remain in camp. Bread had to be well baked. A substitute could be boiled whole wheat to which could be added sugar or molasses.

Cooking utensils were to be washed after each use. Drinking water should be taken from the deepest part of the stream and not near the shore to ensure purity. Water could be tested by dropping oleum tartaric into a glass of water. If a heavy precipitate formed, the water was impure. This could be corrected by the addition of six ounces of vinegar to three quarts of water or with pieces of an aromatic root. Rush took this recommendation almost verbatim from Von Swieten. Soldiers were not to drink cold water when they were perspiring. Rush strongly opposed rum as it weakened soldiers and left them vulnerable to fever, flux, and jaundice. Milk and water were advised instead. Troops were to drink vinegar and water as the Roman legions did. Rum diluted with three parts of water was kept only for sentries in rainy weather. Sentries were to be protected from the environment and relieved from duty often. Crowding was to be avoided to reduce perspiration, which Rush believed led to typhus. Officers had to keep soldiers out of damp clothes as well as damp blankets and straw. The area around camp was to be kept free of offal, animals, and filth. If the camp was near a river, it should be placed so that the wind blew off camp toward the river, not the other way around. Troops were to avoid unnecessary fatigue, and all exercises were to be done in the early morning and evening. A good officer was one who cared for the health of his troops. This was also the advice given by Von Steuben to the officers at Valley Forge. His suggestions suggest that Rush had the soldiers' best interests on his mind despite his troubles with everyone around him.[47]

In addition to this pamphlet, Rush published another pamphlet on his observation about armies, their diseases, and their therapy. Most of its salient features were described in chapter one. However, he also discussed other problems he had observed. Rush believed that the fever and dysentery patients recovered best when they were kept away from the walls in a hospital room, because the walls could reinfect them. Dysentery caused little mortality, and warm baths helped cure it. Some fevers were caused by rubbing in sulfur mixed into lard and used to treat the "itch." Rush recommended the use of dry flowers of sulfur two or three times a day. He recommended amputation for gunshot wounds. Rush felt artillery noise caused deafness, but it could bring back hearing occasionally. Rush also attacked large crowded hospitals and urged that a hospital should be used only for mad patients and those with venereal disease. Other illnesses were best treated in private homes, although he believed the Tilton Hospital was the best for an army. He also reminded officers that enlisted men were children and should be treated as such. These remarks were numbered, and Rush probably wanted the medical officers to memorize them.[48]

After Rush had completed his tour of duty, helped reorganize the medical department of the army, and helped bring down his nemesis Shippen, he returned to private practice, teaching and writing and writing and writing. He wrote about Indian medicine, alcoholism, tetanus, care of disease by removing decayed teeth (a practice used on baseball pitchers earlier in this century when they were in a slump), worms and their therapy, use of arsenicals in the treatment of external cancer, aging, effects of climate on the body, consumption, therapy for blood spitting, gout, dropsy, hydrophobia, and cynanche trachealis. Cynanche trachealis, listed as the cause of Washington's death, is worth some attention at this point. Rush believed the disease could be brought on by a cold or following another illness such as smallpox, measles, scarlet fever, aphthous sore throat, yellow fever, or rheumatism. It came on gradually, got worse, and remitted. It affected mostly children, but occasionally adults were the victims. It lasted three to four days, but sometimes ten. Examination of the trachea showed inflammation with a membrane over it covered by a thick matter. In acute and rapidly fatal cases, there were no findings. The patient complained of hoarseness and a stertorous cough. It was treated by a puke with antimony, tartar emetic, and ipecac, which led to immediate cure. If the disease was fully present, therapy entailed bleeding, then vomits followed by a purge. Calomel (mercury) until salivation was prescribed as well as blisters to the throat and chest and warm baths. As symptoms subsided, laudanum was used to ease the cough. When the cough produced mucous, the danger was over. This disease was described by Cullen. Rush's description sounds like a mixture of diphtheria, croup, and strep throat descending to the larynx or an infected epiglottis due to Hemophilus influenzae.

The intermittent attacks of yellow fever that struck Philadelphia, and particularly the decimating attack of 1793, pushed Rush to extremes of therapy. It caused divisions in the community of physicians of Philadelphia with attacks and counterattacks in the press. Rush's extreme therapy of the disease largely isolated him from the rest of his contemporaries. He believed yellow fever or bilious remitting fever was caused by exercise of the body or mind, heat, intemperance of eating or drinking, fear, grief, cold, sleep, and excessive purging and bleeding (as opposed to what Rush felt was moderate bleeding). He described the general constitution of the air that cooperated with miasmata. Rush believed spoiled coffee on the wharf caused the epidemic of 1793. He knew that people did not spread it to their neighbors. Rush's almost maniacal bleeding of patients during the epidemic was frightening. His great cures were probably of other milder illnesses whose victims could tolerate his therapy of bleed and purge. Rush discounted this idea of other illnesses, because to him all diseases were one disease, just as there was one God who could appear in different ways. Rush's bleeding therapy is partly blamed for the high mortality in the epidemic of 1793. He believed that taking four-fifths of the circulating volume of blood was necessary. Fortunately, his calculation of the total blood volume was off the mark. Rush took 60 to 80 ounces of blood on rare occasions. He might take as much as 200 ounces during the course of an illness. This is twelve pints. He urged a good bleed early in the disease and smaller bleedings two or three times a day during the course. Toward the height of the epidemic, he had no time for repeated bleedings and took a large amount on the first visit.[49] Rush described ten varieties of pulse requiring bleeding. He had learned bleeding from his preceptor, Dr. Redman, who was a "big bleeder." William Cullen used bleedings in inflammatory diseases. Sydenham was a bleeder early in his career, but he cut back on it as he matured.[50]

In addition to his medical practice and his writing career, Rush also became professor of theory and practice of medicine and continued his lectures until 1812.[51] It is said that about 2,872 students passed through his tutelage in addition to his apprentices. Unfortunately, this group accepted Rush's words as though from "on high" and carried his concepts of bleeding, purging, and vomiting to all parts of America. The number of people destroyed at his and his pupils' hands probably ran into the thousands. His rigidity, his disbelief that others might have ideas worth examining, and his reaction to all criticism of his concepts as an attack upon his person are horrifying in retrospect.

Rush took apprentices and depended on this revenue for his family's needs. He charged one hundred guineas to take on an apprentice. Rush had several at a time, some in the house, others lodged nearby. He chose them carefully (sons of friends and those his old students recommended). Some had apprenticed earlier in their own communities, while others had already been in practice. James Hall, one of his apprentices, was subsidized by Rush to continue his education at Edinburgh, and then Rush took him in as a partner. Of these apprentices, fifteen served in the Revolution. Elisha Dick left Rush in the midst of his study to apprentice to Shippen. Another apprentice, James McHenry, gained fame as a regimental surgeon, hospital surgeon, personal secretary to Washington, and secretary of war under Washington and Adams. Two of Rush's sons, James and John, also were his apprentices. Rush continued to take apprentices until 1812, some of them coming from Delaware, Georgia, Kentucky, Maryland, New Hampshire, New Jersey, New York, North Carolina, Pennsylvania, South Carolina, Virginia, Ireland, England, Barbados, and St. Croix.[52]

Rush professed himself to be an expert in all fields of medicine and in his writings on obstetrics recommended that 30 ounces of blood be removed at the start of labor and the bowels be kept open. He placed women on a "low diet" ten to fourteen days before confinement. This therapy was instituted because labor was short and easy in the last stages of a "chronic disease," and he created a medical condition resembling a chronic disease. He gave opium if pains were too weak to expel the fetus. He believed labor was painfree in paroxysms of epilepsy and in drunkenness. Rush believed that a perfect panacea for labor would be one to suspend the sensibility of the nerves without impairing the irritability of the nerves (a block is now the solution).[53]

Some of Rush's most beneficial works were his early writings in psychiatry. He was considered the father of American psychiatry. Rush advocated good care, recreation, hot and cold baths, and occupational therapy. He believed the insane were sick, not possessed. His text on psychiatry was reprinted as late as the Civil War. He was involved in the formation of Dickinson College in Carlisle and was a charter trustee of Franklin and Marshall College in Lancaster. He urged free schools, women's education, and a national university. Rush urged reform of the penal laws and was a strong abolitionist and helped organize the Abolition Society of Pennsylvania. He also helped found the first African Church in Philadelphia. He was a teetotaler and wrote of alcoholism's dangers to society. Rush founded the Philadelphia dispensary for the treatment of the poor. From all this we can see that his contributions to society were great, but it would have been better if he had stayed out of medicine.

While Rush did not believe in research, because "all diseases were one disease," there were many others who were advancing the frontiers of medicine at the time. Morgagni's work in correlating symptoms with pathological changes in organs demonstrated the need for research on the cause and therapy of disease (1761). By 1795, the "Paris School" was pushing ahead in spite of Rush's dicta. Parisian investigators pushed Morgagni's work on morbid anatomy forward. The science of statistics helped destroy another of Rush's aphorisms. In 1830 a Parisian physician divided pneumonia cases into two groups. One group was bled, the other was not. The results showed that bleeding was a useless, if not dangerous, technique. By 1840 leaders of the profession generally discarded Rush's theories.

Rush was a true "Revolutionary Gadfly," the name given to him by his biographer, D. F. Hawke. Like so many doctors of the past and present, he was so sure of his abilities and the correctness of his theories that he brooked no opposition. He probably caused more damage than good because of his insistence on severe bleeding in the therapy of all disease.

— 3 —

Smallpox and the Canadian Invasion

Every American school child knows that the Revolution started at Lexington and Concord that day in April 1775 when British forces were sent from Boston to take Sam Adams and John Hancock prisoners and collect the ordnance stored in Concord — but did it start then?[1] John Adams was heard to say that the American Revolution began with the first plantation in America. It is not necessary to go that far back to trace the beginnings of the War of Independence. The French and Indian War seems a more logical step. The British were finally able to vanquish their historical enemy, France, and clear the French government, if not the people, out of North America. However, they were left with a national debt of 130 million pounds. In addition, they planned to quarter 10,000 regular British troops in the colonies to keep the French out permanently. Naturally, the colonists benefited from the war and would be protected by the British troops, so they should help pay for it. Of course, the "movers and shakers" in parliament forgot the cost in lives and money sustained by the colonists in bringing about this great victory. The true benefit of the war to the colonies was that the French were cleared out of the Trans-Appalachian and Mississippi areas, and the merchants and adventurers could take the land from the Indians who had been allied to the French.

The start of an attempt to raise money for that debt was made with the old Acts of Trade and Navigation. These had been on the books for years but had not been enforced. American shippers dealt with foreign nations directly without going through British ports. They smuggled in foreign goods and evaded import duties. Thus, the British navy was practically converted into a "coast guard" to enforce the importation laws. For example, American shippers traded openly with West Indian planters for molasses, which New England distilleries turned into rum for which there was a huge market in the colonies. Parliament insisted the shippers trade only with the British West Indies and pay an import duty when the cargo arrived. The duty was half of its original amount, but it was now enforced. The British West Indies could not supply all the molasses needed, and because trade was restricted to only these planters, the latter could price their sugar and molasses well above the market rate. This so-called "Sugar Act" was the first linchpin that helped unite the northern mercantile and manufacturing colonies behind a common cause. The enforcement of the "Sugar Act" seemed to be "trampling in the dust" the rights of Englishmen in the colonies. All shippers accused of a violation of the act were to be tried in admiralty courts in Halifax. They were not given a jury trial even though the right to a jury trial by one's peers was a basic tenet of English common law. Also, removal of an indicted malefactor away from his neighbors, who would have served as his jury, was another infringement on the rights of an Englishman.

The next blow was the Stamp Act of 1765. John Brooke, an English historian, felt the Revolution started with the Stamp Act when the colonies challenged the right of parliament to raise revenues. More significant was the fact that parliament buckled to the outcry instead of taking vigorous actions to enforce its decision.

The House of Burgesses passed the Virginia Resolutions proclaiming that only Virginians could tax Virginians. The resolves were distributed among the colonies, and they all concurred that they could not be taxed by a parliament without being represented there. The Massachusetts legislature called for a meeting in New York to consider unified action. Nine colonies sent representatives. They produced the Declaration of Rights and Grievances, which affirmed that only the colonies could tax the colonists. This edict was backed by the crowds who intimidated the men wishing to become stamp officers. The mobs received the uplifting name of "Sons of Liberty." The colonial merchants imposed a greater threat on their counterparts in England. They joined together and refused to import anything from England. This economic attack had its effect on parliament and the Rockingham government repealed the Stamp Tax, which had been passed by the Grenville ministry. However, parliament insisted on its right to tax the colonies. William Pitt, a manic-depressive but firm friend of the colonies, followed Rockingham. He lowered the molasses tax but ruled that all colonial exports must first stop at British ports. One can only imagine the expense of shipping goods from New England to London on their way to their destination in the West Indies.

Meanwhile, Governor Moore of New York requested that the New York legislature raise money to pay for quartering British troops in New York, a request based on the old Mutiny Act. The legislature refused. Across the ocean, Townshend replaced Pitt in parliament and suspended the New York legislature until they raised the money. Townshend, who believed that the colonists resented all internal taxes on them by parliament, passed a series of "external taxes" in the form of levies on imports from England. Items such as glass, lead, tea, and paper were included. To enforce these duties, the Writs of Assistance were passed in parliament. As a result, British officials could search ships without a specific warrant. In addition, a board of customs commissioners, responsible to England, was formed to raise the money necessary to pay the cost of civil government. The colonists recognized this as an attempt to take the fiscal control of colonial government out of their hands. In 1768 Sam Adams prompted the Massachusetts legislature to denounce the Townshend Acts. British parliament, now under Hillsborough, dissolved the Massachusetts assembly. The other colonial legislatures supported Massachusetts, and so they too were dissolved. Further storms of protest developed in Boston Harbor when John Hancock's ship, *The Liberty*, was seized by royal officials. A mob in Boston intervened to save *The Liberty* and physically attacked the officials. Further fuel was added to the fire when British troops landed in Boston in September 1768. The Quartering Acts were passed, requiring any colony to house British troops. The British troops in Boston were forcibly quartered in the State House and Faneuil Hall. The problems in Massachusetts were recognized in the House of Burgesses in Virginia, and they resolved to join Massachusetts in the nonimportation of British goods. They were joined by all the other colonies except Pennsylvania and New Hampshire. This wreaked havoc on British merchants and shippers, and by 1770 the Townshend Acts died except for the tea tax. Nevertheless, Parliament continued to insist on its right to tax.

The Boston Massacre occurred in March 1770. Unemployed workers crowded around a British sentry and abused him with snowballs. Reinforcements were called, and the British opened fire, killing several civilians. Lieutenant Governor Hutchinson ordered the army leader, Captain Preston, and eight soldiers to be tried for murdering civilians. John Adams and Josiah Quincy successfully defended them. Samuel Adams made these victims martyrs in Massachusetts' eyes and gave the incident its name in history.

Overt destruction of royal property took place in Narragansett Bay, Rhode Island, in 1772 when *HMS Gaspee*, in pursuit of smugglers, ran aground. It was set afire by the citizens of the community. A board of inquiry could not find the malefactors, and the case was dropped. In 1773, Governor Hutchinson of Massachusetts announced that he and all judges in Massachusetts would be paid by the crown. This removed them from the control of the locally elected legislature. This concept would eventually spread to all the colonies. The officials naturally supported the party that paid them. Samuel Adams was handed a great propaganda ploy. He activated committees of correspondence to write to all the villages. Similar committees developed in other colonies and eventually linked the entire eastern seaboard. Information could be passed as rapidly as a good rider on a good horse could get to the next community.

In England, Lord North, the new prime minister, added more fuel to the fire on May 10, 1773, when he tried to save the British East India Company. He gave it a tea monopoly in the American colonies. The Prime Minister permitted the company to export tea to the colonies without the remission of ordinary British duties. Americans would get tea at a cheaper price (even cheaper than smuggled tea), the company would be saved from financial ruin (the value of its stock had dropped tremendously on the London stock exchange), and the principle of the right to tax would be vindicated. The colonists distrusted monopolies and strongly urged "tea appointees" to resign their positions and not handle any tea sent to the colonies. Tea ships left England for Boston, New York, Philadelphia, and Charleston with half a million pounds of tea in their holds. Three ships laden with tea arrived in Boston harbor. On December 16, 1773, a total of 342 chests of the material were dumped into the water by three bands of "Mohawk Indians" led by their chiefs—Warren, Revere, Samuel Adams, and Hancock. Dr. Joseph Warren's part in the Tea Party was preserved in the second verse of the Tea Party's rallying song. "Our Warren's there with bold Revere, with hands to do and words to cheer. For liberty and law."[2] New Yorkers followed Massachusetts' lead and dumped their tea in the East River. Philadelphia allowed its allotment of tea to rot. In Charleston, the tea was later sold, and the proceeds went to help arm South Carolina.

The English responded as soon as the news crossed the Atlantic. The Boston Port Bill closed the port of Boston. The Royal Navy sat in Boston harbor. British troops in Boston were reinforced until the cost of the tea and its duties were paid by Boston. The colonies backed Boston with food, money, and strong moral support. Parliament further punished the colonies with the remainder of the "Intolerable Acts." One took crown officials back to England for trial if they killed someone during the suppression of a riot or collecting of revenue. Another act removed from the Massachusetts constitution any subject parliament felt detrimental to Britain. This destroyed the effectiveness of the Charter of Massachusetts, as all high officials in Massachusetts would be appointed by the crown, and the crown's sheriff would pick juries. Town meetings could be held only when the governor gave written consent. Parliament also passed the Quebec Act. While the other Intolerable Acts hurt the colonies economically and politically, the Quebec Act was an attack on the spiritual beliefs of Puritan New England.[3] It was pushed through parliament by Sir Guy Carleton, governor of Canada. The Act did much to assist the acceptance of English rule by the French Canadians. Roman Catholics were given the right to vote and could take an oath on a Catholic bible if appointed to a government office. The Roman Catholic church was free to collect tithes and carry out its services. The Quebec Act sanctioned the civil law of Canada and the system of land tenure, and it increased the size of the governing council to which French Canadians could be appointed. As a sop to the English speakers in Canada, the act did allow them to increase their commercial interests. The colonists to the south of Canada abhorred the bill, because it again created a papist French state on their border. In addition, French civil government was based on laws different from English common law, and the English feared a loss of civil rights. Massachusetts was aghast at the recognition of the Roman Catholic church and the appointed (not elected) council. New York, Pennsylvania, and

Virginia opposed the return of "the western lands" to Canada that they wanted for trade and speculation. George Washington and Patrick Henry, among others in the colonies, were financially involved in the Ohio Company, a group formed to open the area beyond the mountains, but through the Quebec Act the area north of the Ohio River was incorporated into Canada.[4]

The Virginia House of Burgesses called for a congress of all the colonies to discuss the defense of their rights. On September 5, 1774, the first Continental Congress met in Philadelphia. The leaders of the Congress wanted Canadian involvement, and they appealed to the English-speaking minority to send representatives. The merchants refused because they feared a nonimportation agreement against the mother country, which would leave all trade in the hands of the loyal French Canadians. With the outbreak of hostilities the following year, Congress again invited the English Canadians to unite with them for mutual liberty. Among the American colonies, only Georgia refused to send delegates. While the delegates sat in Philadelphia, Congress learned of the "Suffolk Resolves" passed in Suffolk County, Massachusetts. The authors, one of whom was Dr. Joseph Warren, declared the Intolerable Acts null and void. The people of Massachusetts were called upon to form a new government, to collect and keep taxes, and to form militias and arm themselves. The Continental Congress in Philadelphia adopted the resolves and strengthening them by its refusal to import any British goods. In addition, the Congress stopped the slave trade and also passed the Declaration of Rights of Americans based on the English Constitution. The Non-Importation Act was very effective. In 1774 New York imported 437,937 pounds of material from Britain. The following year imports dropped to 1,228 pounds. British merchants petitioned parliament to discontinue the coercion of the colonies, but parliament stood fast. The Continental Congress adjourned in October 1774, with plans to reconvene the next year, but events at Lexington and Concord intervened.

Massachusetts was placed under martial law when Governor Hutchinson was replaced by General Thomas Gage. In February 1775 parliament asked George III to declare Massachusetts to be in a state of rebellion. The monarch gladly acceded to the request. General Gage sent British soldiers to Cambridge and Charlestown in September 1774 to gather up all military supplies concealed in the colony. In February 1775 a similar attempt was made at Salem under British Colonel Leslie, but his contingent was turned back. The "rump" Provincial Congress of Massachusetts met in Cambridge and set up the committee of safety to act as an executive body. This replaced the governor and his council appointed in England and could call out the militia as necessary. Small groups in the militia companies who could respond rapidly to a call were declared "Minutemen." The committee of safety purchased and stored ordnance in Concord.[5]

Meanwhile in the South, Virginia again took the lead when the planters of Fairfax County moved to tighten defenses with the creation of a strong militia to "relieve the mother country of the expense of provincial defense." This act relieved the mother country of the need to tax and maintain a standing army. On March 20, 1775, a convention in Richmond accepted the Fairfax Resolutions. However, on April 20, the governor of Virginia captured the militia's gunpowder in Williamsburg and threatened to free the slaves. He later paid for the expropriated gunpowder. Parliament sent a conciliatory plan, which was rejected by the Burgesses, and Governor Dunmore fled aboard the British warship *HMS Fowey* and bombarded Norfolk. The first actual combat in the South occurred when Virginia militia under William Woodford defeated a group of loyalists at Great Bridge. In North Carolina, Governor Martin left the state on the sloop *Scorpion*.[6]

Meanwhile, in an attempt to further push the colonies against the wall, parliament forbade all New England colonies to engage in commerce anywhere except with England or the British West Indies, and the New England fishing fleet was prohibited from sailing into the North Atlantic fishing grounds.

Fighting Starts

The actual combat between American and British soldiers started when General Gage sent 700 men under Colonel Francis Smith to pick up the leaders of the committee of safety and to seize the ordnance stored in Concord. Dawes, Revere, and Prescott were sent by Dr. Warren on April 18, 1775, to alert Hancock and Adams of their impending arrest. The doctor remained in Boston despite great danger of capture. Captain John Parker and seventy militiamen reached Lexington Green, where they met six companies of redcoats commanded by Major John Pitcairn. There was a cry of "Disperse Ye Rebels," then a pistol shot, two musket shots, more musketry, and the war began. After Lexington, Colonel Smith added his troops to Pitcairn's soldiers and pushed west to Concord.[7] (In the battle at Lexington Green, ten of the Minutemen were physicians.) In Concord the British pushed the Americans aside and were able to destroy some of the hidden ordnance. Colonial arms in Concord included 21,549 firearms, 12 field pieces, 17,441 pounds of powder, 22,191 pounds of lead balls, 15,000 canteens, 10,188 bayonets, 11,979 pouches and 144,699 flints as well as salted fish and rice. Minutemen from around Concord poured into that town and held the North Bridge. They counterattacked, and the British were forced to withdraw to Lexington where they were rescued by a strong column under Lord Percy. The combined group withdrew painfully to Boston. The British suffered 72 killed, 174 wounded, and 26 missing. The Americans surrounded Boston but without artillery they could not take it. This problem would be solved later by actions taken in New York on May 10, 1775.[8]

After he had sent out his riders, Dr. Warren left Boston for Watertown. On May 20 he was asked to organize an army of Massachusetts colonists. On June 14 the doctor was offered the position of physician general of Massachusetts troops, but he asked for hazardous duty instead, and was appointed major general of Massachusetts troops.[9]

The dawn of June 16 found colonists under Colonel Prescott and Major General Israel Putnam digging emplacements on Breeds Hill. This elevation and Bunker Hill stood on the Charlestown peninsula facing Boston, and they were armed to prevent General Gage from an invasion of Charlestown. To the south of Boston, Dorchester Heights was also strengthened. On June 17 British warships bombarded Breeds Hill with no effect on the entrenched infantry. The guns were turned on Charlestown and destroyed part of the city. Dr. Warren made his appearance on the hill and was offered command. He refused because he had not yet received official notice of his rank of general. Rather, he grabbed a rifle and ammunition, and took a position on the hill as a "line infantryman." Gage sent his troops across the water to the foot of the hill. They eventually succeeded in seizing their objective, but it was a pyrrhic victory. In the American retreat from the hill, Warren was killed by a ball through the head. British troops stole the fancy clothes off his corpse and sold them in Boston. The terrible casualties suffered by the British forces led to Gage's replacement by General Howe.

Meanwhile, events of another kind were developing in New York, which was still neutral. Two forces made their way to Fort Ticonderoga across Lake Champlain. One, under Benedict Arnold of Connecticut, was composed of troops from Massachusetts and Connecticut; the second was composed of men from the Hampshire Grants under the command of Ethan Allen, also from Connecticut. They took the fort without a shot. The decrepit fort contained a cache of 100 cannons that would break the stalemate around Boston. Arnold, without orders, took Crown Point. He then went further north into Canada to take St. Johns but turned back. Colonel Henry Knox, a Boston bookseller who had learned how to use artillery from his books at the store, took over the task of moving the cannons across the Berkshires to Boston. Knox, with 45 cannons and 16 mortars arrive in Boston in January 1776. On March 4 General John Thomas occupied Dorchester Heights. On March 16 George Washington, who had been made commander-in-chief after Congress converted the Massachusetts army into the Continental Army, occupied Foster's Hill. Knox's cannon looked down on Boston, and General Howe was forced to evacuate that city. He moved his army to Halifax.[10]

The months spent in Boston were difficult for the British. All food, feed, and forage had to be brought in by ship. Scurvy and smallpox as well as the usual enteric fevers became widespread. Many of the British soldiers who had been pulled from the crowded cities of England had been exposed to smallpox as children. However, the civilians in Boston had been exposed only during epidemics, and they suffered seriously from the disease. It is said that 2,000 British soldiers were sick with smallpox, although a majority were convalescent from inoculation rather than "the natural way." The concept of inoculation was an accepted practice in the British army. Howe, in a conference with Washington, offered to send civilians out of the city. Washington suspected a ploy to spread the disease among his troops who had no immunity, and he refused. Some civilians did leave Boston, but they were thoroughly examined, and their belongings were smoked out. Some authorities believe Washington stayed outside Boston for nine months because smallpox was rampant in the city.[11]

Washington had reason to be suspicious of his enemy; the use of "biological" warfare was not uncommon. The early colonists in Massachusetts wanted to send blankets from smallpox patients to the Indians as a peace offering. Lord Jeffrey Amherst, in the French and Indian War, wanted to decimate his Indian opponents in the same way. Amherst wrote a letter to Colonel Henry Bousquet to suggest that he spread smallpox among Chief Pontiac's Indians to stop their depredations in "the West" (Pennsylvania and Virginia).[12] It is also said that the British defenders of Quebec sent young girls with the infection to "mingle" with the troops besieging the city.[13] Cornwallis is believed to have sent slaves with the illness out of Yorktown to spread it among the Americans and French opposing him. British surgeons inoculated captured slaves and sent them back to their plantations to spread the illness.[14]

When the British evacuated Boston, Washington sent in American troops who had been exposed to smallpox in the past. Eventually Boston was occupied, and Dr. Morgan began to inoculate American troops. It is said that 5,000 men were inoculated by the end of 1776 with only two deaths reported. The low mortality rate was attributed to Morgan's use of Dr. Dimsdale's technique. In the older technique, the physician made two deep incisions in the flesh and inserted a thread steeped in the pus of a ripened pustule. The wound was then covered with a bandage of plaster. The newer technique had been devised by Dr. Sutton and was improved upon by Dr. Dimsdale, who advocated a two-week preparation before inoculation. This included a special diet, rest, and cathartics. Dimsdale inoculated his patients with a shallow puncture into which he inserted serum from a ripened pustule. The wound was left uncovered. The final step was a recuperation period on a mild diet and moderate exercise. The low mortality was also due to the fact that the patients were young, healthy, well-fed, and rested.[15]

After August 19, 1776, American troops guarded ferry wharves and the Boston "neck." They allowed only immunes in or out of the area. By September 19 the epidemic had died down. There had been 5,292 cases of smallpox, 4,988 of them due to inoculation, and 28 deaths from the disease. Towns around Boston started inoculation hospitals. However, twenty families in a community had to have at least one member sick with the disease before inoculation could be started.[16]

When word of the outbreak of hostilities reached England, the British government had to raise an army to put down the rebellion. Many in England felt the colonists were fighting for the rights of all Englishmen. Lord Cavendish, Sir Jeffrey Amherst, General Conway, and Admiral Keppel resigned their commissions. Attempts to raise an army among the common people failed. Attempts to raise an army of fifty thousand out of a population of one million men of fighting age were unsuccessful, and the British press may have contributed to this failure by printing letters and articles from Benjamin Franklin explaining the colonial position. In addition, Thomas Paine's *Common Sense* was published in England, and thousands of copies were sold. Parliament had to turn to the continent to hire soldiers. Catherine of Russia refused as did Frederick the Great of Prussia. Holland had the "Scotch Brigade," which its government refused to rent to the king. George III raised troops from Hanover, the electorate from which his family had been called to the British throne. The Prince of Brunswick-Luneburg (brother-in-law of George III) sold him 4,300 troops for 160,000 pounds. The principality of Hanau as well as the Landgrave of Hesse-Cassel sold men. Hesse-Cassel, with a population of 300,000, sold 20,000 troops for three million pounds. The total German supply was about 30,000 men at a cost of 4.7 million pounds. Of these, 12,000 were killed or remained in America. These men were not German soldiers but largely civilians rounded up to meet the needs of the ruler. In some of the principalities, the ruler received a bonus if his soldier was disabled. He received an extra bonus if the recruit died. With "pounds in their eyes," they urged the British to put their soldiers in the most hazardous positions. Even with foreigners hired to fight them, there was still a strong sentiment for reconciliation among the Americans.[17] The Olive Branch Petition was sent to George III on July 8, 1775. He refused to receive it and to treat the colonies as a group. Furthermore, he declared them in a state of rebellion.[18]

To me, an interesting side issue of the American Revolution has been why the fighting started in Massachusetts. I have always felt most wars were based upon economic problems and needs. I think Massachusetts was ready. In the eighteenth century, the colony spent vast amounts of men and money in support of England's European wars (and their satellite wars fought in America) with little to show for the effort. In 1764 the "Crash of Boston" started with the bankruptcy of Nathaniel Wheelwright, which precipitated a depression that lasted a quarter of a century. People blamed the Stamp Act for the depression. Large numbers of citizens were out of work, and they had time to "talk politics" and discuss problems of government and the question of being ruled from abroad. The unemployed could attack British sentries, tea ships, and the "lobsterbacks" who were an obvious source of their financial problems. The unemployed had time on their hands and had nothing to lose in a radical change.[19]

Attempt at a Fourteenth Colony

In 1775, while Washington was immersed in making an army out of a group of independent militia units, the idea of union with Canada emerged from several quarters. The concept of invasion of the north was not new. In 1690, in response to the frequent raids of the French and their Indian allies on New England, the English colonists had prepared an invasion force. A land force would take Montreal and a sea force would take Quebec. The Montreal force under Fitz John Winthrop landed on the southern end of Lake Champlain. Smallpox broke out among the troops, and they withdrew. A fleet under Sir William Phipps with 2,000 troops was ready to leave for Quebec when smallpox developed on board. The invasion was cancelled. Again, in 1740, New England troops captured the Fortress of Louisberg and were forced to return it after the war (King George's War 1740–1744) ended.[20]

The merchants in Massachusetts still cast covetous glances at the Indian trade in this large new area. The intolerant church leaders of Massachusetts could not abide the presence of a "popish country" on their border. Equally significant was that Roman Catholic French Canadians had been given rights similar to those enjoyed by Englishmen who knew the only right way to achieve heaven's rewards. The Continental Congress felt it had to take Canada to prevent the descent of the French Canadians from Montreal down the Richelieu River, Lake Champlain, Lake George, and the Hudson River to cut off New England from the rest of the colonies. Congress had invited Canada into the rebellion earlier. Add to this the expense of an army that sat around Boston and did nothing except devour the financial reserves of Massachusetts as well as the other New England colonies. Physicians and generals knew that an encamped army was sicker than a moving army. In addition there were the adventurers like Benedict Arnold who could not just "sit on their hands" to wait for something to happen.

Arnold submitted a plan to forcibly seize Canada. The gates to Canada would be opened by the "friends of congress." St. Jean, Chambley, and Quebec would capitulate and actively join in the glorious fight. The plan called for a two-pronged attack on Canada. An army would move up the waterways to Montreal. It would be met by the second prong that marched overland through Maine. The two would meet before Quebec and take that prize without a fight.[21] The command of the "waterways army" was given to Major General Philip Schuyler, a patroon (large landholder) from upstate New York. On July 18, 1775, the general arrived at Ticonderoga to find one-fifth of his army sick due to exposure and poor rations. He pulled his army into shape, and by August 30, 1775, they had started on their trip north. He had 1,500 men from Massachusetts, Connecticut, and New York under his command. Shortly after the start of the expedition, Schuyler was out of action from scurvy and rheumatism. He returned to Fort Ticonderoga, and the general was replaced by Brigadier General Montgomery, a leader beloved and respected by both his troops and his adversaries. Ethan Allen, always ready to seize the limelight, tried to take Montreal before the major American force could reach it. He was captured and sent as a prisoner of war to England. His rash act caused many French and English Canadians to swing to the king's cause. The main "river army" moved up the lakes to the Sorel River. They easily captured Chambley and laid siege to St. Jean, which was taken on November 13, 1775, after an excellent defense by the out-gunned garrison. During this short period, there were about 100 American casualties from the engagement, but 937 were discharged due to illness, typical figures for a novice army. The army fought and slept in wet clothes because of the constant rainfall. In early October, the soldiers were ready to return home, but the timely arrival of 700 troops with tents, provisions, and artillery raised their morale. With Chambley and St. Jean taken, Montgomery with reinforcements of 2,000 troops moved up the Richelieu River and reached Montreal. The city was exposed, and it capitulated on November 13, 1775. The St. Lawrence River was now open to the invaders. Montgomery left General Wooster in charge of Montreal with 200 troops, and he sailed for Quebec at the end of November in ships he had taken at Sorel. Most of his New England troops returned home, and Montgomery was left with 300 effectives when he arrived under the walls of Quebec.[22]

The second or land prong under Colonel (later Brigadier General) Benedict Arnold, an apothecary from New Haven, assembled in September 1775. It consisted of 1,100 men from Pennsylvania, Maryland, Virginia, and New England. In the force were rifle companies of 65 to 75 men. These troops carried rifled guns, tomahawks or small axes, and a long knife. The rifle companies were commanded by Captains William Hendricks, Matthew Smith, and John Morgan. These special units wore ash-colored hunting shirts, leggings, and moccasins. There were ten musket companies whose uniform was a woolen roundabout jacket and buckskin breeches. They also carried a hat, hunting shirt, leggings, moccasins, shoes, and two pairs of stockings. It was assumed that the Canadians and Indians wanted the colonials to invade. George Washington cautioned Arnold about the behavior of his troops. They were to respect the Canadians and their property. They were not to show disrespect for their religion but rather to look with compassion on their errors without insulting them. The army left Cambridge for Maine. From Maine it was 180 miles to Quebec. They believed it would take three weeks for the trip.[23]

The surgeon who accompanied the overland army was Dr. Isaac Senter of Rhode Island, age 22. His mate was Dr. Green. They had two assistants, Mr. Barr and Mr. Jackson. According to Dr. Senter, the army left Cambridge on September 13, 1775, marched to Newburyport, and set sail for the Kennebec River. The first casualty was a soldier shot by another soldier while drunk, and he died of internal bleeding. After the army reached the river, they changed to bateaux. All the medications were in one bateau that leaked. Senter bought another one for four dollars, but he lost most of his supplies. Bread, kept in casks, became wet and had to be discarded along with some dried cod fish. Salt beef and pork were saved. Dysentery broke out, and Captain Williams, leader of a rifle company, almost died. Dr. Green became so ill he had to be left behind at Fort Western in Augusta, Maine. The water was bad and turned yellow. The men cooked with it and drank large quantities of it because of the salted food they consumed. This caused vomiting and diarrhea.[24] Senter was probably the first physician to describe Reiter's Syndrome. One of Morgan's riflemen, Mr. Irvin, had dysentery and recovered. He then developed severe rheumatism of all the joints of his extremities. Two other soldiers had similar problems.[25] The disease is now known to be largely congenital, but it is set off by an external event like dysentery or gonorrhea.

The men could supplement their meager diet with trout caught as the bateaux moved on. On October 22 rations were cut by half. Senter commented that the expedition matched the exploits of Hannibal when he crossed the Pyrenees and the Alps. The very sick were left behind. Healthy men stayed with their sick comrades until they died, buried them, and then rejoined the expedition.

Between September 25 and November 2, almost 80 men died of starvation and hardship. The men were also treated for peripneumony (pneumonia) and angina (throat infection). Senter described the trip through Maine and Canada: "The army was too much fatigued being obliged to carry the bateaux, barrels of provisions and warlike stores, etc., over on their backs through a most terrible piece of woods conceivable. Sometimes the mud knee deep, then over ledgy hills. Diarrhea was widespread."[26] Dr. Irvin of Virginia, Dr. Coates from Pennsylvania, and Dr. Dearborn of New Hampshire were also in the force but served as line officers. This phenomenon of medical practitioners who served as line officers was common in the Revolution. The army had to ascend the Kennebec and the Dead rivers, cross the Height of Land, and descend the Chaudiere River to the St. Lawrence. They then had to cross the St. Lawrence to Quebec. There would be no settlements on the route until they reached the French settlements on the Chaudiere River. The army had one hundred bateaux, but the men frequently had to portage boats and supplies through a "howling wilderness." Scores of men died or fell out and refused to go any further. The weather grew worse with rain, snow, and ice. They reached the Dead River where General Arnold ordered a log hospital built (the Arnold Hospital). Dr. Irvine stayed behind with eight to ten sick. In mid–October, the army was down to 950 effectives, and they had to start on half rations. On October 25, Lieutenant Colonel Enos "threw in the towel" and started back with 300 men. He reached Massachusetts where he was court-martialed and acquitted with honor, because the officers who accompanied him testified in his behalf.

Arnold and his men moved on and were able to supplement their supplies with game, such as deer, moose, and ducks. They ate the fat and marrow because they believed this would sustain life better. Then they started on the meat. There were no vegetables, bread, or salt, and the men became weak. They smoked the meat for jerky, but improper preservation caused diarrhea. When game became scarce, they were forced to eat shoe leather, shaving soap, candles, as well as a dog that accompanied them. On October 31, they reached the Chaudiere River without food. Arnold moved forward with a small unit and reached the French settlements at Sartegen. He sent food back to the main army. The men gorged on the new supplies, and three of them died in the process. Several of the soldiers became sick and were turned over to the French Canadians who nursed them back to health. They were returned to their companions without charge. The food revived them, and they reassembled to march on to reach their leader. On November 9, these soldiers, who two or three months earlier had been farmers, fishermen, and store clerks, reached the St. Lawrence opposite Quebec practically without clothes. The men had had neither training in frigid warfare nor any special winter gear. During World War II, men were trained for a year or more as ski or mountain troops with proper winter clothing. The results of the time spent and cost of the training could not compare with the achievements of this small band.

On the night of November 13–14, five hundred men crossed the St. Lawrence to Wolf's Cove. The remainder crossed the following night. Many were sick with pneumonia and sore throat. They demanded the surrender of Quebec, which was refused in the form of an artillery barrage. One soldier received a cannonball injury to his leg. Dr. Senter amputated, but the man died the following day. The American force had no artillery, so the walls of Quebec were impregnable to them. The army pulled back to Pointe Aux Trembles. Within the walls of Quebec, the French lieutenant governor tried to strengthen his defenses. He had 1,126 men, among them veterans, militia, raw recruits, and seamen from ships frozen in the St. Lawrence River. His veterans were the Royal Highland Emigrants (Scots) who emigrated to Canada and the Mohawk Valley. Their commander was Colonel MacLean, a veteran of the Seven Years War.[27] The lieutenant governor was replaced by Governor Carleton, who forced out a potential fifth column of English-speaking merchants whose sympathies were with the invading forces.

Smallpox Breaks Out

Montgomery, who brought some artillery, joined Arnold at Pointe Aux Trembles on December 1, and they proceeded to blockade Quebec. The combined force began to bombard the city on December 9 without any visible effect. The troops outside of Quebec tried to dig protective fortifications, but the ground was frozen solid, so they tried to build forts of snow turned into ice with water, but these forts could not withstand cannon fire, and several Americans died from the cannonading. Many suffered frostbite of their hands and feet, which was treated by rubbing in snow until circulation was restored. One American sergeant, Singleton, deserted to the British and told them of the plans of attack. Montgomery had to attack regardless because his New England troops' enlistments ended January 1, 1776. He had 300 infantry, some artillery, and a few Canadians. More important, he carried clothing he had captured at St. Jean and Montreal. Total effectives in both groups numbered 800 including Livingston with 200 Canadians as well as a "pick-up" force of an additional 100 to 200 Canadians from the environs of Quebec. A convent of the Recollarts on the St. Charles River was set up as a hospital. A few cases of smallpox developed by December 18, but most of the patients were sick with pneumonia and pleurisy. The smallpox cases were placed in isolation. For some unknown reason, men in the army with early signs of the disease were not removed from duty and were able to spread the disease to the healthy. By mid–February, 100 men were sick with smallpox. Inoculation was started by Dr. Senter who also inoculated himself.

Dr. Senter wished to lead one assault company to the gates, but he was turned down by Arnold even though three captains of the line had previously refused to lead their companies in the attack.[28] On December 31, 1775, Montgomery attacked from the right; Arnold from the left. Montgomery was able to reach the lower town with the defenders in retreat. A primed cannon filled with grape stood in their path. A drunken seaman, while in retreat with the rest of the defenders, put fire to the touch hole. Montgomery, most of his aides, and other leaders of the attack were killed or maimed by this last discharge. Many of the wounded died because they were lying in the snow without help and froze to death. The remainder of the force, dispirited by their loss, pulled back instead of joining Arnold in his drive.

Arnold's force did no better. Arnold was led off the field with a gunshot wound in his leg. The shot passed between the tibia and fibula in his foreleg and embedded itself in the gastrocnemius, from where it was removed by Senter. The doctor believed that Arnold's men could have carried Sault Aux Matelot and taken Quebec if not for that wound. The troops lost their spirit and retreated. Captain Morgan of the Virginia Rifles took over the command. However, the defenders rallied and captured Morgan and his force.[29] The invading Americans suffered 150 killed and wounded and about 300 prisoners. Most of the officers were killed or captured.

Smallpox broke out among the prisoners of war taken in the attack on Quebec. Private Simon Forbes described the problems:

> When the pock was coming out on 70–80 of our number, a fever very high and no water to drink, the men drank their own urine which made the fever rage too violently to be endured. Our flesh seemed a mass of corruption. At the same time we were covered with vermin. When we were a little recovered, we were moved back to our former prison without any cleansing or changing of our apparel. Our clothing was stiff with corrupted matter.[30]

Many of the prisoners died of smallpox that winter. In the spring they developed diarrhea and scurvy. The dead were collected and stored in the Dead House until spring thaw when graves could be dug. The prisoners who were born in Great Britain were given the opportunity to join the British forces. Some did because if they were returned to England as prisoners, they faced trial for treason, and would be hanged. The prisoners received the same rations as their captors: one biscuit, a half pound of pork or three-quarters of a pound of salted beef, butter, molasses, and vinegar. They were given candles for night use. In general, the prisoners of war were treated well by Carleton. Eventually, they were sent to New York on parole to await exchange.

The survivors of the attack who managed to avoid capture retreated back across the river and "laid siege" to Quebec in six feet of snow. They were joined by reinforcements from Massachusetts and New Hampshire in March 1776. The command of all forces was taken over by General David Wooster, and he in turn was replaced by General John Thomas, a physician from Massachusetts.

By early April 700 men were sick with smallpox. This represented half of the force besieging Quebec. Thomas was supposed to have 1,900 effectives, but he could count on only 1,000 troops who were really fit to fight. Reinforcements arrived, and on May 1, 1776, there were 7,000 men outside the city; 900 were sick, most with smallpox. Massive numbers had deserted. Two hundred were inoculated against smallpox and would be unfit for line duty. General Thomas ordered all inoculation to be stopped on pain of death, but the men started to inoculate themselves by injecting pus under their fingernails. The inoculees could not quarantine themselves, and thus they spread the disease to those who obeyed orders. In early May, the ice in the river began to break up and British ships with 1,000 reinforcements could reach Quebec. On May 6 the reinforced British army attacked the American lines while they were decamping. American forces were scattered. Smallpox patients retreated as best they could, and they reached safety with disastrous results to the healthy. The colonial army was forced to retreat back to Duchambault. They next pulled back to the Sorel River between Quebec and Montreal on the St. Lawrence. At the Sorel, 3,300 men were sick with smallpox.[31]

Meanwhile, the other "prong" of the American forces who had moved up the waterways arrived to reinforce the small group around Quebec. Captain Lemuel Roberts was part of a detachment that arrived in April 1776 and recorded his trip from Massachusetts to Bennington, Castleton, Ticonderoga, and Crown Point. His force then boarded boats for the trip to St. Jean, the Chambley River, the St. Lawrence, Three Rivers, Wolf's Cove, and the Plains of Abraham. He commented that all civilian houses had smallpox patients. Some of the men in the regiment inoculated themselves. This activity forced the regiment to be sent back to receive proper inoculation and isolation.

Dr. Senter was ordered to Montreal to set up a hospital for the ever increasing number of sick. In addition to riflemen, surgeons were sent north to support Dr. Senter. One such was Dr. Samuel Fisk Merrick. Examination of his medical chest gives us an idea of what was considered important in caring for sick troops. He carried elixir of camphor, hiera pera (a powder of aloes and carella) used as a tonic and stomachic, powdered rhei (rhubarb) for diarrhea, and jalap, a cathartic that was a remedy of the Indians in Mexico. He also had a supply of powdered ipecacuanha and tartar emetic, pills of cathartic salts, and artemisia (a wormwood from Europe used as an anthelminthic). The doctor described the illnesses he saw. In addition to "the smallpox there was bilious and intermittent fevers with some of the putrid kind," dysentery, diarrhea, and rheumatic complaints.[32]

Benjamin Franklin was sent by the Continental Congress both to investigate the debacle in March 1776 and to try again to bring the Canadians over to the American side. He was accompanied by Samuel Chase and Charles Carroll, both Roman Catholics, and a Catholic priest, Father John Carroll. They were unsuccessful and had to return south prematurely because Franklin developed dropsy.[33] Franklin urged the inoculation of all troops gradually despite General Thomas's earlier order. Arnold agreed with Franklin. He wrote a letter to Congress for permission to inoculate 500 to 1,000 soldiers at a time. A new group could be brought in every five days until the army would be fit in about four weeks. Dr. Senter started to inoculate the troops a regiment at a time. In his diary, the doctor noted that New England troops had no immunity to that disease. He also put troops recovering from inoculation on garrison duty, which they could perform. General Thomas developed smallpox the "natural way," and he died.[34] The army was then forced to pull back to St. Jean at the northern tip of Lake Champlain.

By then it was a dispirited army without discipline or supplies. In an attempt to rescue the scattered and defeated army, 5,500 fresh troops under Generals Sullivan and Thompson were sent. They brought weapons and provisions and planned another attack on Canada. On June 8 Thompson with 2,000 Americans blundered into a force of 6,000 British reinforcements, and they were destroyed. General Sullivan was now in total command, and he pulled the army back. There were now 4,000 sick in the camps at St. Jean and Chambley on the Richelieu River. Mortality statistics listed 30 deaths daily. Some regiments had no men fit for duty. By June 12, about one third of the army had become unfit. The sick were loaded into bateaux and transported to Lake Champlain, then to Isle Aux Noit, the last piece of Canadian soil held by the Americans. This was ten miles north of the New York border. Of the sick, 2,000 had smallpox, and an equal number had malaria and/or dysentery.[35] British ships followed the retreating army.

The army in front of Quebec started its retreat, and Captain Roberts's regiment joined the army around Quebec in time to embark on bateaux and row to keep ahead of the pursuing British troops. In the retreat, they left their wounded and hospital equipment. Senter was sent to Albany to start a hospital. General Arnold gave him a house belonging to the East India Company. Meanwhile, Captain Roberts became sick with the pox, but he and the others still continued to row to avoid capture. Fortunately, the wind blew against the pursuing British who were in sailing vessels, and the bateaux could pull away. They crossed to Sorel, forty miles south of Montreal. By this time Roberts's clothes stuck to his body from the pus. He was able to rest at Sorel and recovered his strength. By that time Arnold had recovered from his wound, and he and Sullivan joined the remnants of the American force on their retreat. However, Roberts developed dysentery, and although he was in the rear guard, he could not keep up with his unit because of frequent stops to relieve himself. He became delirious and was placed in a boat. By the following day, Roberts had improved, was able to take medication, including "bokea" tea, and was able to rest at Chambley. They continued their retreat to St. Jean then to Isle Aux Noit, Crown Point, Ticonderoga, and Mt. Independence. The men were forced to fortify Mt. Independence, and many died at night after a day of extreme labor. Roberts again developed a fever and turned as "yellow as saffron." He still did his duty; relapsed, then improved. He moved south to Albany and from there to New Jersey. A surgeon found him unfit for duty and wanted him discharged. The captain begged to stay on. His wish was granted, and he was shipped to "The Highlands" in New York state, then to Kings Ferry, then to the Jersey shore. Roberts marched to Morristown, Connecticut Farms, Elizabethtown, Brunswick, and Amboy. Finally his term of enlistment ended.[36] His loyalty and devotion to the cause despite hardships was impressive. The same devotion was demonstrated among the Tories, of course.

Upon arrival at Crown Point in July 1776, General Gates was appointed commander of the army, and he retreated further south to Ticonderoga. Gates received 10,000 reinforcements from New York and New England. Many of these troops became sick when exposed to the veterans, and many died.[37] Arnold tried unsuccessfully to stop the British fleet's pursuit by rapidly building a lake fleet at the Skenesborough shipyards. The ships were of poor quality, however, and built of green timber, and the American navy was composed of soldiers from the retreating army. They fought Pringle at Valcour Island in Lake Champlain, but the entire fleet was either sunk by the British or scuttled by their American crew near Crown Point. Arnold destroyed the remains of his fleet to prevent it from falling into British hands.[38]

Despite this total defeat at the hands of the British navy, he had succeeded in slowing their advance, so that on November 2, 1776, Carleton ordered his troops back to Canada after he had reached the foot of Lake George. The battle at Valcour Island caused some damage to the British, and they required a month to refit. It may have been this month of delay that held Carleton back from a move down to New York City to cut off New England from the rest of colonies.[39] The campaign ended with an estimated American casualty rate of forty percent. Over 5,000 men were captured, perished, or rendered unfit for service, and Canada was lost forever. The army that retreated from Canada carried smallpox with it. Deserters and discharged patients carried the disease to their communities, causing widespread epidemics. Potential recruits refused to join for fear of contracting smallpox. Many colonies were forced to give bounties to get replacements for the service.

John Adams wrote that smallpox was ten times more terrible than the British and was the cause of the retreat from Quebec. This has been picked up by historians to explain our failure to take Canada. In all honesty, smallpox was of little consequence in the unfortunate attack on Quebec. There were few sick with smallpox at the converted convent. Smallpox created disaster in the retreat of the army from Canada after the arrival of British reinforcements. Dr. Potts, sent north by Dr. Morgan with medical supplies for the army, described the horrible picture of more than 1,000 sick without clothing or shelter from the elements. The causes of these deaths were dysentery, bilious and putrid fevers, and smallpox as well as exposure. There were four surgeons and four mates to care for the army, and they had no medicine.[40]

The army eventually settled in at Ticonderoga, Skenesborough, Fort George, and Crown Point. General Gates enforced sanitation at these bases, and smallpox patients were quarantined. He met with the surgeons to try to improve care and raise the morale of his shattered troops. New recruits were screened for smallpox. Skenesborough was set up as an inoculation hospital. Self-inoculation was forbidden. On August 28, 1776, Gates was able to report to Washington that smallpox was eradicated and that he could defend Ticonderoga. With the eradication of smallpox, Ticonderoga became the "Gibraltar of the North." General hospitals were set up at Fort George and Albany. The surgeons had their full share of smallpox, putrid fever (probably typhus), malaria, dysentery, and jaundice. Dr. Potts worked with the Fort George installation, but this was evacuated and the casualties were transported to Albany. The Fort George hospital could handle 300 patients, but it was inundated with 1,497 casualties. In September 1776 there were 5,247 effectives with about as many in the hospitals, despite Gates's optimistic report to his superior.[41]

Saratoga

As 1776 drew to a close, Gates had a healthy army of veterans. In January 1777 Dr. Stringer, more a politician than a doctor, was replaced by Dr. Potts as director of the Northern Department. Dr. Potts was a well-trained physician whose primary interest was the health of his troops. Unlike the physicians in Philadelphia who were sparring for position in the army and control of medicine after the war, Potts paid attention to his job. The results were obvious in the next campaign when he received a commendation from Congress for keeping medical casualties to a minimum.

The winter of 1776–77 was spent in camp by both the British and the Americans. Major General John Burgoyne was occupied with his campaign to again try to split New England from the other colonies. He was to lead an army from Canada and knock out Ticonderoga on Lake George, cross the land and reach the Hudson, then proceed down to Albany. At Albany he was to meet Lieutenant Colonel Barry St. Leger with a column moving east from Oswego along the Mohawk River. Howe was to sail up the Hudson from New York City and join them. It was hoped that news of the battle would pull Washington up from New Jersey so he could be destroyed and the war ended. On paper the plan was excellent, and certainly a professional army under professional leadership could carry it out. However, deficiencies developed. The British leaders failed to raise adequate numbers of Tories to join the assault, and so felt it necessary to use Indians against "English colonists," a weapon previously used by the French and looked upon with great distaste. The savagery of the Indians was known in London, and including them lost the English many friends on both sides of the Atlantic. However, only 400 Indians "joined" the army. The Canadians did not join the army, nor did they sell their horses to the British forces that were needed to haul supplies and artillery for the army. Burgoyne also carried excessive amounts of artillery for the anticipated campaign. He obviously had no idea of the wilderness of the Adirondack Mountains. Worst of all, Howe believed the war could be ended in the south rather than in the north, and he was more interested in a plan to take Philadelphia, the capital of the colonies.

Burgoyne headed west along the St. Lawrence and picked up his army at Crown Point on July 1, 1777. They sailed down Lake Champlain to a point above Ticonderoga. The Hessians went ashore on the east side and the British on the west side. The Hessians took Mt. Independence on the eastern shore, where they found an impenetrable wilderness. On the west side, a road of felled trees had to be laid to make it possible for the British to place artillery on Mt. Defiance, which looked down into Ticonderoga. The American General St. Clair saw his danger and left Ticonderoga. He crossed to Mt. Independence, then he pulled all troops down to Skenesborough. They were pursued by General Simon Fraser and his light infantry. Meanwhile, the Hessians were lost in the wilderness. On July 7 Fraser ran into the American rear guard. Fraser's force was almost beaten by the colonists until he was rescued by a force of Hessians; action ceased, and the battle of Hubbardton entered the history books. The Americans joined St. Clair while the British and Hessians joined their main army at Skenesborough. Burgoyne was now twenty miles above the Hudson, and rather than using his navy on Lake George to reach the land between the lake and the Hudson, he chose to go overland. He had to build a road of felled trees to cover the twenty miles. General Schuyler, with the help of woodsmen, blocked his trail with massive felled trees that also dammed up waterways. This made the land marshy and more difficult to cross. It took Burgoyne 26 days to cross the twenty miles. They still had to haul the heavy artillery down. On August 3 Burgoyne learned that Howe had sailed to Philadelphia.

Meanwhile, St. Leger had his problems. He was stopped at Ft. Stanwix on the Mohawk River. His Indians and Tories fought a bloody battle with Herkimer's militia at Oriskany, and the Indians started to desert. The fort could not be taken, and St. Leger learned that General Benedict Arnold was approaching with a massive force of Continentals. He gave up the siege and returned to Oswego. The area between Oswego and Stanwix remained a bloody battleground between Tories and Indians on one side and the settlers on the other throughout the war.

Burgoyne on the west side of the Hudson heard of large stores of horses and wagons on the east side in Vermont. He dispatched a group of heavily weighted down Germans, some light British infantry, and Indians under the command of Lieutenant Colonel Baum. Their destination was Bennington. Baum and his forces were wiped out, and his reinforcements were badly battered by General John Stark. All of Burgoyne's Indians deserted. Burgoyne's only thought was to push to Albany without help of the other two wings. They moved south at a snail's pace until they arrived at Freeman's Farm. The battle started when Daniel Morgan's riflemen picked off all of the British officers in the point. Morgan was joined by New Hampshire Continentals. The British were saved from destruction by the intervention of a German regiment. The British dug in and were sniped at by American riflemen. On October 7, 1777, Burgoyne tried an offensive move with 1,500 men who were largely destroyed by troops led by Enoch Poor, David Morgan, and Henry Dearborn. The British pulled back to their fortifications. Then Benedict Arnold led a charge that broke through the line, but he received a musket ball in the same leg that had been wounded in Canada and was out of action.

Meanwhile in New York City, Sir Henry Clinton offered to relieve the pressure on Burgoyne with a move up the Hudson to Fort Montgomery below West Point. This achieved nothing. On October 8 Burgoyne pulled his army together to try to reach Ticonderoga in the north. He reached Saratoga Heights and dug in with Gates in command of the American troops opposing him. Burgoyne left his wounded at his furthest penetration south when he retreated.[42] They were taken to the hospital in Albany where British and Hessian surgeons worked on them. It was in Albany that Dr. Rush and Dr. Thacher watched them work. They were impressed with the skill of the British surgeons, but they felt the Germans were heartless bumblers. Thacher described that war wounds that had not been treated for several days were full of maggots, which he removed with tincture of myrrh. Thacher cared for 20 casualties, one of whom was Captain Gregg, scalped and left for dead by the Indians. His dog licked the wounds and then brought help. The captain's scalp had been completely removed, and he had tomahawk wounds to the skull, back, and side. Gregg also sustained a musket ball wound in the arm, but he survived.[43]

The Americans were able to encircle the British at Saratoga, and Burgoyne surrendered and signed the "Convention of Saratoga." This agreement was also signed by Gates without the consent of Congress, which later repudiated it. According to the convention, Burgoyne's army of 6,350 men was to be allowed to embark for Europe and never fight in North America. However, they were able to go to other theaters and replace other troops who could be sent to America. Every American school child has since learned that this victory brought the French openly into the war. In Great Britain the opposition press urged the cessation of hostilities to prevent this dangerous alliance. A second consequence of the victory was the Conway Cabal. It was an attempt to replace the plodding Washington with the victorious Gates. The end of 1777 saw the British holding New York City, Philadelphia, and Newport, Rhode Island.[44]

Of significance to our discussion is the low mortality of casualties once they had reached the hospitals of the Northern Department. From March 1 to November 10, 1777, there were only 250 deaths, including wound fatalities. General Gates and Congress commended Dr. Potts for the care he gave his charges.[45]

Smallpox played no part in this watershed battle of the Revolution. Many of the troops who had survived the expedition to Canada were inoculated. In addition, when Washington wintered in Morristown, New Jersey, in January 1777, he requested from Congress and was granted the right to inoculate his troops. His army was inoculated under the supervision of Dr. Nathaniel Bond. In addition, three inoculation hospitals were set up in the south to inoculate the troops coming from that area to join the war. Also, Washington wrote to Dr. Shippen in Philadelphia to order him to inoculate the troops in Philadelphia. As a result of this wholesale inoculation program, smallpox never played a major nor even a minor part in any further battle. Occasional cases broke out at Valley Forge and on board the prison ships off New York and Charleston, but the disease never regained its destructive capacity on massed armies. Smallpox inoculation early in the century was a major surgical procedure requiring considerable care both before and after the operation. During the Revolution, much of the preliminary care was disregarded with equally good results. To inoculate 100 servicemen, the physician used six ounces of calomel, two pounds of jalap, three pounds of nitre, elixir of vitriol, one pound of Peruvian bark, and one pound of Virginia snakeroot.[46]

History of Smallpox

Smallpox has been a companion to humanity for thousands of years. It is probable that the smallpox virus was originally a harmless virus of animals. When humans became farmers about 12,000 years ago, and animals became domesticated, the organism evolved and adapted to a new host. Medical writings of thousands of years ago already described the disease. Writings in Sanskrit depict a disease that resembles smallpox. There was also a description of true vaccination used 2,000 years before Jenner. The fluid of a pock on a cow's udder was placed on the tip of a sharp instrument and scratched into the upper arm of a patient until blood appeared. India, with a long history of exposure to smallpox, has an almost equally long history of inoculation. However, the patients also depended on spiritual help, and in India's pantheon, there is a goddess of smallpox.

Ancient Egypt was plagued by the disease. Reifer described a mummy of the twentieth dynasty with scars of smallpox. It was believed to have struck down Alexander's army in India in 327 B.C. The disease may have been introduced into China about 250 B.C. by barbarians invading from the north. China had a second introduction when its army invaded Hunan Province in the south while an epidemic was raging there in 48 A.D. Historians of smallpox believe the plague in Athens during the Peloponesian War was smallpox. It was believed to have destroyed one quarter of the army and caused the downfall of the Athenian city state. (One should view this theory skeptically. Every medical historian writing about his favorite disease points to the devastation in Athens as due to that disease.) The disease may have been responsible for disbanding the Carthaginians when they besieged Syracuse in Sicily in 395 B.C. An epidemic in Syria in 302 A.D., described by Eusebius, probably was smallpox. This contagion left many of its survivors blind. Smallpox can cause ulceration and scarring of the cornea.

There are several contenders for the dubious honor of introducing smallpox to the world. It was believed to have been endemic in India at least 3,000 years ago, and it spread from there to Egypt, then to the Hittites of Turkey, and on to Persia and Greece. From Persia, it passed to the Huns who carried it to China. The Chinese carried the virus to Japan in the sixth century A.D. when they introduced Buddhism to the islands off the Chinese coast. The Roman armies, while subjugating the Parthians in 164 A.D., picked up the virus along with the spoils of victory and brought it back to Rome. This caused the plague under Emperor Marcus Aurelius Antoninus. From Rome it was reintroduced to Europe (after the initial Greek introduction), and it raged there for fifteen years. Historians believe it killed between three and a half and seven million people. Another reintroduction to Europe came with the returning crusaders. This reintroduction spread to Scandinavia, Ireland, and then to Greenland where the virus wiped out a colony in the fifteenth century. Greenland remained free of European settlements for 300 years after this attack.[47]

A second, younger contender for the honor was Ethiopia. In the sixth century A.D., smallpox was spread by Ethiopian soldiers to Arabia. It is believed that Ethiopian soldiers, the Aksumites, may have brought it to their homeland in 370 A.D. Arabian armies spread the word of Allah and probably also smallpox to North Africa and Asia.[48] The final contender for the honor was tropical

Africa. From here it spread to the Arabs with slavery. The sub–Saharan Africans had an extensive relationship with the disease. Like the Asiatic Indians they had a god of smallpox, whom they called Shapona.[49]

Smallpox became an endemic disease in European population centers in the fifteenth century. Children developed the disease without too great a mortality rate. There were, however, occasional virulent epidemics that destroyed children. In Naples in 1544, as many as 5,000 to 6,000 children died in one year from the virus. Venice in 1570–1571 lost 10,000 citizens, mostly children. It is possible that the "mild disease" affecting children may have been chickenpox. Paré treated smallpox as a minimal problem. The English, in the early sixteenth century, called it smallpox to differentiate it from the great pox (pockes, pocks) of syphilis. (*Potakes* in Old English was a skin eruption.) In France, *petite vérole* as opposed to *grande vérole* distinguished the two diseases. In the mid-seventeenth century, the virulence of smallpox increased and led to great mortality among adults. (Deaths among children were not seriously counted, because they were expected.) The disease was first listed in the London Bills of Mortality in 1629. In 1632 the London Bills showed sizable numbers of deaths from smallpox. It was responsible for more than eight percent of total mortality after 1649. In normal years in London, mortality ranged between 1,000 and 1,200. Epidemic years raised the death rate to 2,500 to 3,000. The facial disfigurement of smallpox was first described in England in the seventeenth century.[50] (An interesting aside to the history of the disease is the failure of Shakespeare to describe smallpox in any of his plays. He described many other illnesses as well as the degenerative processes that prey upon humanity.)

The contagious nature of smallpox was first recognized by Jean Baptiste Van Helmont of Belgium (1578–1614) and later by Boerhaave of the Netherlands (1688–1738). By the mid-eighteenth century most scholars had accepted the theory of contagion.[51]

Treatment of the disease varied. Europeans in the eighteenth century still believed in bleeding and purging. In West Africa, palm oil ointments and herbal liniments were used. Brazilians used powdered horse manure to drive out the spirits causing the disease. The fat of the jackass was a favorite of Arabian physicians. Japanese bathed in warm water with sake, rice water, red beans, and salt. It was believed that the color red in the patient's surroundings was vital for the complete treatment. In India, the family was forbidden to fry or season any food meant for the patient during the illness, and pustules were opened with a gold or silver needle.[52] In Germany, patients wore a "lapis variolitis" (a type of amulet), a green stone with flecks running into each other and resembling the smallpox lesions. This particular concept is based on the doctrine of signatures, that is, the therapy of a disease by objects resembling the disease or the organ in which it manifests itself. In Great Britain, drinking tar water was a universal panacea and was tried in smallpox. Tar water became a specific in Barbados. From there it spread to Charleston, South Carolina. The North American Indians heated their bodies to create a sweat, then jumped into a cold river, which probably increased the mortality. Among the colonists in America, the concept of bringing the body and mind to the most perfect state of health so that the disease would be mild was developed. This was accomplished by light diet, calomel, and purges. When the colonists were in the best condition possible, they exposed themselves to the mildest case in the community in hopes that their good health as well as the mild disease in the carrier would cause a mild disease in the individual.[53] Sydenham was sensible enough to treat his patients in a cool room with cool drinks.[54] The concept of "the wrath of God" as the cause of the disease was treated by prayers, sacrifices, and supplications.

The "red treatment" started in Japan in the tenth century and continued until the nineteenth century. The windows in a room were painted red; all furniture and bedding in the room were red, as were the garments the patient wore. Averroes, a twelfth-century doctor, believed red had a warming property that brought the smallpox humors to the skin's surface so that the body could excrete them. In 1893 a physician in Denmark urged the therapy of smallpox with a red light. The red concept existed in Europe until 1925.[55]

The fatality of the disease was probably not as severe as that of the plague, but smallpox was more consistent in its destruction. In the London Bills of Mortality from 1647–1700 there were 210 deaths per 100,000 population per year. From 1701–1800, the rate jumped to 300 per 100,000. In London, smallpox deaths varied between four and seventeen percent of total deaths, averaging nine percent. In Manchester, a community the size of Boston, fifteen percent of mortality was due to this disease that affected children under ten predominantly. By 1800 it had caused one-third of all blindness and killed 400,000 Europeans per year. It is believed that sixty million Europeans died of smallpox in the seventeenth century.[56] Overall probability statistics claimed that the virus was responsible for the death of one quarter of each generation.[57]

Surprisingly, the death rate was higher among the nobility than among the common people. The probable explanation is that the poor could not afford the care of the physician. The illness killed two Japanese Emperors, the King of Burma and Siam, a Pharaoh, a Caliph, and a Roman Emperor. In France, the son and grandson of Louis XIV died of smallpox. His great-grandson became Louis XV, and he in turn died of the disease. Louis XVI, after his ascent to the throne, was inoculated. In the Hapsburg family, smallpox caused several shifts in the line of succession. Members of the ruling families of England were repeatedly carried off by smallpox. Charles II survived an attack of the virus, but his brother, the Duke of Gloucester, died of smallpox. Queen

Mary died of smallpox and left no children; her husband, William III, ruled for eight years without a consort and died. Queen Anne's only surviving child of seventeen died of the virus. There were no further Stuarts, and the House of Hanover was called to rule Great Britain.[58]

Inoculation in the Old World

The introduction of inoculation in the eighteenth century was as important an innovation as antibiotics were to the twentieth century. Inoculation, not vaccination, was the introduction of the live virus into the body of the recipient by pus or scabs. This deliberately caused the infection, hopefully in a milder form. The patient became ill and developed a rash, usually around the inoculation site. It conferred lifelong immunity, unlike vaccination. The main drawback was that it could spread virulent smallpox to anyone in contact with the inoculee. The process had a one to three percent mortality rate. Various techniques had been used in Asia and Africa for centuries before it was introduced into Europe. The technique used in China was to harvest the scabs from a mild case, dry them, and crush them into powder. This was blown into the patient's nose and caused a milder form of the illness. It was called "Planting the Heavenly Flowers." This technique was tried in England in 1721 on a woman prisoner who became deathly ill. Although she survived, the procedure was judged too dangerous for further use.[59]

Inoculation of the skin was introduced into Constantinople from Persia in 1672. It was known to peasants around the Caspian Sea before this time and found its way to Poland in 1670 ("burying the smallpox"). Turkey had a severe epidemic in 1706, probably spread from Greece. A Greek woman inoculated 4,000 patients in Constantinople. As a result of her excellent results, the Europeans living in Turkey had their children treated. Robert Sutton, ambassador from Britain to Turkey, had the sons of his secretary inoculated. These two were the first English patients to receive inoculation. Dr. Timoni, a graduate of Padua, described the technique of inoculation in letters to eminent physicians in England, Sweden, and Austria. According to descriptions, pus was taken from a recovering boy on the twelfth or thirteenth day. It was placed in a vial and kept warm. The material was injected in the forearm or upper arm. Sometimes, the superstitious had it inserted in an incision in the form of a cross. Seven days after infection pustules developed in the area around the incision.[60]

Princess Caroline influenced King George I to order a trial of the inoculation process in England, which was conducted on August 9, 1721, on six Newgate prisoners and ten children from the charity ward of the Parish of St. James. All felons who survived were pardoned. As a proof of her immunity, after her recovery one of the women was sent to care for a patient with smallpox in Hereford. She also slept in a bed with a ten-year-old boy with the active disease. She did not become sick. Statistical studies of results by Secretary Jurin of the Royal Society showed the value of inoculation over becoming infected naturally. The Royal Society favored and backed the procedure; however, most people tended to fear it and stayed away. Some clergymen opposed the technique because they believed it contravened God's will. After the epidemic of 1721 in England, the disease seemed to take a milder turn for the remainder of the decade.[61]

The technique of inoculation fell out of favor until Dr. Killpatrick (or Kirkpatrick) of Charleston, South Carolina, went to England to describe his results in the epidemic of 1738. The American doctor experimented with attenuation of the virus. He passed it through humans and diluted it with water. He also used the virus in an unripe state. The physician reported a one percent mortality rate in 800 inoculations. The concept gradually grew in acceptance so that by 1743 all residents of the Foundling Hospital of London were inoculated.[62]

Worry about the poor working classes who could not afford the entire inoculation process resulted in the founding of a county smallpox hospital in Middlesex for treatment of patients who had contracted the disease naturally as well as those who had been inoculated. Inoculated patients were admitted free. Those with the naturally acquired disease had to post 16 shillings to pay for burial if this became necessary. Gradually, smallpox inoculation hospitals were opened throughout the provinces. Many physicians volunteered their services to perform the operation. The wealthy contributed to the upkeep of the hospital. The inoculation of the poor was not completely altruistic. The ruling classes realized they could cut pauperism by keeping the breadwinner alive. In 1746, the London Smallpox Inoculation Group was endowed to care for inoculated people while they were infectious and to care for the poor if they acquired it in the "natural way."[63]

In 1752 a virulent epidemic of the disease struck England. Inoculation was urged by physicians, and this time they were aided by the clergy. Private inoculation hospitals were opened outside of a town's limits, because its citizens still feared the process. In 1755 the prestigious Royal College of Physicians supported the technique. Inoculation was still practiced in England after the discovery by Jenner. Finally, in 1830 Parliament passed a law prohibiting the use of inoculation instead of vaccination.[64]

Europe failed to follow England's lead in its acceptance of inoculation. Only Hanover, the Netherlands, and the Republic of Geneva adopted the idea, but at a slower pace. It took 15 to 20 years for general approval. The French delayed because of the fear of new foreign ideas. The Acadamie Royale eventually backed inoculation, but it could not overcome the inherent prejudice of the people.[65]

The method of inoculation was far from uniform. In some areas in Scotland, a piece of thread dipped into the pus from a mild case was wrapped on the wrist of a child. "Buying the Pox" was another method practiced in Scotland and Wales. Children bought the material from pustules in a mild case for between one and three pence and this was rubbed into their skin without incisions.[66] In Ethiopia, during an epidemic, all adolescents who had never been exposed were gathered together and marched to a community where smallpox existed. A man, not a slave, who was free of all disease except smallpox was chosen. He was kept isolated until the pox ripened. Material was collected in an eggshell by a lay priest. Butter or honey was added to the material. A cross was cut on the forearm of the recipient four fingers above the wrist with a razor. The virus was placed in the incision with a magic stick and bound with a rag. The lay priest received a gift from the inoculees in the form of grain or salt. This was shared with the donor. Many inoculees died from the procedure. Others developed syphilis from the material. (It may have been "great pox" that was injected instead of "smallpox.")[67]

After inoculation, patients had to be isolated from the community, because of the danger of spreading the disease to the susceptibles in the population. Often, the spread produced a particularly virulent attack. The inoculees could remain in their own homes if everyone at home had previously been exposed to the illness. The alternative was the creation of smallpox hospitals, either private or public. The patient had to stay isolated until all pustules dried and the scabs fell off. This took about two weeks, and it served a legitimate purpose. The preparation phase was another story. As Lady Montague, wife of the British ambassador to Turkey, pointed out, preparation really was not necessary. She saw inoculation in Turkey without preparation, and she had her daughter inoculated this way. Nonetheless, a true "cottage industry" grew up in England for the preparation of inoculees. People were kept up to two weeks on various diets and medications before the operation.[68]

The greatest smallpox entrepreneur was Robert Sutton, who learned the inoculation technique from John Rodbard and improved on it. In 1757 he rented a large house to inoculate for smallpox. The doctor supplied room, nursing, tea, wine, fish, and fowl for seven pounds, seven shillings per month. He lowered the price for farmers to five pounds, five shillings, and charged ten shillings, six pence for the non-boarders. The cost was paid on admission in case there were any unforeseen problems. To his credit, Sutton also treated the poor without a fee. He inoculated patients in their own home if they lived within 20 miles of his establishment. He had a bargain fee of one pound, one shilling per person for ten or more people together. For 30 people the cost was ten shillings, six pence. If a town paid for 100 poor, it was five shillings, three pence per patient. The rich, on the other hand, paid twenty to twenty-five pounds. Business grew, and he acquired two more houses. Sutton started advertising in the newspapers. The doctor claimed that he never lost a patient nor had one go blind. By 1760 he began to franchise his method. Sutton also opened a house for "lower classes" on easier terms. His next development was inoculation without incision. This technique made people sick for only two days. He also took in people who had contracted smallpox "the natural way."

Sutton then took his son Daniel into the business.[69] Daniel Sutton was no slouch when it came to "turning a pound." In 1764 the elder Dr. Sutton inoculated the entire village of Maldon without mortality. In 1766 Daniel claimed only six deaths in 40,000 inoculations. The doctor built a chapel for his patients and hired a minister to hold services and sing his employer's praises. Doctors came from all over England and the continent to learn Sutton's technique. As Sutton's other sons came of age, they joined the enterprise without studying medicine, all performing the operation.

Sutton's technique caused minimal trauma. The site of the inoculation was not visible for 48 hours until it "took." He placed the inoculum on the point of a lancet and laid it on the skin tangentially. Sutton applied pressure so that the point probably entered about one-sixteenth of an inch. The site was not covered. The patient was kept in his hospital for two weeks before the treatment on a diet free of animal food and liquor. (This was a cost-saving as well as healthy idea.) The patient was exercised in the fresh air until the fever developed. Fever was treated with cold water, warm tea, and thin gruel. When the eruption developed, the patient was urged to walk in the garden. The inoculee received purges and a secret remedy containing mercury and antimony to control the symptoms. According to Benjamin Rush, Sutton did not use pus. He took clear serum from an early lesion before it was contaminated by pus. The patient was kept cool rather than made to sweat, and he was kept on a largely liquid diet. The Suttons eventually discarded the preparation before surgery. This cut the cost to the patient, and the doctors were able to inoculate an entire isolated community at one sitting.[70]

Sutton was not the only practitioner who prepared his patients for inoculation. The venerable teacher, Boerhaave, placed his patients on a mixture of mercury and antimony prior to the procedure. This was supposed to be an antidote against the poison causing smallpox. Another practitioner, Freiven, published a handbook on preparation. He advised strict regularity of diet including only the lightest of animal foods for two weeks before inoculation. People with florid complexions were bled, and given emetics and purges. A weaker appearing individual was given a vomit or a purge and then a dose of bark. An obese patient was given "Aethiops mineral" or Cinnabar (mercury) with a milk diet for four to six weeks. His patients received moderate exercise and were rested.[71]

SMALLPOX IN THE NEW WORLD

With the advent of the white people, the New World was introduced to the destructiveness of smallpox. About 15 years after the first landfall on Hispaniola, smallpox struck. One third of the population of the island perished;

one half of Puerto Rico's natives died. There were repeated epidemics of small-pox in the West Indies as the Spaniards brought in African slaves infected with the disease. Every shipload of black humanity brought another group of nonimmunes. Haiti originally had a population of perhaps half a million. After 22 years, the population shrank to 14,000. By 1574, only two native villages remained. Cuba was left with 300 Indian families. In Jamaica the Indian population disappeared completely. The virus was introduced into Mexico by a black slave who accompanied Cortez. One half of the population is believed to have perished in the first six months—a total of three and a half million.[72] (This figure seems unbelievably high.) Among the casualties was Cuitlahuac, brother of Montezuma. It must be remembered that smallpox was not the virulent disease for whites that it became in the eighteenth century. It was an endemic disease in Europe with children the primary targets. The disease spread to South America and to the Incan Empire. The virus killed the emperor, Huayna Capac, and his son and heir. A war of succession followed, and Atahualpa became the monarch and was later executed by Pizarro. The population of Peru dropped to less than one million in 150 years.

By 1620, Mexico's population had dropped to 1.6 million due to deaths largely caused by smallpox. The Spaniards in their areas and the Portuguese in Brazil deplored its effect as it left them with a smaller pool of laborers. The Catholic missionaries accompanying the conquistadores tried to save Indian souls by converting them to Christianity, and they ministered to their bodies as well. In Brazil during the severe epidemic of 1728, which killed every Indian affected, a Carmelite missionary, with little knowledge of inoculation, started to inoculate the natives and saved many in this way.

The English came to Virginia in the early seventeenth century and brought with them smallpox, measles, and probably typhoid. These illnesses likely were responsible for the destruction of the Powhatan Confederacy of tribes followed by the movement of the native population beyond the mountains. In New England, an epidemic of smallpox from 1617 to 1619 (just before Pilgrims landed) wiped out most of the Massachusetts Indians. The English pilgrims, unlike the Spanish missionaries to the south, thanked God for sending an avenging angel to kill off the heathen and give them room to expand. The religious Puritans were not above giving God a little help. They gave the Indians garments infected with smallpox pus. In 1633 another smallpox epidemic practically wiped out the few remaining Indians of Massachusetts. It was also responsible for the death of Samuel Fuller, the first physician who had arrived on the Mayflower. A total of 20 whites died in the Plymouth Plantation. In 1634 the virus spread to the Narraganset Indians of Rhode Island and then to Connecticut. The disease spread to Canada as the Indians fled north to avoid the destruction. The French brought their share of smallpox to the Canadian Indians as well. The Indians referred to the disease as "medicine of the black robes" in honor of the missionaries. One hundred years after its introduction to Canada, the disease was reported on the west coast. Another outbreak occurred in Massachusetts in 1638. Between 1662 and 1663 the virus almost destroyed the Iroquois Confederacy to the west. In 1667 smallpox was reintroduced into Virginia by a sick sailor.[73]

The ports on the eastern seaboard were the avenues of reintroduction of smallpox. Boston early on tried isolation and quarantine. All cases had to be reported, and patients were required to stay at home with guards stationed at the door until all members of the household had been exposed and had recovered from the illness. Alternatively, the patient was sent to a pest house outside of town where he received little more than shelter. Another law required that a red flag be hung outside of a house with smallpox patients. The victims at home were kept heavily covered. Heat and stimulating drinks were applied with a view to bring out the eruption by causing a diffuse perspiration.[74] The first medical article about the disease was published by a "clergyman physician," Thomas Thacher, and entitled "A Brief Rule to Guide the Common People of New England How to Order Themselves and Others in the Small Pockes and Measles." Most of the material was based on Sydenham's writings.[75]

Inoculation in the Colonies

The most serious epidemic in Boston occurred in 1721. It demonstrated to the Bostonians that quarantine and isolation were useless. The epidemic was brought in by the ship *Sea Horse* from the Tortugas. Of a population of 11,000, as many as 5,984 caught the disease, and 894 of those died (about fourteen percent). This epidemic led to the inoculation controversy in the city.[76] Cotton Mather was a cleric of the North Church, but like all educated men, he had a profound interest in medicine and was widely read on that subject. Mather considered the concept of inoculation very sensible and theorized that it caused the milder disease because in "natural acquisition" the "virus" passed through the lungs, then to the blood, then to the organs while it was still strong. When smallpox was given on the limb, the "virus" had to pass through solid structures before reaching the blood, heart, lungs, and other organs. This longer passage weakened it and resulted in a milder illness. Some physicians in Europe had hypothesized that the "virus" was somehow weakened before it was inoculated. Mather also explained the lifelong immunity it produced because the "virus" (living animalcula) ate up all the material in the body needed for its support. If a similar animalcula invaded, it starved and died. He therefore propounded a germ theory of disease. It is interesting to note that Mather used virus in its proper meaning while physicians of his time used virus to mean toxin.[77]

The story is told about Mather's black slave who had scars of inoculation only. He questioned the boy who described the process used in Africa for generations. It was generally similar to the technique described by Timoni. Mather wrote to the physicians of Boston to urge them to start inoculation. The only physician to believe in its effectiveness was Zabdiel Boyleston, an apprentice-trained physician. On June 21, 1721, he inoculated his son and two slaves, and all three survived. Boyleston was pilloried by the physicians and laymen, and he was threatened with lynching. A council of selectmen forbade him to do any more inoculations. The physician disregarded their order, and doctors in neighboring communities also started inoculation, but his only other allies were a few clerics who respected Mather's religious faith. Mather published a pamphlet describing the process. He was rewarded for his effort with a "Granado" (Molotov Cocktail) thrown into his house on July 21, 1721. Fortunately, it did not go off. The leader of the opposition was Dr. William Douglass who had been educated in Edinburgh, Leyden, and Paris and had an M.D. degree. It was said "he was always positive and occasionally right." The doctors opposed inoculation because of the danger of spreading the disease throughout the community. They also disdained the advice of the cleric and an apprentice-trained doctor. Boston suffered a "War of Pamphlets," some even urging the death penalty for the inoculators. Some religious people felt it was an act of the devil to rid the world of Christians. Besides, they believed it thwarted God's will.[78] After the epidemic subsided, the results were tabulated. One of 48 inoculated people died of the disease; one of nine who caught it naturally died.[79] Douglass eventually recognized the benefit of the process. Boyleston went to London in 1724 and was lionized by the British medical establishment. He became the first American member of the Royal Society.

Colman had published a description of the technique in 1721 in Boston. The doctor made an incision on the arm or leg but only skin deep. A small drop of variolous matter on a bit of lint was applied. After 24 hours, the lint was discarded and replaced with a dressing of a cabbage leaf, which was changed daily. After six to eight days, a gentle fever developed with all the symptoms of smallpox in minor degree — with aching head and back along with pain in the bones. This made the patient "heavy" for one to two days. He then felt well, and the pock appeared, rose, turned, and went off without any more illness or pain except the soreness of the pock itself and some external fever. As the pock appeared on the skin, the incision opened and discharged. As the pock ripened, more drainage occurred from the incision. The turning of a pock on the sixth or seventh day caused the fullest flowing. Then flowing decreased and stopped, and the incision healed. A nurse was needed to watch the patient during the day, but no one was needed during the night. The patient ate, drank, and slept well. The second, usually fatal fever was prevented because the oil or putrid matter that was fuel for the fever was lost through the incision. Also, the body was not covered with pocks and scabs, so that perspiration was free, and there was no foul mass upon the skin to return it and mix with the juices of the blood. The patient had no boils on his body as seen in the confluent form of smallpox

—again due to free running of ill humors from the incision. Four to five months later the patients were completely well—in fact, better than before with better complexion and stomach. These patients did not have the "smell of sickness" about them. The issue from the incision had little or no odor. In the natural infection of the fluxy sort, the smell was overwhelming and lasted for days. If a person acquired smallpox in the natural way and was then given inoculation by incision, the drainage of material produced a milder case. It also brought out the infection at the proper time (seven to eight days) instead of lying in the body sometimes for up to a month.[80]

The concept of inoculation was accepted in most of the colonies after the epidemic of 1721. Smallpox houses or hospitals were started, and friends formed groups to be inoculated together, so they could be isolated together. They chose an otherwise healthy person as the donor. On the twelfth or thirteenth day of the disease, the doctor pricked his pustule and squeezed the matter into a stoppered glass container. It was carried in the bosom of a courier to keep it warm. A three-pronged lancet or needle was used for the inoculum. Two or more sites were chosen to ensure a take and the incision was made deep enough to bring blood to the surface. A drop from the container was mixed with the blood at each site. It was covered with a half walnut shell or other concave vessel (this walnut technique had also been used by the Greek woman in Constantinople), and it was bound in place. The patient stayed in the house and remained warm and abstained from animal flesh and broth for 20 days. The operation was best performed at the beginning of winter or spring.[81]

The acceptance of inoculation in Boston grew with each new epidemic. Two percent were inoculated in 1721, and by 1764 87 percent of the population were so protected. The mortality rate diminished so much in 1764 that it was the first epidemic year without a big jump in reported mortality statistics. The epidemic of 1764 showed the benefit of inoculation vividly. While 699 Bostonians caught the disease the "natural way," and 124 of them died, 4,977 received inoculation and only 46 of those died. The patients were inoculated at Castle William and Point Shirley, the areas originally used to quarantine ships' crews. Castle William was a barracks with 48 wards, each containing ten beds. Food, inoculation, and lodging were given free to the poor, but they had to share beds. Before inoculation, patients received antimony and mercury. After the surgery, they were kept indoors in bed, covered, and given "heating and stimulating medication" to induce diffuse perspiration in order to get the "eruption out." Bedding was not changed during the entire stay. People were frequently well in less than a week unless they had been debilitated prior to the treatment.[82] Even with the obvious benefits of inoculation, the selectmen were still wary of the process, and it was considered a last resort.

In July 1776, after Boston was retaken from the British and during the smallpox epidemic of that year, inoculation hospitals were given permission to open. However, strict rules had to be followed: the community had to agree to its presence; each hospital had to have a "cleansing room"; there were "cleaners" and guards on duty to keep the patients within the bounds of the hospital; three weeks after inoculation, the patient went to a "shifting room" under the supervision of a cleaner. There the inoculee removed his clothes, washed himself down completely while his clothes were washed in rum or vinegar, then fumigated, and then he entered a clean room where he was given his clean clothes and was discharged. Preference for admission was given to local inhabitants and soldiers about to engage in a campaign. Patients put up a bond of ten pounds and the doctor added a 100-pound bond, "to assure their obedience to regulations." The patient was prepared with a diet of pudding, gruel, sago, milk, fruit, and vegetables for nine to fourteen days before the operation. He refrained from meat, butter, cheese, liquor, and spices. The inoculee was given mild doses of mercury, antimony, and Glauber's salts. An incision, one-eighth of an inch long, was made through the epidermis with a lancet dipped in fresh "virus." No cover was applied. The patient was kept on a spare diet with mild purges. When the eruption came with a fever, he walked around outdoors and drank cold water. The cases were mild and fatalities few.[83] The cost of inoculation in Boston was one pound five shillings four pence including medicine and treatment. The cost of food and bed were extra. The poor workers of Boston were against inoculation and the hospital. They could not afford the cost of the procedure and they could not be out of work without an income during the infectious period. They were also concerned about developing smallpox the "natural way" from inoculees who were let out of hospitals too early. The poor occasionally set fire to the hospitals.[84]

After massive inoculations, new cases occurred in Boston only sporadically. A mild epidemic in 1788 was immediately ended with only a few deaths due to early inoculations. In 1782 a group of doctors including John Warren petitioned a town meeting to set up an inoculation hospital away from Boston to inoculate people when no epidemic was present. This was approved by the people at the meeting.

The developments in Boston generally mirrored the problems in the other port cities where exposure was greater and population was more dense. In New York, the Dutch and then the English were constantly made aware of epidemics. Early sanitation laws and ordinances were passed. The relationship of smallpox epidemics to ships docking, particularly from the West Indies, led to the first isolation legislation in 1689. However, it was not until May 3, 1755, that a true quarantine act was passed in New York. Isolation and quarantine were generally useless against smallpox, because sailors could incubate the disease without overt signs. New York suffered a severe epidemic in 1731. It was so generalized that business almost came to a dead stop. In two and a half months, 549 residents died. Governor Clinton of New York, fearful of inoculation because it could spread disease, outlawed the process. Residents had to go to other colonies for the treatment.[85] Dr. William Bennett of New Jersey opened the first private inoculation hospital in America in 1759—perhaps to catch the New York crowd.

Philadelphia differed somewhat in that it had Ben Franklin, a respected voice in the community. His son had died of smallpox contracted in the natural way in 1736, and he became a firm believer in inoculation. While in London in 1759, he asked the eminent Dr. Heberden to write a pamphlet about inoculation and the post-operative care of the patient. Heberden believed the best time to harvest the pus was just before it dried completely. This was a wise decision because by then the organism was probably less virulent. The head of the pock was opened with a needle and a thread was passed through the material until it was saturated. The thread was placed in a pillbox to dry. It was used as soon as it was dry, or it could be stored in a closed vial and used several days later. About half an inch of thread was used as the inoculum, and an incision in the skin about half an inch long was made deep enough to draw blood. The thread was placed in the incision and covered with plaster.

Dr. Heberden's pamphlet was printed and widely distributed in America. Indirectly, Franklin's discovery of the lightning rod was used to encourage inoculation. People feared that they would be tempting God by "giving illness through man," a right that God alone supposedly possessed. However, they would install a lightning rod to put aside God's wishes to destroy a house. In the 1750s, inoculation was widely practiced in Philadelphia. However, in 1775, a severe epidemic of smallpox in Philadelphia carried off many of the young children of the poor. Eight doctors in the city formed a society to inoculate and care for the poor gratis. Inoculation in Philadelphia was stopped when the first meeting of the Continental Congress met there. Many of the delegates from sparsely populated areas had had no exposure to smallpox, and Philadelphia's authorities did not want to run the risk of causing the disease among representatives sent to this important body. Despite this decision, many potential delegates refused to go to Philadelphia for fear of the contagion. For example, of the Connecticut delegation, Wolcott and Law resigned because of this fear.[86]

On April 13, 1738, the *London Frigate* brought a shipload of slaves and smallpox from Guinea to Charleston, South Carolina. The ship passed quarantine inspection. The disease spread through the population, and Mr. Mowbray, a surgeon on a British man-of-war in the harbor, started to inoculate civilians. Dr. James Killpatrick was enthusiastic about its benefits. The *South Carolina Gazette* published a study on October 5, 1738, which called attention to a 17.6 percent mortality rate in the naturally acquired disease compared to 3.6 percent mortality among inoculees. The newspaper tried to explain the difference between natural and surgically acquired smallpox. The natural infection was dangerous because it resulted from inspiration into the lungs or by smell where the brain or nerves were immediately disordered from the assault of the "pocky effluvia." A milder case developed if the disease was sucked into the pores and admitted to the "Road of Circulation" first. On September 21, the South Carolina Assembly passed an act prohibiting inoculation in and around Charleston. Dr. Killpatrick left Charleston for England where he again demonstrated the benefit of inoculation, just as Dr. Boyleston had fifteen years earlier. The concept had fallen into disuse after the initial acclaim of Boyleston, but Killpatrick rekindled the interest. He used material from an inoculated patient, and he made sure the recipient was in good health before the operation.[87] Throughout the discussion, I have referred to the procedure as an operation. Those of us who can remember vaccination know it to be a simple procedure in a doctor's office performed in a minute or less. In colonial times it was an operation.

The inoculation controversy was put to rest with the work of Dr. Jenner. While still an apprentice, he treated a young girl moderately ill with cowpox. She told him it would protect her from smallpox. The expression "having the complexion of a milk maid" must come from the protection afforded these girls by cowpox, while so many in society were scarred for life. In 1796 Jenner took material from Sarah Nelmes' pustule and inoculated James Phipps, age eight. He developed cowpox and was mildly ill about nine days later. When he recovered, Jenner tried to inoculate him with smallpox pus, and the boy had no reaction to the material. Jenner published his results in 1798. It took years before this procedure was accepted universally.[88] Unlike inoculation, it did not give lifelong immunity, but it was responsible for the almost complete disappearance of the disease from the earth.

−4−

Disease and Medical Care in the Navy

The health of a sailor was in constant jeopardy even in peacetime. During the period under discussion here, he suffered malnutrition, avitaminoses, respiratory disease, and multiple enteric diseases from contaminated water as well as injuries and death from falls, fires, sinking, and bad weather. Overall, the life expectancy of a seaman was ten years shorter than that of his brother ashore. During wartime, these hazards increased due to fire, explosion of gun powder, steel and wooden splinters, and small arms fire.[1]

Ship's Surgeons

The need for a ship's surgeon was recognized when large numbers of men sailed beyond the limits of their native shores. From Homer we know physicians accompanied the Greek soldiers to Troy. The two sons of Aesculapius, Machaon, a surgeon, and Podalirius, a physician, accompanied the expedition. The Romans, too, had surgeons on board their ships. They were "immunes"—exempt from military duty. There was one medical man for every 200 soldiers and sailors. The surgeon was usually a young man, rarely older than 21. His salary was minimal, though on occasion double pay was offered to attract a surgeon. The surgeon carried his own equipment and medicine when he boarded. He was responsible for enforcing general and personal hygiene aboard ship. No alcohol was allowed during a campaign. The Greeks and Romans probably had hospital ships that accompanied the fleet. Their writings describe ships named *Therapeia* and *Aesculapius*, which at least suggest a "medical care" function.

In the Middle Ages, Venice, Genoa, the Order of St. Stephen, and the Knights of Rhodes had navies to keep the Moors at bay. They had surgeons on board their ships as well as at shore installations to care for their sick and wounded. The Black Death of the Middle Ages resulted in the need for shore physicians to prevent the spread of this alarmingly fatal disease in the ports.

It was spread to Europe from Africa and the Middle East by ships' commerce. Three public health officers were appointed in Venice in 1348 to examine ships and crews for possible plague before ships were permitted to dock. Florence, Lombardy, and Milan followed Venice's example. At first, incoming ships were isolated for 30 days. This was raised to 40 days (hence the term "quarantine"). Marseilles developed the concept of a bill of health in the latter part of the fifteenth century. Before embarkation, a ship and crew were thoroughly examined. A responsible official of the port gave the captain a bill of health if there were no findings of disease. A ship with this certificate was not quarantined at its next port of call.[2]

The earliest description of a ship's surgeon in the British navy dates from 1512, during the reign of Henry VIII. Many years later the medical service of the Royal Navy started under Dr. Roger Morbeck, a fellow of the Royal College of Physicians. He was appointed to attend Admiral Howard on his expedition to Cadiz in 1596. In 1597 Henry Atkins was appointed to an expedition with the Earl of Sussex, also to Spain. However, he developed seasickness and disembarked at Plymouth. In Cromwell's Protectorate, physicians were appointed to foreign expeditions to care for the crews' health. Physicians and surgeons were then appointed to major commissioned warships. By the early eighteenth century, medical affairs were under the control of the "Sick and Hurt Board," which was composed of medical and lay members. Overall, there was little official attention paid to the health of seamen. It depended primarily upon the conscientiousness of the surgeon whose education, however, was limited.[3]

On board ship, convalescent sailors nursed the others. The "ship's boy" became an attendant to the sick. He was the "lob-lolly boy," so called after a porridge he carried to the sick. A cannon occupied an area called a bay. In the forward part of the ship, where no cannon were kept, was the area where the sick were treated and confined. This became the "sick bay." This bay was on the gun deck and was exposed to enemy fire. During combat, the sick were removed to the cockpit, below the gun deck, where surgery was performed. The cockpit was the living quarters of the midshipmen, surgeon's mates, and purser between battles. Their mess table was also the operating table.[4]

At sea the British naval surgeon was also a physician and apothecary to the crew. He was a craftsman, not an officer and a gentleman, and he received about five pounds per month and held the rank of a warrant officer, about equal to that of a purser. He was not a commissioned officer of quarter-deck rank, and he wore no uniform. The surgeon received his warrant from the Navy Board after an examination by a court of examiners of the Company of Barber-Surgeons. In 1747 the Association of the Navy Surgeons of the Royal Navy of Great Britain was organized. Its purpose was to lecture naval surgeons on anatomy and surgery at a cost of one guinea per year.[5]

Regulations spelled out the duties and responsibilities of the naval surgeon in detail. He had to supply his own instruments and chest of medicines.

These were examined by proper authorities, and if found adequate, they were sealed and sent on board (probably to prevent the surgeon from selling the contents before they arrived on board). The surgeon was to carry "smart tickets" on board. These were passes to send the sick and injured ashore. He was responsible for the "necessaries" used for the sick. The surgeon visited the sick twice a day and sent a sick list to the captain daily. If a sailor had to be sent to a hospital on shore, the surgeon sent an account of the illness and treatment received. During battle, the surgeon remained in the cockpit with his mates to care for the injured. He was required to keep two journals. One was to cover illness, the other surgery. These were examined by proper authorities on shore. He also prepared his dressings for anticipated surgery and lectured the crew in first aid—predominantly about how to control hemorrhage.[6]

During battle, a platform, usually the mess table, was placed in the cockpit that was the rear of the orlop deck near a hatchway. The orlop deck was the first deck above the hold and below the gun deck and the water line. The platform was covered with sailcloth, as were the berths of the seamen who were normally quartered there. They were dispossessed during battle, and their places were taken by the wounded before and after surgery. A cleared area about twelve feet square served as operating room. Near the table were placed a chest containing the surgeon's operating tools, a bucket of water for rinsing the bloody sponges, an empty bucket to catch the blood, and a bucket of sand for spreading on the deck to keep it from getting slippery from the blood. Dry swabs were within reach to keep the table dry. A few medications were also within reach, including vinegar and wine. For a wounded officer, the surgeon's and purser's beds were kept available. After the battle, the injured seamen were moved to the sick bay and the officers to expropriated quarters, usually below the forecastle (the forward part of the ship under the deck).[7]

The surgeon's mate was very low in the hierarchy. His pay was less than that of carpenters, gunners or sail makers. His duties were to help the surgeon visit the sick, clean up after the surgeon, make the bandages, and make some of the simple ointments for skin lesions and wounds. He also boiled gruel, washed towels, mixed plasters, filled water buckets for patients, and dumped the patients' commodes. The mate also held a walk-in sick call each morning. His berth was in the cockpit.[8]

A civilian surgeon without naval experience always started as a mate. To receive this rating, he was examined in all aspects of surgery and physic with which he might come into contact. Life on board was very relaxing when not in actual combat. James Ker, a naval surgeon, described his day. He awakened at 7:30 A.M., breakfasted at 8:00. Starting at 9:00 A.M., he saw patients for thirty to sixty minutes. The surgeon had to write out a report to the captain on the sick once a day. Following this, he could read, write letters, or walk around the ship until lunch. Following lunch, there was more time for reading, writing, walking, games of backgammon, cards, and good conversation. The surgeon had his evening meal at 8:00 P.M. After that he relaxed with officers over grog. This idyllic life occurred on short trips. On longer trips, particularly to the West Indies, more of his time was occupied with sickness. For example, on one trip to Barbados, this surgeon had four or five cases of scurvy. He described the multitude of mosquitoes and the presence of yellow fever. The sailors started to develop remitting fever (a fever that was high and low, but did not come down to normal), perhaps typhus, ague (malaria), flux (dysentery), or bilious fever (yellow fever). Fifty of his crew were sick and tents had to be erected on shore to care for them. The number of sick increased to 260 out of a complement of 600. This included three of the surgeon's mates. Men who recovered from the fevers on shore came back on board and became sick with the flux from "hard salted meat and indigestible food." Gradually the men recovered and took up their duties. The ship visited St. Lucia where "putrid fever" existed. Those whose resistance was low from previous illnesses died of this. If the sailor had been involved in debauchery, he would always get the putrid fever and die of it (the wages of sin). Ker's treatment for putrid fever was to induce more vomiting with tartar emetic than the natural occurrence caused by the disease. This was followed by an opiate that caused sweating and broke the fever. Cathartics, if given early in the disease, were helpful. If given late, they caused debility. If debility was great, clysters were used instead of cathartics. If the patient showed a remission, he was given cinchona bark (quinine) in wine. If no remission was observed, bark was given any time during the illness. Convalescents received cold baths. In recruits, mortality from yellow fever was thirty percent. He believed the illness could be caused by miasmata, filth, putrescence, or the moon. Ker developed ague with frequent recurrences, and he had to be returned to England.[9]

Aftercare of Casualties

The few medical doctors in the Royal Navy were usually senior surgeons who later took a medical degree. The physician in the navy was usually stationed aboard a hospital ship at sea. He was predominantly an inspector and administrator. He examined other ships, the surgeon's journals, and the medical chests. The concept of a hospital ship was adopted by the Royal Navy after the continental powers developed a well-organized system. Cromwell had hospital ships during the Protectorate, but these were abolished in the Restoration. The Spanish Armada had hospital ships with 85 physicians and surgeons on board. The French had hospital ships in a ratio of one to ten with ships of the line. A floating hospital had a 100-bed capacity in the seventeenth and eighteenth centuries. It carried no cannon. There were large ports cut in the sides for ventilation below deck.

The British navy added hospital ships in the eighteenth century. They were reconditioned old fighting ships that carried a special, recognizable flag on the mizzenmast. The medical crew included one physician, one surgeon, three surgeon's mates, six nurses, a dispenser of medicine, and auxiliary servants. The ship was usually divided into wards for fevers, fluxes, itch, etc. The dead were housed forward until they could be brought ashore. The British navy, unlike that of the Catholic powers, buried their dead at sea during long voyages. The French and Spanish placed their dead (as well as amputated parts) in the hold of the ship with the sand and gravel ballast until they could be entombed back home.[10]

There is no historical evidence that ancient navies had special hospitals on shore for their sick and injured sailors. During the Middle Ages, sick seamen were cared for in churches, almshouses, or civilian hospitals in port cities. These were supported by charity and the church. In England, Henry VIII appropriated church property that had been used to care for the sick and poor and replaced it with nothing. At times, sick seamen went to contract houses, which were private homes in port. Here they were fed and cared for in return for a specified fee. The casualties of the Royal Navy and the merchant marine were treated identically.

Venice established a seamen's hospital in 1318. In 1666 Colbert, minister to Louis XIV of France, commissioned a marine hospital at the naval base of Rochefort. He appropriated the monastery of St. Eloy to serve this purpose. It had eight wards with 50 beds in each. In 1695, William and Mary inaugurated the first English naval hospital at Greenwich. The building had originally been planned as a palace for Charles II, but it was converted into a hospital and old sailor's home in 1705. It could house 2,700 seamen. Funds were available for 6,000 more to be boarded outside the hospital. The British built their second marine hospital in Portsmouth, the Haslar Hospital, in 1761. With the growth of the British Empire, hospitals were built in Gibraltar, Alexandria, and Halifax. The nature of the illnesses treated at these hospitals can be seen from statistics compiled by Dr. Lind when he became head of the Haslar Hospital. In 1760 he admitted 2,174 with fever, 1,146 with scurvy, 360 with consumption, 350 with rheumatism, 245 with dysentery, 80 with old injuries, 73 with skin disease, and 52 with ague.[11]

Needs of Seamen

In peacetime, requirements for acceptance into the Royal Navy and the merchant marine were maintained at a responsible level: The men had to be able-bodied, healthy in all limbs and sight, of sound health; and free of rupture and other visible infirmities. Able seamen, not ship's boys, had to be above five feet four inches and between 16 and 50 years old. They had to be clean, with clean clothes and short hair when they came on board, or their hair would be cut and the men washed once on board. If they were above 40, they had to have a robust constitution.[12] During wartime, all health specifications were put aside. Press gangs could take anyone they caught for Royal Navy sea duty. If not enough warm bodies were obtained, jails were thrown open, and vagrants and criminals were conscripted. They were either packed into guard ships or sent directly to the ship on which they would serve. This was an excellent way of spreading typhus on board.[13]

The environmental problems faced by the sailors can be divided into air, water, and food. Prior to the development of multideck ships, air was no problem. The sailors worked, slept, and ate in the open. With the increase of the size of ships and the number of men and provisions aboard, decks were added. Oxygen in adequate amounts could not reach the lower decks, and the sick might suffocate, because they were not able to get topside. Inventors developed windsails and windscoops, canvas tubes with the large end open into the wind. The wind forced air down the hatchway. Further tubes carried the air to lower decks. This system was not effective in calm weather or in heavy weather when hatches were battened down. Attempts were made to force air down mechanically. In 1737 a wooden fan wheel, invented by Desquiliers of France, was tried in England. It required manpower to operate and was discarded. Stephen Hales of England in 1741 invented a bellows operated by a pump handle similar to a railroad hand car. This too required manpower and was discarded. The need for manpower to run the wind machines required that more men had to be carried on board who were fed and paid. This cut into the profits of the owners. In the early nineteenth century, Robert Perkins developed an air pump that employed the roll of the ship for power. With the development of steam engines, the attachment of mechanical power to a rotary fan solved the problem. Another technique was to cut holes into the sides of the ship. In addition, there were ports in the gun deck that were kept open in calm seas and when the ship prepared for action. However, the ports could not be cut too near the water line, because excessive rolling in bad weather would cause them to ship water.

In addition to the need to get air into the ship, a means was needed to get the odors out. The bilge was a serious source of odor production. The smell in French and Spanish ships would have been unbearable. The British used gravel for ballast which was less of a problem than sand. However, the addition of water and heat could lead to bacterial and algae growth with the smell one associates with marshes. By the end of the eighteenth century, Sir Richard Lipping introduced pig iron for ballast instead of gravel with definite improvement. In addition, he introduced vents from the bilge to the weather deck to allow odor to escape.

The smell of poorly washed or unwashed bodies was difficult to eradicate. Again, if quarters were reasonably high above the water line, vents in the side would help. Since Elizabethan times, able seamen slept in hammocks, a device copied from the American Indians. The hammocks could be taken down and aired during the day. The men frequently ate in the areas where hammocks had been hung. (I can attest to the odors personally. I was sent to Europe during World War II on an English troop ship. Our outfit was packed into one hold, and we slept and ate in the same place. Because of the danger of submarines, we were told to sleep in our clothes and socks with our shoes hung from the hammock. We tried to bathe in seawater with "salt soap," but this was not truly effective. The odor still persists in my nostrils.)

The ship's crew drank grog, small beer, and water. Small or little beer had a low alcohol content and was fermented and could be produced aboard ship. Little beer was the major beer on board and in some reports, the sailor was issued as much as one gallon per day. Rum or brandy had been issued in the British navy since 1700. Each able seaman received a half pint per day. It was issued straight until 1740 when Admiral Vernon (for whom Mount Vernon was named) ordered it cut with water. Vernon was called "Old Grog" after the cloth named grogram used in his cloak. Grog was the liquor ration cut with water. It was issued this way to try to cut down on drunkenness and the associated accidents in a rolling sailing vessel.[14]

Water was stored in aged casks with the staves burned to produce a layer of charcoal. Water was "purified" by filtering it through charcoal or adding quicklime to the water for three days. This was done to destroy the vermin. Passage of water through filters of charcoal and sand cleared it as well. The water was also aerated to remove the offensive smell. In the early nineteenth century, the British used the "Osbridge machine" for aeration. Water had to be loaded at each port of call. Rules were prescribed for the collection of water. In tropical climates, ships were anchored away from shore. If this was not possible, all portholes were closed. The water gang was sent to shore during daylight hours. If the gang had to sleep on shore, large fires were kept burning during the night, and the men were kept covered. The ship's surgeon was aware that these regulations avoided the "ague," which usually broke out after the ship was at sea.

Water was stored in casks in the hold of the ship. After two weeks of storage it became cloudy and smelly due to bacterial overgrowth. By the end of six weeks, the water cleared. This was a result of algae growth and self-destruction of bacteria by overproduction. The "old salt" would advise the recruit to drink from the "older water." Water was the prime cause of gastroenteric diseases and fevers on board. Water consumption was minimal; about two quarts per day for drinking and cooking, but more if the men were in the tropics.[15] In an attempt to obviate the need to store water and its associated problems, scientists worked on ways to produce potable water from seawater. Dr. Lind in England and Poissonier in France tried distillation on board ship. Dr. Lind felt the copper cauldrons used in the galley could be used. For smaller amounts of water, he used a tea kettle, a musket barrel to convert the steam back to water, and a kettle to collect it. To assist in the distillation process, an apothecary in Durban, England, added calcined bones and silver nitrate. The water was not only fresh, but it was sterile as well (a fact not understood at the time). The main drawback was the taste. Distilled water is tasteless, but this could be improved by aeration.

An important consideration in view of the frequency and severity of diarrhea was stool disposal. Planners figured on one seat for 40 men. The seats led to wooden troughs then to scuppers, closed pipes fitted with valves, to prevent backwash in rough seas. The stool went into the ocean from the scupper with the help of a flush of seawater. (With the frequency of diarrhea, I would think one seat for 40 men was inadequate, but the British shipbuilders and traders were not known for their humanity toward the common seaman.)

Food had to be taken on board and stored for prolonged periods. It was of the poorest quality, and it was usually of less weight than listed on the manifest. The supplier could bribe the purser to accept the short weight. In addition, the sailor received "fourteen ounces to the pound." The extra two ounces went to the purser. This was credited to his pay. The seaman's diet varied according to national taste, time of the year that the food was loaded, and the port where it was purchased. In Queen Anne's reign, around 1700, a sailor received one pound of biscuit daily, two pounds of salt beef twice a week, one pound of salt pork twice a week, two ounces of dried fish three times a week, two ounces of butter three times a week, four ounces of cheese three times a week, and four ounces of peas every four days. This provided the sailor with 3,700 calories daily. Other foods included "burgoo" (oatmeal sweetened with molasses), plum duff (pickled suet pudding with raisins for Sunday dessert), peas made into a soup, and "lobscouse" (a combination of soup and stew). The week's food was collected by one man who represented his mess mates and also did the cooking. Fifteen to twenty men were grouped into a mess.

The biscuit was usually old, hard, and full of weevils. During a meal the men would bang the biscuit against the table to shake the weevils out. A biscuit without weevils was suspect. "If it's not good enough for weevils, it's not good enough for me." Salted beef and pork lost some of their nourishment; it was believed that cured meat was better. The use of black pepper, red pepper, and saltpeter cut down on the amount of salt needed. It was believed that meat packed with clay, sugar, and pimento would keep better and avoid scurvy. The scorbutic effects of salted meat could be prevented by using molasses, sauerkraut, lemon juice, oatmeal, raisins, and rice. In warm weather sauerkraut stank. It could be replaced by beans and cucumbers in vinegar. Butter could be kept from becoming rancid if stored in salt water, which was changed frequently. In general, the diet led to avitaminoses of the water soluble vitamins, particularly vitamin C. The need to avoid scurvy was never far from the surgeon's thoughts. He urged the purser to stock up on cabbages, onions, greens, and other vegetables as soon as the ship landed in port. The antiscorbutic effect of vegetables had been known for centuries.[16]

Physicians and surgeons trained in the theories of the time believed that "bad air" caused illness on board. Attempts to alleviate this problem included anchoring the ship as far from shore as possible, because people knew a ship at sea was healthier than one in port. If near land, the side that faced land was closed to keep the bad air out. The sailor spent much of his day below deck in the cold, damp darkness. The surgeon associated this dampness with an effluvium that poisoned the air and led to a malignant fever, which may have been typhus. If the dampness was cold, this cut the exudation from the skin and predisposed the individual to scurvy. To keep moisture out of the ship, the surgeon urged the captain to cut back on washing the deck. Ports were kept open for ventilation. Fires were started between decks to move the air and dry the area. Windsails were set in every hatchway to force fresh air down. The sailors were kept as clean and dry of sweat as possible. If men did not wash themselves and their clothing, they would be scrubbed down in the presence of the crew.[17] (This punishment was used in more recent basic training in the service. If a man did not wash, he was undressed and held down while others in the barracks used scrubbing brushes to clean him. He soon learned to wash himself.)

Scurvy and Other Disorders

The sailor could be afflicted with any, several, or all of the diseases known to man, but the great killers of seamen were yellow fever, scurvy, and typhus. Scurvy became a disease of the seafarer when he covered his ships with decks and used new navigational instruments to explore the unknown sea. When he left sight of shore, scurvy became his constant companion. Signs of scurvy usually appeared any time between two and six weeks after leaving shore. However, scurvy also had a long history on land, and one possible derivation of the term is from Old Norse "skyr," which means sour milk, and "byn," which is the word for edema. This would describe a typical patient's appearance. The Ebers papyrus described a disease resembling scurvy. Hippocrates described soldiers with pain in their legs, perhaps due to hemorrhage, as well as gangrene of their gums accompanied by the loss of teeth. Jacques de Vety described the illness among the crusaders at Damietta in 1318. De Joinville described scurvy among the crusaders in St. Louis's army in 1250 in Egypt. He wrote about surgeons cutting away dead flesh from the gums so men could chew and swallow. Scurvy also developed among English troops in front of Quebec in 1759, and in our Civil War, there were 30,714 probable cases of scurvy with 338 deaths. Scurvy was common in armies on the Eastern Front and in the Middle East during World War I.

The morbidity and mortality of scurvy on land, while awesome, cannot hold a candle to the destruction caused by scurvy at sea. Vasco da Gama, in his search for the Indies around the Cape of Good Hope, lost 100 of his crew of 160 apparently to scurvy. Magellan, in his circumnavigation of the globe, lost a similar number to this disease. Anson left England in 1740 to attack the Spanish possessions in the Pacific, starting with 1,200 men but returning with only 335 plus three million in loot.[18]

The cause of scurvy is a lack of vitamin C. This is a six carbon compound closely related to glucose. It acts as a reducing agent in the hydroxylation of reactions of lysine and proline (amino acids) in protocollagen. If these amino acids are not hydroxylated, the protocollagen cannot crosslink into proper collagen fibrils. Collagen is the main constituent of connective tissue and is most important in wound healing. It is involved in bone formation, because the organic matrix of bone is collagen. Collagen is a component of the ground substance surrounding the capillary walls. Vitamin C is stored in the adrenals and is involved in the hydroxylation process needed for the production of corticosteroids. It has other functions that are not related to its action as an enzyme. Vitamin C aids in the absorption of iron in the gut by converting it from the ferric to the ferrous form. It spares vitamin A and E and some of the B vitamins by protecting them from oxidation. The vitamin helps in the utilization of folic acid. The body's requirement for vitamin C is increased in stress and trauma because the level drops in the serum in these states. Collagen is found in almost all tissues and organs. Therefore, an aberration in collagen production results in a multisystem disease, including cardiovascular, musculo-skeletal, skin, and eye. In scurvy, there is a decrease in hydroxyproline synthesis. Collagen with decreased hydroxyproline is unstable at body temperature.[19]

The pathological changes in the body resulting from a lack of vitamin C can be determined from its function. Skin hemorrhage occurs, either as petechiae (pinhead size spots) or as massive extravasations. The hemorrhages are worse in areas of trauma. There is hemorrhage into the muscles and along fascial planes in areas of mechanical stress. Infants develop massive subperiosteal (below the membrane enveloping bone) hemorrhages. Children suffer these hemorrhages particularly in the legs. These may become infected and break down. Ulcers develop in the gums with associated loosening and loss of teeth. Massive hemorrhage can occur in the gums in adults. Anemia is common due to both hemorrhage and folic acid deficiency. Death can result from acute heart failure, which is sudden. Sudden death can also occur in an Addisonian (adrenal) crisis as a result of increased physical activity associated with a lack of cortisone. Death may follow fulminant infection because of the patient's inability to lay down a bodily defense. This is seen particularly in tuberculosis where collagen is normally laid down to encapsulate the bacteria.[20]

Dr. Lind, of the British Royal Navy, did the best early experimental work on scurvy. He had joined the navy as a surgeon's mate. After nine years he became a naval surgeon, did his study in 1747, then left the navy. He returned to Edinburgh where he received an M.D. degree in 1748. In 1754 he published his treatise on scurvy. In 1757 he also published "Preserving the Health of Seamen in the Royal Navy." Dr. Lind was then made physician to the Royal Hospital at Haslar. In 1758 he was elected a fellow of the College of Physicians of Edinburgh.[21] In 1768 Lind published a manual on tropical diseases.

Dr. Lind gave an accurate description of the subjective symptoms and objective findings in scurvy when he reported that the patient's face becomes bloated and pale and a lassitude develops. Scurvy destroyed morale with associated mental and emotional deterioration. The individual became gloomy, morose, and apathetic. He could become maniacal or melancholic. The victim refused all physical activity, his appetite was still good early in the disease, but his face later became livid, his knees stiffened and contracted, and he developed breathlessness and panting. His gums became itchy, swelled, bled, and became red and spongy with associated bad breath. The gums then became putrid and developed fungous growths. His face became smooth and shining like the "sour milk" described by the Norsemen. The victim's skin was covered with red, blue, and black spots (the petechiae). These coalesced and could become very large but rarely affected the face. The patient's ankles swelled, and the edema proceeded up the leg. The legs remained puffy longer than with true edema. His skin broke down, and ulcers developed that produced a thin liquid. The tissue beneath the ulcer was soft and spongy. Fungous growths developed in the ulcers, and if removed, they recurred. Any bruise developed into an ulcer. When the patient moved, he could suddenly expire. Old wounds and fractures broke down. The skin could burst from swelling. The patients started to bleed from all orifices and they developed jaundice, dropsy, melancholia, colic, pain in the chest and dyspnea, and ultimately died.[22]

Baron Von Swieten, one of Boerhaave's students from Vienna, whose "cookbook" for military surgeons with numbered treatments for the various illnesses the surgeon might see was discussed in an earlier chapter. He described the soldier with scurvy as follows: numb limbs and lassitude with weak, painful muscles; respiration became difficult, and the legs swelled. The patient's face became brown and spotted, and his mouth smelled. His teeth loosened, and as the gums swelled, they became painful and started to bleed. He developed hemorrhages and ulcers on the thighs with shooting pains in the limbs. The sufferer's body was covered with black spots. He developed fevers, then hemorrhages from the nose, mouth, and anus, and then death. Von Swieten felt scurvy occurred in winter quarters from noisome vapors, inaction, scarcity of greens and vegetables, drinking stagnant water, and eating smoked and salted meat and fish as well as old cheese. He believed that damp lodgings contributed their share to the development of symptoms, which were exacerbated by fear and sorrow. The patient's humors were putrid, acrimonious, and condensed. Therapy required correction of putrefaction and dimunition of viscosity. The specific therapy advised by Von Swieten was to correct the patient's drinking water by adding two ounces of vinegar and two ounces of brandy per pot of water. If these were not available, calamus aeromaticus was to be added to the water. This plant was found in marshy areas. He urged doctors not to use strong purges, vomits, or bleedings and gave the patient broth in which chervil, sorrel, spinach, lettuce, endive, red cabbage, young nettle buds, and tender greens had been boiled. (Boiling, of course, destroyed much of the vitamin C present in these vegetables.) He urged ripe fruit. If this was unavailable, barley and oat broth were substituted. The doctor then prescribed an antiscorbutic. Ripe fruits, such as roasted apples and pears, were part of the therapy. This treatment had to be carried on over a long period. The patient also received an elixir in wine and water.[23]

The physician in practice saw scurvy in lean years. Buchan devoted a section in his book to scurvy, stating that it occurred in northern countries in damp areas and that land scurvy was different from sea scurvy, because there were no putrid symptoms. It was due to lack of exercise, confined air, poor diet, exposure to cold moist air, the use of salted or smoked food, and suppression of evacuations (sweat and menses) as well as heredity. Therapy included removal of the patient to warm air, exercise, and fresh air and efforts to keep him amused. If scurvy was caused by salted provisions, the patient received certain foods including vegetables, oranges, apples, lemons, limes, water cress, scurvy grass, milk, freshly baked bread, fresh beer, and cider. If fresh vegetables were unobtainable, preserved vegetables could be substituted. Chemical acids (cream of tartar, elixir of vitriol, vinegar, and spirits of sea salt) were prescribed as well. For land scurvy, the physician prescribed a milk diet. The patient had to drink whey or buttermilk. If this was unavailable, the patient could substitute cider, spruce beer, decoctions of mucilaginous vegetables such as sarsaparilla, and tar water. Tar water was believed to be the universal panacea much as chicken soup today. Also prescribed was Harrowgate water, from a spa in fashion at the time. This water had large concentrations of sulfur and smelled accordingly, but it was to be consumed regardless and bathed in. The patient also received salad greens.[24]

William Northcote, in his *Extracts from the Marine Practice of Physic and Surgery*, published in Philadelphia, also discussed scurvy.[25] His theory was that scurvy could be prevented by liberal use of acids, particularly vegetable, with decreased intake of salted provisions. He advised friction daily with a brush or coarse cloth. Nortcote also urged that the patient be kept clean, in dry linen, and should exercise. He knew oranges and lemons cured the disease and that oranges were better than lemons. If the patient did not get well on oranges, he did not have scurvy. Fresh vegetables were given as well. Oranges could spoil, but their juice could be preserved. His recipe called for removal of the pulp from the juice by sedimenting; then the juice was poured into a china or stoneware vessel wider at the top so that it could evaporate. The vessel was placed in a pan of water on a fire, and the water was brought almost to a boil. The process was finished when juice was of a thick syrupy consistency when cold. Slow evaporation, twelve to fourteen hours, was better than fast. He advised that a little rind should be added to the material before removing it from the fire. This gave the juice the taste and smell of the fresh fruit (if not the vitamin content). Then, it was placed in a bottle and corked. This way, the juice of a dozen oranges could be stored in a quart bottle for several years. When used, it was diluted with water as a punch. One quart could serve one man for years at sea. Seamen were advised to carry this with their gear. They were also to bring aboard bullace (a wild plum), aloes, hips, elderberries, and gooseberries preserved in bottles. Cabbage and French beans, stored between layers of salt and compressed, were also effective. The salt was washed off before use. The sailor was urged to keep a supply of onions, mustard, and Greenland scurvy grass stored in salt. Dutch sailors preferred pickled cabbage. A soup of pickled cabbage and onions could cure early scurvy. If the sailor had to eat salted provisions, vinegar, mustard, and onions were added. Meat was used in moderation. Those who were sick with obvious symptoms were given a diet of boiled biscuit, plus orange evaporate and wine, oatmeal, rice gruel, flummery, stewed barley with raisins and currants, pickled green cabbage, or beans and small onions. The food was made acid with orange evaporate and the juice of turnips. Water dock, berries, apples, and pears preserved in sugar or brought to a rob (jellied evaporate) or sliced apples and pears were recommended. These would keep in dry casks. Slices of fruit could be dried and stored. Good wine and spruce beer were effective. Common beer (small beer) was made more therapeutic with the addition of wormwood, camomile flowers, and gentian. Black spruce of America also made a wholesome drink. The tops, cones, leaves, and green bark were all antiscorbutic. If the spruce mixture was fermented, it was more effective (spruce beer). (The use of spruce beer in scurvy had a long history by the time this monograph was published in the late eighteenth century.) Sassafras chips were very good for scurvy. All fermented liquors, particularly cider at least three months old, were excellent antiscorbutics. Each sailor was given a pint of cider per day along with beer and water. Northcote urged that ventilators should operate on the ship, and decks were to be kept clean with water and vinegar. Vinegar, lemon juice, or elixir of vitriol added to drinking water made it more wholesome. Garlic brandy or tincture of bark had to be taken daily. Cream of tartar, an excellent acidifier, was used if oranges were not available. The material was very cheap. One shilling's worth would keep a sailor free of scurvy for one year. Cream of tartar plus rum and sugar in water was better than grog. Every man was expected to have his own stores of pickled vegetables, particularly onions, as well as acid fruits.

One wonders about the constant references to acid fruits, inorganic acids (vitriol), the acid properties of cream of tartar, etc. Could this be related to Galen's humors and Boerhaave's "acid and alkaline acrimonies"? In other words, did physicians back then think that scurvy was a disease due to an alkaline state in the humors of the body? Another interesting therapeutic measure was the use of tincture of bark. Cinchona bark (quinine) was introduced to Europe more than one hundred years before Northcote published his monograph. It was a specific for intermittent fever or ague (malaria). The results in malaria were so phenomenal that it was used in other illnesses. This resembled the use of cortisone for many of the unusual illnesses today. Fortunately, we employ the science of medical statistics today to determine the effectiveness of drugs.

The therapy described was used in the seventeenth and eighteenth centuries. The ancients apparently had tried to deal with this disease as well. It was recorded that the Phoenicians interrupted long voyages to keep their sailors healthy. They made frequent stops to allow the men to go ashore and harvest fresh fruit. The French navy treated scurvy with a tea brewed from pine needles as early as 1537.[26] James Woodall, surgeon to Queen Elizabeth I, in his publication of 1612, "The Surgeon's Mate," argued that lemons, limes, tamarinds, and oranges were antiscorbutic. The Dutch favored sauerkraut for scurvy. It could be stored on board ships for prolonged periods if well salted. The Dutch also cultivated vegetable patches on board some of their larger merchant ships, as had the Phoenicians. They established settlements such as Capetown and St. Helena on trade routes to the Indies where their ships could dock and pick up fresh vegetables.[27]

In 1757 John Travis, a surgeon, suggested that scurvy was due to boiling foods in copper pots, and he urged the British navy to discard them. He believed copper had a toxic agent that was transmitted to the food. However, he found iron pots acceptable. British sailors usually ate their vegetables cooked in a soup or stew. As was common at the time, his observations were good, but his explanation of the observation was faulty. Copper ions are catalysts in the aerobic breakdown of vitamin C; ferric ions are less effective. This was tested in the preparation of cabbage soup, a good source of vitamin C. When cooked in a copper pot for forty minutes, the vitamin C content dropped to 25 percent of the initial value. In an iron pot, the vitamin C content only dropped to about half of the initial value.[28]

The definitive work on scurvy was done by Dr. Lind aboard the sixty-gun ship *Salisbury* in 1747. He isolated twelve sailors with scurvy and gave them all the same diet. In addition, two were given cider; two were given 25 drops of elixir of vitriol; two received vinegar; two received sea water, and two received a combination of garlic, mustard, horseradish, balsam, and gum myrrh. The last two received two oranges and one lemon daily. The two who ate citrus fruit were fit for duty in six days. In 1753 Dr. Lind published his work, but the British navy did not act on his recommendation of citrus fruit until 1795, after 40 years of useless deaths. In the French and Indian War, 185,000 seamen were deployed. Of these, 130,000 died of disease. A major killer was scurvy. It is difficult to understand this lapse of 40 years. The most likely explanation was the expense of preparing and storing the citrus fruit. The suppliers to the British navy were more interested in cost and profits than in the lives of the seamen who could easily be replaced. In an attempt to demonstrate to the admiralty and the owners of the merchant fleet the low cost involved of preventing scurvy, Lind explained how to concentrate the juice, advised the use of gooseberries and other fruits dried by heat. He recommended fermented cider, spruce beer, onions, and soup of boiled cabbage. The method used to make juice lost half of the vitamin C content of the oranges through heat and evaporation. Storage resulted in further loss. After 28 days of storage at room temperature, juice retained only about thirteen percent of its original content of vitamin C. Gooseberries had a C content of 65 milligrams per 100 grams. Dried and stored according to Lind's technique, they had no vitamin C any more at all. Cider had 33 milligrams of vitamin C per 100 cc. Spruce beer stored 14 days lost all of its antiscorbutic effect. Onions stored for two months had four to five milligrams per 100 grams compared to fresh onions with twenty. Lind advised pickles to replace onions if necessary, but pickling removed all the antiscorbutic effect. The body requires five to ten milligrams of vitamin C per day to prevent scurvy.[29]

Dr. Lind did not restrict his pragmatism and observations to scurvy alone. His common sense observations about ship's fever would have conquered another destroyer of seamen. He observed that seamen rounded up by press gangs were immediately placed aboard the ship on which they would do their sea duty. Typhus epidemics usually followed. He did not realize that the epidemics occurred because the men were infected with lice. However, he suggested that the new men be kept separated. They were washed down, and their clothing was baked or burned. He recommended uniforms for seamen—not to instill martial spirit, but to get rid of their regular clothing. His suggestions were not accepted. The doctor's treatment of typhus, once it started on board, was based on the beliefs of his time. Therapy included bark, which was useless. The patient then received a vomit daily. If the patient was bled, the vomit was given a few hours later. He also received antimony. The next day he received an ounce of salts, and the antimony was repeated that evening. After this, he received bark every hour until he was out of danger, and then it was given less frequently.

Dr. Lind was not as wise when he theorized rather than observed. Like the learned physicians of his time, he feared miasmas, and he described steps to prevent them from affecting a ship in port. He also advised doctors about the best way to protect their health when they visited the sick. Prior to a visit, the physician was advised to drink a mixture of wine, lemon, and sugar. During his visit, he chewed on the root of calamus aeromaticus dipped in vinegar and he was urged to spit frequently.[30]

Sir Gilbert Blaine and Dr. John Harness were responsible for the acceptance of Lind's observations on scurvy by the British navy. Sir Gilbert was physician to the fleet, appointed by the fleet commander, Lord Rodney. The doctor served in the navy in the West Indies between 1780 and 1783. (It must be remembered that the American Revolution was part of a World War involving Britain, France, Spain, and Holland, and that the war continued after the victory at Yorktown. It became then largely a war at sea, fought predominantly in the West Indies.) In 1781 scurvy broke out on the British ships that had been at sea for a prolonged period. The disease usually developed within six weeks of leaving port, sooner if the sailor was stressed by hard work, danger, wet clothes and hammock, and exposure to the elements. The physician to the fleet accepted Lind's work, and he urged the admiralty under Lord Spencer to supply lemon juice to the crews of naval vessels. Dr. John Harness was fleet physician to Admiral Hook in the Mediterranean Sea in 1793. He had lemons supplied to all the ships in his fleet.[31] By the end of the century, deaths of seamen in the Royal Navy dropped to 32 per thousand per year. It was probably the defeat of scurvy that allowed Britain to successfully blockade Napoleon in Europe. The British could keep their ships at sea for a prolonged period. In 1844 Parliament ordered lemon juice on board the ships of the merchant marine as well.[32]

Before we leave this section on scurvy, a word on why British sailors are called "Limeys" is in order. Lime juice, in the early nineteenth century, collectively referred to lemon juice from Malta and to the juice of the sweet lime from other parts of the Mediterranean littoral, both of which were rich in vitamin C, and the sailor received a mandatory amount each day. After 1860 juice from the sweet lime grown in Monserrat in the West Indies was used, though it was low in antiscorbutic properties and lost what vitamin C it had with storage.[33]

Royal and Colonial Navies

The purpose of the British navy and merchant marine was to sink or capture enemy ships, fire on ports and harbors, and transport ordnance and other equipment. They were also responsible for convoying soldiers across 3,000 miles of ocean. When the troops arrived, they were expected to be fit for duty. The Naval Transport Board used chartered merchantmen to convoy men and material. Naval agents examined ships at the royal shipyards and checked hulls, masts, yardarms, and timbers. They also determined the ships' tonnage, which could be falsified with a bribe to the inspector. The owner of a ship fitted, armed, and manned the ship, and he had to have it inspected periodically to be certain of its seaworthiness. If tonnage was falsified, passengers and crew found themselves in cramped quarters as space reserved for troops was often filled with mercantile goods.

Small vessels (150 to 300 tons) were used for American destinations, and the troops were packed in like herring. Space was divided into two-tiered wooden berths with six men in a berth normally used for four. Food was scarce and sickening, and the soldiers were allowed only two-thirds of the ration of a sailor, because they were not working. A week's supply for six soldiers included 18 pounds of bread, 18 pounds of beef, eight pounds of pork, two pounds of rice, two pounds of cheese, one pound of butter, 12 pints of peas, eight pints of oatmeal, and half a pint of rum and water per man per day. However, the meat was old and spoiled, and the bread and biscuits were maggoty. Sometimes livestock was carried for fresh meat or delivery at the new port. The soldiers could fish to supplement their diets. Water was dirty and spread disease, and baths were infrequent. Uncounted passengers included an abundance of rodents, lice, and other vermin. Overall, the passage to America carried a mortality rate of eight percent; to the Caribbean eleven percent. The mortality was so high because the soldiers were from the slums of the city and from jails; they were poorly nourished before the trip, and many had consumption or were maimed or insane before they boarded the ships. On board there was no space to isolate the sick, no hospital ships as part of the convoy, and drugs and medicine were not easily available. The captains of these ships tried to maintain some appearance of hygiene—if for no other reason than to protect their crew. The decks were washed, sometimes daily, but usually weekly. They were rubbed with vinegar, sand, or pumice stones. If moisture increased below decks, portable fires ("bogies") were brought down. Bedding and hammocks were "cleaned frequently," and berths were scoured with vinegar. For fumigation the men used a lime wash or vitriol with potassium nitrate. They also set fires sprinkled with brimstone, vinegar, arsenic, tar, tobacco, or gunpowder. Cloths soaked in vinegar hung from the rafters. The ship owners were urged, but not forced, by the admiralty to put in scuttles above the gun ports, brass air tubes and wood funnels before the foremast, and "wind machines" at the hatchways.[34]

Upon reaching their destination, English surgeons were assigned to inspect all those on board and allow only the healthy to disembark. However, to please their regimental commanders, the surgeons overlooked illnesses and let a full complement leave the ship. This led to fresh epidemics in and around the ports as the infected and sick mingled with the healthy.

The Colonial navy was the beneficiary of the experience and tradition of the Royal Navy. The colonists had 150 years of their own maritime tradition as well. The earliest settlements were along the coasts of the ocean, rivers, and bays. The safest means of communication was by water. The soil of New England was rocky and not particularly productive agriculturally, but it did have

virgin forests with straight trees for masts, and pitch and turpentine were readily available from southern forests. The colonists thus turned back to the sea
to gain their livelihood.[35] This resulted in a major shipbuilding and seagoing
population. The first ships were launched off the coast of New England in the
early seventeenth century. By the mid-seventeenth century, Boston and Salem
were building oceangoing vessels and so was New York. The Navigation Acts
made it mandatory that all goods sent to English ports and colonies had to be
carried in British bottoms. This resulted in many new orders, and the shipbuilding industry grew, becoming the largest industry in the American
colonies. By the outbreak of the Revolution, a third of all ships built for the
British Empire were fabricated in colonial shipyards.

The production of a substantial merchantman required one year of labor.
The colonials preferred to build the smaller and faster sloops and schooners,
which were also cheaper to operate and easier to sail. A ship could be produced
thirty to fifty percent cheaper in American than in English shipyards because
of the easy availability of raw materials. However, they were of inferior quality, because timbers were not adequately seasoned and therefore rotted
more rapidly. In addition, colonial workers left greater spaces between the
timbers. Four warships were built for the British admiralty, but they did not
last long enough in service, so this work was discontinued.[36] A major ship of
the line was the biggest, most heavily armed vessel built. It could withstand
the onslaught of a fleet of enemy ships. The monster was 200 feet long and
50 feet at its widest, and it drew 22 feet of water. This was needed to keep it
upright against the push of the wind on the sails. Two thousand stout trees
were used in its construction at a cost of $1.5 million. It was built of hard British
oak with a hull four inches thick. By the 1770s, the ship had a copper sheath-
ing on the hull to protect it against sea worms, barnacles, and seaweed. These
caused a drag and slowed the ship's speed. Tall American pine was used for
masts and spars. (During the Revolution, the British had to obtain these
from the Baltic states.) Ships of this size carried 100 guns on three gun
decks. On a 74 gunner, there was a crew of 650. A ship of the line had
three masts, the fore, main, and mizzen. Spars held the square sails to the
masts. During battle, only the top sails were used, the others were kept furled.
The ship did six knots with the wind and one knot against it by tacking. The
British captain fought "by the book." The frigate was a smaller ship with
three masts, and one- or two-gun decks with 20 to 44 guns. The sloop was
still smaller, and only about 110 feet long, but it also had three masts and
carried 29-pound cannon. A 70-foot, single-masted sloop was also afloat, and
the navy also had brigs, brigantines, and ketches. The guns were measured
by the size of the shot they threw and could reach up to 42 pounds. The
carronade, introduced into British ships in 1779, could throw a 68 pound
shot.[37]

The colonists, however, continued to produce competent vessels for lake and river work as well as fast ships to chase smugglers (as well as to smuggle). They were of shoal draft, and they could withstand bad weather. Although British ships of the line were not built here, they were sent to American ports for repairs and refitting, which gave our shipwrights an opportunity to study their construction. By 1713 Massachusetts had 3,493 seamen and 492 vessels owned by local merchants. Trade was far from peaceful. The major European powers had colonies in the New World, and their citizens were encouraged to prey on the shipping of rival nations. Pirates were a constant source of danger, and a ship's crew required considerable fighting ability to withstand their depredations. The pirate had a special position in the Western Hemisphere. If he refrained from attacking your vessels, and he came to your ports to spend his loot, he was a welcome guest. If he preyed on your ships, he was labeled a pirate, hunted down, and executed. If a pirate was brought to a friendly port and sent to trial, he was defended by reputable lawyers, and juries rarely convicted him. If convicted, he could put down security money to promise good behavior and was soon pardoned. Many privateers turned to pirating if pickings were not good among the enemy. In addition to raiding, privateering, and pirating, there were many periods of formal warfare in the eighteenth century. In declared and undeclared wars, French and Indian incursions into New England forced the colonists to retaliate. Massachusetts, covetous of French Canada, sent several expeditions to capture key areas. Some were successful, some were disastrous, but all led to a heavy debt in New England. It was an armada from New England that captured Louisberg in 1745.[38]

The year 1775 saw 30,000 colonials working as merchant seamen. The colonial merchant ship carried a medical complement in peaceful commerce as well as during the wars of the century. A surgeon and/or a mate, depending on the size of the ship, was chosen by the captain. The contract lasted while the ship was at sea.

There were several sites along the New England coast that could lay claim to being the first site of the war at sea between Britain and her colonies. The action at Buzzard's Bay on Cape Cod was my choice. H.M. sloop *Falcon* seized a colonial ship and sent it toward Boston with a prize crew. Local citizens re-seized the ship, as well as a British tender, at Martha's Vineyard. They sent the British prisoners to Cambridge, Massachusetts. A second contender for the title occurred in June 1775. Americans in Machias, Maine, took the first British ship, the sloop *Margaretta*, in actual warfare. The *Margaretta* was sent to Maine for lumber to supply Boston. The ship was converted into a "warship" with the local people's money. The "Machias Pirates" captured two more British sloops by subterfuge and used them as privateers along the coast. Around Boston, civilians in whale boats burned and destroyed the *Diana*. This represented the third possibility as the start of naval warfare. In the period from November 13, 1775, to March 3, 1776, when the British fleet left Boston, 31 British ships were taken as they tried to land in that city.[39]

Naval Warfare

My choice for the father of the navy was George Washington. The general was commander-in-chief of troops around Boston. When Washington took command, he was immediately aware of two important problems. First, the troops around the city were in encampment, and it was well known that troops in camp became lazy, sloppy, and sick; in addition, they were receiving payment from a tightly budgeted economy and were completely unproductive. Second, ships moved in and out of Boston and kept the British garrison adequately supplied with food, fuel, and armament. Washington could solve both problems by creating a navy. He turned to Colonel Glover, a regimental leader from Marblehead, Massachusetts. Glover rented his ship *Hannah* with Nicholas Broughton as captain to the new government. The colonel chose its officers, and the able seamen would be members of the militia from Marblehead who were competent sailors. They received their first salaries as sailors on August 24, 1775, and were also to receive a third of any prize taken. On September 2, 1775, Washington sent them to sea. They seized the *Unity* almost immediately. The ship was seized originally by the British from a New Hampshire patriot and so was not considered a prize. The *Unity* later went aground and was saved from destruction by the British ship *Nautilus*.

Washington again turned to Glover to find other ships for his navy. The *Speedwell* and *Elizabeth* were obtained and commissioned. Washington then "borrowed" two ships from Massachusetts, the *Lynch* and the *Franklin,* and he sent them into the Gulf of St. Lawrence to intercept military supplies. They missed the Gulf and ended up at the Bay of Fundy where they took ten prizes. In the spring of 1776 the *Franklin* captured the *Hope* with 1,500 barrels of powder, entrenching tools and gun carriages. Washington also personally commissioned the *Lee,* the *Harrison,* and the *Warren;* all were schooners. The brigantine *Washington* also joined the embryonic fleet. After the retirement of the *Hannah,* Washington had a fleet of six vessels. The *Lee,* John Manly captain, captured the *Nancy* with a cargo of muskets, bayonets, 32 tons of shot for cannon, and gunpowder. He captured nine other prizes and was promoted to commodore. He was given command of the *Hancock* which was not yet completed. Washington's navy functioned until the end of 1776. He left Boston earlier in 1776 for New York City where he created a similar navy.[40]

The Continental Congress passed a resolution on July 18, 1775, that authorized the separate colonies to protect their own harbors and navigation. The colonies, particularly those engaged in active trade, commissioned their own navies. The largest state navies belonged to Massachusetts, Pennsylvania, and South Carolina. New Jersey and Delaware had no navy. The state navy was under the control of the Committee of Safety (the executive branch) of each state. While predominantly for coastal defense, some ships were very large.

South Carolina commissioned ships larger than those commissioned for the Continental navy.

The development of a Continental navy came at the request of the delegates from Rhode Island.[41] Silas Deane, John Adams (later replaced by Christopher Gadsden), and John Langston were appointed as a committee by the Continental Congress on October 13, 1775, to outfit two-armed sailing vessels to intercept two British ships that transported guns and ammunition to Quebec. The "Naval Committee of Three" became six with the addition of Stephen Hopkins, Joseph Hewes, and Richard Henry Lee. The committee was given executive powers. Congress expected its ships' captains to refrain from acts of violence when they took British ships (an oxymoron). However, when the British burned Falmouth (now Portland), Maine, and seized colonial vessels, Congress ended its "double-talk." It authorized the capture of any British ship employed against the colonies, or one that carried munitions. (How could the captain determine that it was carrying munitions until it was taken?)

On December 13, 1775, Congress ordered the construction of thirteen frigates, one per colony, to be afloat by April 1776. These were to be 115 to 160 feet long and would carry 220 to 350 seamen and 24 to 50 guns. The workmanship was not too good; the timber was "green," and the few that went to sea accomplished little. In addition to the new construction, Congress authorized the purchase of vessels that could be converted to cruisers. These ships were named the *Alfred, Columbus, Andrea Doria,* and the *Cabot*. The commission authorized an expenditure of $100,000 for this project, and the ships were to be used for the "protection and defense of the United Colonies."[42] On November 28, 1775, the Continental Congress adopted "Rules and Regulations of the Navy of the United Colonies," written by John Adams. The rules were based on Britain's naval regulations.[43] On November 9, 1775, Congress ordered that two battalions of marines be raised. They were to be oceangoing soldiers who had previous experience with the sea. They were expected to serve as sailors at sea if that became necessary. As the year of independence approached, four more vessels were purchased: *Hornet, Providence, Fly,* and *Wasp*. Congress also posted pay scales for the new navy. Salaries ranged from $125 per month for the commander in charge to eight dollars for the able seaman. Prize money was also regulated. The captain of a ship received six parts; the surgeon and the lieutenant each received four parts, and the able seaman one part.

In January 1776, Captain Esek Hopkins stepped aboard the *Alfred,* and Lieutenant John Paul Jones raised the Pine Tree and Rattlesnake flag with the motto "Don't Tread on Me." The flotilla left in mid–February 1777 with orders to clear Governor Dunmore's ships out of Chesapeake Bay, then clear the seas along the southern colonies, and finally return to do the same duty around Rhode Island. (Governor Dunmore was the ousted Tory governor of Virginia.) Hopkins disobeyed orders and instead attacked New Providence in the

Bahamas. He then sailed north and encountered the *Glasgow*. His flotilla of eight ships damaged the *Glasgow*, but they could not capture or sink her. Hopkins was dismissed and his title was retired.[44]

Early in 1776, Congress retired the naval committee and formed the marine committee. It was composed of thirteen men, one from each colony. Congress also appointed a navy board of three to run the business of the navy and report back to the committee of thirteen. On April 19, 1777, another board of three, appointed from the New England area, replaced the original three who became the board of the middle department (Pennsylvania). On October 28, 1779, a board of admiralty was formed, composed of two congressmen plus three commissioners. The marine committee was phased out, and the board of admiralty itself died quietly two years later. During its tenure, the board passed regulations about surgeons and mates on ships. They were chosen according to the number of guns on board. A ship of 20 guns had one surgeon, less than 20, a mate; a 44-gun frigate had one surgeon and two mates, a 36-gunner, one surgeon and one mate. On February 7, 1781, all naval affairs were transferred to one person, a secretary of marine. This post was never filled, and Robert Morris, superintendent of finances, gradually assumed control of naval affairs. All naval boards were abolished, and Morris, as agent of marine, ran the navy until the end of the war. Naval affairs overseas were under the control of three commissioners in France: Ben Franklin, Silas Deane, and Arthur Lee. These men operated from a naval office in Paris. They controlled agents in Spain and Holland. They bought, fitted, and manned ships, and the committee commissioned officers, disposed of prizes, commissioned privateers, and exchanged prisoners.[45]

The third leg of the "troika" of naval affairs, after the Continental Congress with its boards and navy and the overseas commissioners, was the privateers. The concept of privateers had been recognized for centuries. It was used extensively by England in the middle of the seventeenth century. During the Seven Years War, the French commissioned many privateers who almost destroyed British trade around the home island. The British reciprocated and sent their own privateers out. It was a financially rewarding business, but British merchants still felt uncomfortable with the idea. Early in the Revolution, the British did not use privateers against colonial shipping. However, after the entrance of France into the war, they launched a fleet of privateers against France. The seamen aboard the British privateers were "gentlemen sailors of good background" who sought adventure and quick profits. They did the fighting rather than the routine seaman's duties. The ship owner received a commission (a letter of marque) from a governor, a king, or other executive of a nation. Often the only difference between a privateer and a pirate was that a privateer had a commission while a pirate was on his own. The privateer had no cargo; his ship was built for speed, and it carried ordnance predominantly for offensive action. The ship could travel without national flags, and it could approach a merchantman with gun ports closed. When it was within haling distance of its prey, colors would go up, and gun ports were opened. The merchantman often surrendered without a fight. The crew of the merchantman was kept below decks, and a prize crew was placed on board. The ship was then sailed to the nearest prize court. The crew of the privateer had to be large when it left port. The mission of the privateer ended when its crew was depleted to sail the prizes taken, or it was captured by a warship.[46]

Massachusetts held the first prize court of the Revolution. Fifteen days before a trial, a description of the vessel was printed in the local papers with the date of the trial. On that date, people testified and supplied reasons why the ship should not be condemned and sold (i.e., it belonged originally to a patriot). There were up to twelve jurors in the court of justice. If the ship was proven to be a prize property, it could be sold. If it had belonged to a patriot and had previously been taken by the British, it was returned to its original owner rather than sold as a prize. The cost of the trial was taken out of the prize money. The officers and crew of the privateer received between 25 and 33 percent of the prize money. The owner who outfitted the privateer took the rest of the money.[47] A merchantman and cargo might bring $30,000 on the auction block. Privateers were responsible for the great increase of insurance rates in England, and merchants turned to neutral shipping to carry their products. In addition, they demanded and received Royal Navy protection for their shipping. In peacetime, insurance rates were two percent of the value of the ship and cargo to the colonies; two and a half percent to Jamaica. These rates were doubled during the war if the ship went in a convoy, and they jumped to 15 percent if the ship was unescorted. In a large convoy of approximately a hundred merchantmen, the lead escort might be a ship of the line (the largest "battleship") under the control of an admiral. Frigates, sloops, and brigs kept the convoy together.

Not all American privateers were Whigs. The Tories in New York City and Newport, Rhode Island, fitted out privateers that preyed on patriot shipping. The number of privateers increased from 136 in 1776 to 323 in 1782. In the first two years of the war, patriot privateers took 733 ships with a value of 2.2 million pounds. About 180 of these were retaken by the British. The privateers took 10,995 seamen as prisoners. Some privateers fought British warships, and 18 British warships were taken during the war. Almost half of the privateers were from Massachusetts. The Continental Congress authorized privateers on March 23, 1776, and sent commissioners to all the colonies to authorize Continental privateers. Congress authorized 1,700 commissions for ships that would carry 15,000 guns and 59,000 men. There were also 1,400 state letters. Congress also appointed commissioners in the West Indies to issue letters, as did those in Europe. The overseas commissioners and state commissioners issued about 2,000 letters for ships with 18,000 guns. The British had the same number of privateers with 70,000 men.

Sailors preferred privateer duty to Continental navy duty. Profits were greater, and discipline was milder. A Continental cruiser that captured a prize received half of its value if the ship was a British warship and a third if it was a merchantman. The rest went to the Continental treasury. The percentages were raised on October 26, 1776, to entice men into the navy. The crew received all the money for a British battleship and half for a merchantman. This could not compete with the "take" of the privateersman with a state letter. The lack of volunteers for Continental ships forced Congress to put an embargo on privateersmen until all berths were filled on a Continental ship in the port. The deficiency of privateer duty was the lack of coverage that those men in the navy had in the event of injury, sickness, or death. In illness or injury with permanent disability, the government owed the privateersman nothing. In the event of death, his family was not eligible to receive widow's and orphan's benefits. Privateers ran the risk of hanging if they were caught. However, this never happened, presumably because colonials held British prisoners as well.

During the war, privateers captured or destroyed 16 major warships and 2,980 merchantmen worth $150 million. The merchant ship was large and clumsy. It was built to carry as much tonnage as possible and still stay afloat. The American privateer was built for speed. These ships were in service before the war for the purpose of illegal trading and smuggling in the face of the British Navigation Acts. They had to outrace British frigates to avoid capture. No privateer was more than 120 feet long. Toward the end of the war, in addition to its crew, the privateer carried a marine contingent. The marines acted as police on board, enforced the captain's orders, served as the boarding party, and guarded prisoners.

Officers and seamen could transfer back and forth from one service to the other. If awaiting a berth on a Continental ship, the sailor could sign on as a privateer for a short period of duty, frequently a matter of weeks. The pay in the Continental navy was set by Congress on November 15, 1776. The surgeon's pay varied with the number of guns, and in July 1777 the surgeon's income was raised to equal the lieutenant's. The surgeon's quarters were in the wardroom, and he belonged to the wardroom mess. His mate was with the midshipmen in steerage, the cockpit, or on deck. The appointment of a ship's surgeon and mate was standardized by Congress on September 3, 1776, when Congress resolved that all state legislatures appoint examiners to examine and certify all applicants for positions of surgeon or mate in the army or navy.[48]

The purpose of the Continental navy was to convoy merchantmen, deliver mail to keep the colonies in contact with the West Indies and Europe, take prizes, and try to fight the British navy. The fleet carried out the first three functions reasonably well, but the last was a complete fiasco. The Continental navy faced an enemy in 1775 that comprised 270 ships (131 were ships of the line and carried 60 or more guns on two or more decks). To oppose them, the U.S. Navy had 50 to 60 vessels at most. These included frigates of 32 guns down to schooners, sloops, and some ships of the states' navies. The Americans were outgunned, outmaneuvered, and outfought. At no time did the Continental navy have more than 3,000 able seamen or 340 naval and marine officers.[49] The British navy had a tradition of superiority. Its commanders and seamen had long experience and expertise. However, they had problems as well. The first lord of the admiralty, the Earl of Sandwich, was interested only in lining his pocket. Seventy-six vessels built for the navy capsized or foundered. Poor food purchased by pursers led to malnutrition and scurvy. Forty-two thousand men deserted, and 18,000 died of disease. There was embezzlement at all levels. The food and ordnance were frequently shortchanged. Men were in positions of command because of family and money. The enlisted men were impressed criminals and foreigners with no particular loyalty to Great Britain. Furthermore, they had to sail 3,000 miles before they could approach the Continental navy.[50]

The only real engagement between a British fleet and a colonial fleet occurred on Lake Champlain in 1776. The Continental force was composed of 15 ships whose timbers were as green as the crews and that carried 88 guns and a total crew of 811 soldiers pulled from Fort Ticonderoga. The British squadron under Captain Pringle had better ships, seamen, and Royal Navy officers. A five-hour battle took place off Valcour Island in Lake Champlain on October 13, 1776. The Continental fleet was overwhelmingly defeated and withdrew to Fort Ticonderoga, and the remnant was scuttled.[51]

The Continental navy fared no better during the rest of the war. In 1777 the Continental ships *Reprisal, Lexington,* and *Dolphin* sailed around Great Britain and captured prizes, which they took to French ports illegally (France was still overtly neutral). By the end of the year, all three ships were lost. The *Revenge,* under the command of Captain Cunningham, captured or destroyed 33 ships. The year 1778 was an equally bad one. The frigate *Randall* blew up and killed Captain Bedde. The frigates *Warner* and *Providence* became ordnance transports. The frigate *Virginia,* with Captain James Nicholson, surrendered. The frigates *Hancock* and *Delaware* were captured. Five frigates were burned or scuttled to prevent their capture by the British. At the end of 1778 there were five frigates in Boston. The famous *Ranger* was in port. Only the *Alliance* and *Providence* were at sea. At this point the entire Continental navy was reduced to 14 ships with 332 guns. In July 1779 three cruisers assisted the Massachusetts navy in its attempt to take a fort on the Penobscot River in Maine. The British had a colony of displaced Tories that occupied the area. The attack was to be a combined operation of the army, navy, and marines. The colonials were defeated and 14 of their ships were burned by their own crews. Five hundred men were killed or captured. Seven million dollars were wasted. Commodore Saltonstall was court-martialed and dismissed from the service. At the end of 1779 the Continental navy was reduced to only six cruisers after four had been captured or destroyed in the fall of Charleston,

South Carolina. The only encouraging news for the Americans that year was Commodore Whipple's capture of 11 prizes from the Jamaican fleet. A few ships of the Continental navy were bottled up in port until the end of the war when the navy was completely disbanded by the sale of those ships that were still seaworthy.[52]

The only bright spot in the war fought by the Continental navy was the exploits of John Paul Jones. On December 7, 1775, Jones was commissioned a first lieutenant and given command of the *Alfred*, which he turned over to Captain Saltonstall shortly thereafter. He signed on as the captain's lieutenant. The *Alfred* accompanied the fleet under Esek Hopkins to the Bahamas and on its return trip engaged the *Glasgow* in battle before returning to New London, Connecticut. Captain Hazard of the sloop *Providence* was removed for embezzlement and Jones was given his command. Two hundred seamen from the flotilla were sent to shore for medical care. They suffered from illnesses and alcoholism developed in the Bahamas. Jones took the *Providence* out for transport and escort service. His surgeon was Henry Tillinghost of Providence, Rhode Island. In October 1776 Jones was again given command of the *Alfred* with orders to capture prizes and coal ships and rescue American prisoners of war who were forced to work in the coal mines of Cape Breton.[53]

On June 14, 1777, Jones was given command of the sloop of war *Ranger* with 20 guns. The surgeon was Dr. Ezra Green, and Jacob Walten was the surgeon's mate. Both were from New Hampshire. The mate's medical experience came from his duties in an apothecary shop. The *Ranger* left for France on November 1, 1777 to be refitted. When the ship left for its return trip on February 13, 1778, the captain had to turn back because one of the ship's boys showed evidence of smallpox. The ship again set sail from France on April 10, 1778, for Whitehaven, Scotland. Jones burned some ships in port with little damage except to English prestige (much like the Doolittle raid on Tokyo in 1942). He then tried to kidnap Lord Selkirk at St. Mary's Isle, but Selkirk was out of town "taking the waters." The crew compromised by instead taking the silver from Selkirk manor, which Jones bought back and returned to the owner. Selkirk was to be taken as a hostage to force an exchange of prisoners of war. On April 24 the *Ranger* defeated the *Drake*, and the crew sailed it plus two merchantmen back to Brest, France.[54] Dr. Ezra Green left a diary with his description of a battle at sea aboard the *Ranger*. His duty was primarily to give first aid to the wounded until they could be transferred to a facility in France. The seriously injured frequently died before they reached shore. The doctor had little use for Jones, whom he considered a poor commander, and believing the raid on Whitehaven to have been rash and of little consequence.[55] After his return to Brest, Jones sat in France for nine months until February 1779. The captain traded his prisoners for American seamen. This was a first, because Great Britain looked upon American seamen as pirates and refused to exchange them. The *Ranger* was taken from Jones's command and returned to America. It was captured at the capitulation of Charleston, South Carolina, where America lost half of its remaining frigates. The ship ended the war under British colors.[56]

The King of France purchased an East Indies merchantman, the *Duc de Duras*, and converted it into a fighting ship, the *Bonhomme Richard*, for $44,000. The ship was placed under Jones's command. The captain received four other ships to complete his armada, one American and three French. The armada was to attack northern England or southern Scotland as a diversion to keep British troops occupied while a combined French and Spanish fleet attacked southern England and landed an invasion force of 20,000 soldiers. John Paul Jones did his part, but the French and Spanish ships ran into difficulties. The French fleet under D'Orvillier left Brest on June 3, 1779, to meet with the Spanish fleet and invade England. The combined fleet would have 64 ships with 4,774 guns. Admiral Hardy of the British fleet had 38 ships with 2,968 guns. Hardy stayed in protected ports and would not fight. The Spanish fleet joined the French in July 1779, seven weeks after the French were at sea. By this time scurvy (as well as typhus and smallpox) had spread throughout the French fleet and invading army. The allied fleet lingered around the British Isles until the end of August. Finally, after many soldiers and sailors had died, the French returned to Brest with 7,000 sick.[57]

After the invasion fiasco was played out, Jones received additional orders to destroy or capture British shipping. His armada was increased to seven ships and left France on August 14, 1779. The surgeon on board the *Bonhomme Richard* was Dr. Lawrence Brooke of Virginia. The officers were largely American, with three Irishmen, and the crew came from many different countries. They sailed around Scotland. Off Flamborough Head on the North Sea, *Richard*, *Alliance*, and *Pallas* fell upon *HMS Serapis* and the *Countess of Scarborough* as they escorted ships from Scandinavia. The *Serapis* was faster and carried more ordnance than the *Richard*. The *Alliance* gave no help, and the *Pallas* fought and defeated the *Scarborough*. The *Richard* and the *Serapis* fought and collided; the *Richard* grappled. The French ship under Captain Landers (because of jealousy) fired three broadsides into the *Richard* that caused tremendous damage. On board the *Richard*, three gunners believed all American officers were killed and called for "quarters." Jones, incensed, threw his pistols at them. He struck one in the head and fractured his skull. Later, the gunner was trepanned, and he survived. Finally, the *Serapis* struck its colors, and the *Richard*'s men boarded. The *Richard* and *Serapis* were kept together until the *Richard* was cut loose and allowed to sink on September 25.[58] Fanning, one of the crew of the *Richard*, left an eyewitness report of the battle. He said 165 men were killed, and 137 were wounded or missing. Of the wounded, almost 100 died due to the "unskillfulness of surgeons who amputated them."

Only one surgeon in the whole squadron, Dr. Brooke of Virginia, was actually able to perform his duties. He was as bloody as a butcher from the commencement of the battle until nightfall of the day after the battle. The greater part of the wounded had arms and legs shot away or bones so badly fractured that they required amputation. Men were amputated by unskilled doctors and had to be reamputated by Dr. Brooke two or three days later. He worked on the *Serapis* after it was taken, but a gale after the battle kept him from visiting the wounded on the other ships. The British on board the *Serapis* lost 137 dead and 67 wounded. Twenty who were badly burned by a grenade that exploded gunpowder died two or three days later in agony.[59] The armada went to Holland and stayed there the rest of the year. Jones switched to the *Alliance* and left Holland on December 28. For his share of the prizes, Jones received $2,658 in gold. Jones went to Paris where he was feted as a hero. On October 17, 1780, he left France on board the *Ariel* with arms for the Continental army. The ship was savaged by gales and returned to France for refitting. It reached Philadelphia on February 18, 1781.

After the dismantling of the Continental navy at the end of 1779, the *Alliance* under Captain Barry served as a transport and dispatch ship to the French. The frigate *Trumbull* with J. Nicholson as captain was also active. The frigate *Deane* cruised for prizes under the command of S. Nicholson. The others were in port for repairs or bottled up by the British fleet. At this time Robert Morris asked Jones to captain the *America*, the largest ship to be built in Portsmouth. He wanted to give Jones the rank of admiral. Jones went to Portsmouth, but the *America* was turned over to the French as a present in gratitude. (The ship had an ignominious end. In 1786 it was broken up because of dry rot.) Jones went on board the French ship *Le Triomphant* to the Caribbean where he developed malaria. He returned to Philadelphia and spent the summer in the sanitorium of the Moravians at Bethlehem, to take cold baths for the aftereffects of the fevers.

There are a few postscripts before leaving Jones and the navy. He did become an admiral, but in the fleet of Catherine the Great of Russia, against Turkey.[60] He toured Europe and then returned to France where he died on July 18, 1792, of nephritis, jaundice, and pneumonia. Jones was buried in St. Louis Cemetery. The body was preserved in a linen winding sheet soaked in straw and alcohol and sealed in a lead casket filled to the brim with alcohol. When the casket was opened, the body was so well preserved that researchers were able to make a positive identification of his face by comparing it to a medal struck by the United States Congress and from a bust by Howdon. The body was autopsied in 1905, and he was found to have interstitial nephritis. Teddy Roosevelt had the body transported home in a cortege of United States naval units. John Paul Jones was reburied at Annapolis.[61]

While the Continental navy came to an ignominious end at the cessation of hostilities, the entrance of France and its navy into the war in 1778 was responsible for the success at Yorktown. The Comte de Grasse was able to keep the British out of Chesapeake Bay so they were unable to rescue Cornwallis's troops at Yorktown and Gloucester, and this resulted in the capture of the British army. The French navy, like the British, did amphibious duty. They landed, picked up, and delivered troops where they were needed. An attempt to combine amphibious French troops with a Continental army under Sullivan at Newport was a failure and resulted in recriminations and suspicions that persisted for years. The French fleet, unhappily, was seriously defeated by the British under Admiral Rodney in the West Indies on April 12, 1782.[62]

Naval Surgeon

The surgeon on board a colonial ship, like his counterpart on a British ship, had to be physician and apothecary. However, his problems with sickness were not terribly time consuming. The reason, I believe, was because his ship was not at sea long enough to get into the problems of malnutrition, avitaminosis, and communicable diseases. Colonial ships operated mostly out of colonial seaports. British ships had to cross an ocean before engaging the enemy, while colonial ships could be back in port before serious signs of scurvy developed. Also, as was seen in the case of John Paul Jones, when his ship's boy showed signs of smallpox, the ship could easily return to shore to discharge patients before diseases could spread. Writings from ship's surgeons are meager, but I saw no mention of typhus aboard colonial privateers or Continental navy ships. There is evidence that the colonials used press-gangs to a degree, but they did not clear out jails to fill the ship's complement as did the British.

The colonial surgeon was faced with the results of accidents and battle wounds. Article 16 of Naval Regulations called for a convenient place for the care of the sick and injured, and casualties were to be moved there with their hammocks and bedding when the surgeon considered this necessary. "Some of the crew shall be appointed to attend and serve them and keep the area clean. The cooper shall make buckets with covers and cradles if necessary for their use. The buckets to be used for expectoration, vomitus, and other products from the patients."[63] Compared to the British surgeon, the American one was inexperienced. As a civilian he had perhaps treated accidents due to farming, but he was a novice at sea unless he had served aboard merchantmen before the war. Fortunately, there were books he could turn to, including the writings of John Ranby. As so much written at the time, much of the material was didactic and specific, with little theory and philosophy. For example, to stop vein wounds from bleeding, the application of lint and styptic was advised. In arterial wounds, the use of a ligature of waxed thread with a curved needle was recommended. Ranby also advised the use of a tourniquet to control bleeding temporarily. If a tourniquet was not available, he advised compression of the artery against the bone. If the artery was in the bone, it could be compressed with lint. He warned against the use of styptic or cautery on an arterial wound if other means were available. (The discoveries of Ambrose Paré had filtered down.) Ranby also described nerve damage. If a nerve was divided, there would be pain and inflammation, paralysis would develop, and the part would atrophy, or it would be consumed by mortification. This occurred because the arteries could not propel their contained fluids, since the nerves no longer supplied the arterial wall. The humors accumulated, stagnated, corrupted, and mortified the part. If a nerve was partially cut, inflammation developed and spread with excruciating pain, fever, delirium, convulsions, and a thick ferous discharge, so-called gleet. To treat this condition, one dilated the wound, dressed it with warm balsam peruviana on a pledget of soft digestive and an emollient poultice and bandage. Wounds of tendons and ligaments were to be treated the same way.

According to Ranby's observations, gunshot wounds were difficult because fibers and vessels were lacerated, juices extravasated, and the texture destroyed. This required extensive digestion or suppuration to remove injured parts before the wound healed. Wounds were worse if they reached bones, viscera, or joints, particularly if they carried in wadding, clothes, and splinters, which could result in inflammation and gangrene, followed by amputation. Gunshot wounds of the cranium were most apt to be malignant and fatal. They were treated by extracting the ball and other extraneous material. One had to tie off the arteries if they were injured. The surgeon was advised to probe as little as possible, using his finger as a probe. If the ball was beyond the finger's reach, he was not to use long forceps but leave the ball in place because it usually worked its way out. A wound of a musket or pistol was small and had to be dilated. However, if it was near a tendon or joint, the surgeon was kept from excessive use of the knife and produced an opening just large enough for drainage. Wounds of joints, membranous, and tendinous parts were dangerous, because they were exposed to the air. If a ball went clean through, Ranby advised the surgeon to open both orifices and keep them open, particularly the dependent one. A light dressing was applied with a thin flannel bandage. If not too much blood was lost, the patient was bled heavily for the first three days to decrease pain and inflammation, to promote digestion, and to prevent complications. The operator was to observe a cooling regimen for twelve days and to produce a bowel movement daily by clyster or laxative. A dressing of dry lint was applied with a light bandage. This was followed by a digestive covered by a bread and milk poultice with oil to keep it moist. If the wound was large, a fomentation was applied. This was continued until the lesion was clean. Lint was moistened with oil because that way it held better to contused wounds, prevented drying, and allowed drainage. If inflammation occurred due to a foreign body (a ball), Ranby advised doctors not to try to remove it until the swelling was decreased and the inflammation had subsided. The ball could be removed in the face of inflammation only if it was near the surface and easily removed. If a ball had entered a joint, the limb was amputated immediately before inflammation set in. If amputation was delayed, it was useless. Wounds near a big artery bled again on motion and when slough began to separate. (The surgeon had to expect this.) The patient then complained of weight and fullness of the limb with pulsations in the area. This problem was handled with bleeding and bark. Sudden arterial bleeding could cause death by a gush of as little as twelve ounces because this was added to the loss from surgery, and "it put a check on the circulation." The doctor should have tied off all arteries and performed regular bleedings to prevent fevers and "imposthumations" (suppurations). The body was kept open with a laxative and opium was used for pain, "a sovereign and almost divine power." Also bark was advised. It might help when opium did not.

In large wounds, as those from cannon, he continued, there was severe pain with a discharge of gleety matter, which had to be restrained. Bark was given as often as the stomach tolerated it. Elixir of vitriol was added to the regimen. Rhubarb was added to the bark if the patient was costive (constipated). If bark caused diarrhea, laudanum was added. If a gleety matter was discharged, bark would thicken and lessen it. In scorbutic patients who had lost a limb, after eight days the wound looked bad, and a gleety discharge developed, and the patient often died. This type of wound was treated with bark to constrict the blood vessels and prevent the small blood vessels from being dissolved by the acrimony of matter absorbed and returned to the blood. This also preserved the texture of the blood from becoming too watery. Watery blood often led to a fatal outcome and "colliquative hectic" (consumptive melting away).

The surgeon was to keep his instruments clean and in good order. He had to have tourniquets ready, and Pettit's was best, because the patient could control it after application. Crooked or curved needles were threaded with ligatures. The surgeon needed enough lint, some of it mixed with flour. There had to be bandages of all sizes. For slight wounds, bandages made of bunting were good. Linen rollers or bandages were kept for amputations and fractures. The surgeon had common needles and thread, pins, pledgets of tow (flax or hemp), wet with water or oxycrate, then dried. Splints of all sizes lined with linen cloth, bolsters or compresses of cloth, and yards of incle or strong tape to secure splints were kept handy. All of this preparation encouraged the men on board to have confidence in their surgeon.[64]

Cutbush, in his monograph *Preserving the Health of Seamen*, had more advice. He recommended that the surgeon refrain from preparing medications as tinctures because the men wanted them for the alcoholic content. He also advised that medication be kept to a minimum and to prepare fresh ointments. He advised sick call every morning on a specific deck, and then the surgeon was expected to visit his patients in their berths. A list of sick was then sent to the captain and the deck officer to excuse the sick from duty.

At the start of action, the surgeon went to the cockpit with his assistants as well as the chaplain and the purser. Seriously wounded were sent to the gunroom or berth deck. Slightly wounded were sent to their quarters, or they could assist in caring for the seriously wounded. The seriously wounded were checked frequently by the surgeon's mates to watch for complications. In deep bullet wounds, the ball was left in place, because they healed reasonably well. If the ball was near the surface, it was removed with the index finger as a probe. A musket ball made a narrow opening with a bruised appearance. If the sides of the wounds were tense and inflamed, the orifice was dilated, and the patient was bled. A simple thin pledget was placed over the wound, and an emollient poultice made of linseed meal was then applied. No poultice was applied when suppuration started and an eschar separated. The opening was dressed. Overgrowth of tissue was removed with nitrate of mercury, and moderately tight compresses were applied. Throbbing in the wound suggested that a hemorrhage would start. Splinter wounds of the flesh were cleaned with a sponge and water. Arterial bleeding was controlled with forceps or with a needle. If bleeding was diffuse, the patient probably had scurvy. The site was covered with lint and compressed. It was not removed until it suppurated. The patient was well fed to maintain his strength. He was not to receive excessive amounts of bark, because this cut his appetite, nor was he to be bled or purged. Emollients, poultices, and fomentations for inflammation were advised. Applications of acetatus cooled the inflammation and relieved pain. The patient was fed animal products in jellies. The surgeon might have to feed the patient through his rectum. When the wound granulated, dressings were tightened so that escharotics were not necessary. If there was a severe injury with tendon, nerve, muscle tears, or bone splinters, the limb was amputated promptly. In milder injuries, the thumb and forefinger were used to remove the fragments of bone and foreign matter. This was less painful than their removal when inflammation occurred. The surgeon removed all fragments, or the patient would die of trismus (lockjaw). If a wound or stump mortified (gangrene), niter was sprinkled at every dressing change, and it was washed with vinegar. Bark in port wine was given. If a limb was removed by shot, it was amputated further back to create a cover of skin. In wounds of the thorax or abdomen, tincture of digitalis was used to decrease arterial action and allow the vessels to heal. In joint wounds, amputation was indicated. If the patient developed tetanus, which was more common in hot climates, calomel and opium were given. In puncture wounds, two or three grains of calomel twice a day were used until salivation occurred to prevent tetanus. Cautery, wine, porter, and cold baths could also be tried for tetanus.

Early in the war, with men inexperienced with gunpowder, there were many burn accidents due to explosives. The incidents decreased as men learned how to handle them. Burns were treated with linseed oil mixed with lime water or cerise (an ointment of lead carbonate and hydrate), and opium was administered orally. About one fourth of the deaths caused by injuries were due to burns. Another serious problem was wood splinters. When a cannonball struck the side of a ship, it threw out massive amounts of wooden projectiles. These frequently destroyed the gun crew on the opposite side of the ship. Splinter screens were put up behind the gun crew to prevent this catastrophe. Men also died from hemorrhage due to massive wounds. All seamen were advised to carry rope or a garter to use as a tourniquet until the surgeon could treat them properly.

When the ship was not in action, those men not involved in the daily operation of the ship (marines and soldiers) tended to get sloppy and melancholic, and they became prone to scurvy. They had to be kept active with musters, dancing, exercises, fencing, and other forms of amusement. Strict discipline with humanity was advised to keep all on board in a healthy state.

Cutbush also gave instructions for the operation of a hospital ship with a complement of one surgeon and three mates. The colonials had none, but the British adopted this idea. The ship had to be large, dry, and commodious. It was to be fitted with cradles and bunks or cots well supplied with bedding. There were tubs on board for bathing the patient when he came on board, and his linen was changed without cost to the casualty. The ship had a baker to make fresh bread as well as a barber. Wives of soldiers could serve as nurses. Cleanliness was vital, and the interior should be whitewashed with lime frequently.[65]

John Jones, in his monograph published at the start of the Revolution, gave advice to army and navy surgeons. His suggestions were clear and straightforward. Like most trained doctors of his time, his work was marred by theories of medicine devised by thinkers and taught to young students. However, when he relied on observation and experience, his instructions were frequently ahead of their time. He believed slight puncture wounds needed no treatment. Tortuous ones had to be incised and enlarged. Inflammation was countered by gentle laxatives, cataplasms, sudorific anodynes, bleeding, and warm baths. Opium was an essential adjunct to therapy. The appearance of gangrene signified the need for a more nourishing diet, spontaneous fomentations, and more intensive use of bark. Abscesses required immediate incision and drainage. Transverse wounds were sutured with interrupted sutures with a needle dipped in oil. Plaster was then applied over the wound for two or three days. In gunshot wounds, the ball was removed carefully to control hemorrhage. A light dressing was applied with another on top. Major compound fractures required amputation. Soft, dry lint was applied to all recent wounds. It restrained hemorrhage with less injury than styptic medicine. It also absorbed the matter which was at first thin and acrimonious and it became, in effect, the best digestive. During granulation it was the softest medication that could be applied between the roller and the tender granulations. At the same time it acted as an easy compress on the sprouting fungus. Generally, ointments used to cover recent wounds were detrimental. When a wound disintegrated into so bad a state that it resisted this simple mode of treatment and lost that healthy appearance of a recent wound, it was then called an ulcer.

Jones also considered cardiac, aortic, cerebellar, medullary, and receptaculum chyli wounds fatal; chest, abdomen, hepatic, intestinal, and renal wounds were very serious. It was advisable to dilate the external wounds and then to bleed the patient profusely and frequently, followed by emollient clysters, cooling nitrous drinks, anodynes, a most rigid diet consisting solely of thin diluting drinks, complete quiet, and proper posture.[66]

The naval surgeon used the same instruments as the land-based surgeon. These included surgical retractors, surgical hooks and forceps, ball extractors, amputation knives and saws, and phlebotomy lancets. His medical chest matched those on shore and included cathartics, emetics, cinchona bark, opium, and blisters. He may have had a European pharmacopoeia or, after 1778, a copy of Dr. William Brown's pharmacopoeia titled, *Formulary of Simple Yet Efficacious Remedies.* This was the so-called Lititz pharmacopoeia, essentially a compendium of the formulas of the pharmacopoeias of Edinburgh, the Royal Hospital of Edinburgh, and the London pharmacopoeia. Dr. Brown had been educated in Edinburgh and naturally favored the Edinburgh material. There were 84 internal medications, including medicines taken orally, gargles, eye washes, as well as preparations applied to the skin, douches, and enemas. There were 16 surgical or external medications. These included water mixed with wine, barley water, rice water, lime water, material from Peruvian bark, sarsaparilla root, material that worked like the recently developed dried mustard plaster (a counterirritant), emetic solutions such as tartar emetic, cathartic solutions such as Epsom salts and Glauber salts, as well as tincture of opium. One of the most important staples on board ship was cinchona bark, which was used for pain, fever, and as a specific for malaria. Rum was also an important medication.[67]

How did the colonials treat the sick and injured seaman who survived the ship and landed in port? In one word, poorly. The men were left ashore in private homes or almshouses. Private local doctors were contracted to care for them. Care was poor, haphazard, and expensive; many men, as soon as they were able, deserted from these places. On February 27, 1777, the medical committee of the Continental Congress placed care in the hands of the states. In October 1783 Congress debated a general hospital for sick and maimed soldiers and sailors. The proposal was dropped due to bickering about who would pay for the hospital. It was not until 1830 that the United States built its first permanent naval hospital at Norfolk, Virginia.[68]

Books on the medical aspects of war described how illness affected the outcome of a battle or war. Typhus was frequently used to explain the relief of sieges and the defeat of armies. The degree to which scurvy affected the outcome of the war at sea is difficult to judge. It is clear, however, that the failure to invade England by the combined French and Spanish fleets was caused in part by the outbreak of scurvy and other illnesses aboard the French and Spanish ships.

− 5 −

Syphilis and the
Loss of New York

With the final evacuation of Boston on March 17, 1776, by the British and the entrance of the Colonials in their place, the commander-in-chief next turned his eyes south to New York. He knew a British seaborne expedition from Halifax would try to take that city. The danger of splitting the colonies in such an event was self-evident. Washington ordered the New England regiments and those of Pennsylvania, Virginia, and Maryland (8,000 men) to proceed south. When Washington reached New York, he was aware it would be impossible to defend it against an enemy with control of the seas. The enemy could pick a time and place to land, and it would be impossible to defend the entire area with his army of 20,000 men. Part of his army was militia—largely from the local area where the fighting would occur. In the battle for New York and in many subsequent battles, the militia was often useless. The militiamen often left their positions on the line at the first salvo from the enemy, thus leaving a gap in the front the enemy could use to advantage. Also, they stole vehicles and supplies to make their retreat. The Continental Congress demanded that Washington defend New York, and unlike many military men who came after him, Washington recognized the authority of the civilian Congress over the military, and he did the best he could with an indefensible position. A third of his army crossed to Brooklyn, and the rest remained in Manhattan. Many of these men who had lived through the Battle of Bunker Hill recognized the benefits of trenches and earthen fortifications. Needless to say, they fell with vigor to digging fortifications necessary for the defense of the city.[1]

While the men of the line prepared to defend the city, the medical department tried to cope with the medical needs of the army. New York was no exception to the usual problems of no supplies and no money to purchase them. Morgan had a limited supply of material, but he refused to turn over to the wasteful regimental surgeons any of his precious stores kept at the general hospital. He advised the regimental surgeons to meet and send formal applications to Congress to describe their needs, and he sent them lists of material they could put in their requests. Some of these requests were actually granted by

Congress. He also sent the surgeons copies of diets they could use to treat the diseases they would face. The surgeons and their patients represented a block of votes that Congress could not overlook. The regimental surgeons set up hospitals in barns and houses behind the lines. They treated the sick before the battle in these makeshift places with their limited stores. Their colonels, as well as their sick charges, joined the surgeons in their refusal to send the casualties to the general hospital. The sick brought their own blankets to the regimental "hospital," placed them on some straw, and hoped for the best.[2]

The provincial committee of safety of New York ordered the medical college authorities to vacate the hall at King's College and on April 16, 1776, this became the main general hospital in New York City. Unlike patriotic Boston, the population of New York City was predominantly Loyalist. Whereas the population of Massachusetts welcomed the largely New England troops, the New Yorkers did not care for the invasion of their city by soldiers from seven different colonies. Bay Staters supplied food, gifts, clothing, and medical equipment when called upon. New York citizens, except for the prostitutes, kept their distance from the army. Some New England troops had been inoculated against smallpox during the blockade of Boston. The southern troops, however, brought smallpox as well as typhoid or typhus and dysentery to the growing army.

Prior to the army's occupation, the streets were cleaned under the control of the vestry men of the city. However, these were powerless to prevent the troops from throwing body wastes and other debris into the streets. Sanitary control broke down. On May 4, 1776, Washington ordered the regimental colonels to order their quartermasters to clean the streets of the encampments and to dig "necessaries," which were to be covered each morning with fresh earth and to be filled in at set intervals. New ones were to be dug immediately to replace them. The quartermasters were to burn all "filth and carrion." Since orders are on paper, and soldiers do as they wish, enteric disease became rampant. In addition, the water supplies were contaminated. The soldiers washed themselves and their clothing in the ponds that served as drinking water for the city. In New York, the weather cast a baleful eye on the inept work of the colonials. It was a hot and dry spring and summer, with little or no rainfall for three months, which further limited the drinking water for the city. Camp fever broke out. Washington believed this came from food, and he ordered that meat was not to be boiled or fried. Others felt it came from bathing while the body was overheated, so the men were forbidden to bathe during the heat of the day. The men were permitted to bathe their bodies in the cool of the morning and evening when the soldiers felt it was not necessary.

By the end of July, the results of the breakdown in sanitation were seen. Deaths and disability from dysentery and "putrid fever" increased. To this was added smallpox. Approximately a third of Washington's army was ineffective due to disease before hostilities started. On August 27, 1776, Washington wrote

Congress that in some regiments none of the field officers were medically fit for duty. General Greene, one of Washington's most competent officers, was out of action due to disease, and he was replaced on Long Island by old General Israel Putnam of Connecticut. By September 1776 the Continental sick were such a drain on the army that it was decided to discharge the sick if they could make their way home. The rest of the sick would come under the care of the director general, Morgan. Dr. Morgan sent scouts to New Jersey to look for hospital sites. Several were set up at Newark and Hackensack. In mid–September the colonials were pushed out of New York. The were replaced by the British who found it to be one vast stinkhole.

The opposing British forces were not free of disease. However, they had fewer casualties than the Americans. The Hessians suffered from scurvy, and the British had fevers and sore throats. One Englishman commented. "If any author had an inclination to write a treatise upon stinks and ill smells, he never could meet with more subject matter than in New York."[3]

The British from Halifax were joined by troops ferried from the south under Clinton and Cornwallis returning from their unsuccessful attempt to take Charleston, South Carolina. Troops also arrived directly from England under General Richard Howe. These were predominantly hired Hessians. A flotilla of at least one hundred British ships anchored in New York Bay. The fleet took Staten Island without opposition, and the troops reformed. On May 22, 1776, 88 barges full of British and Hessians left Staten Island under naval protection. Fifteen thousand men were landed at present-day Fort Hamilton, Brooklyn. Washington further cut his New York army to reinforce Long Island. Now half of his force was in Brooklyn, and half in Manhattan, separated by water controlled by the British fleet. On August 26 the British moved around the colonial defenses on Long Island and rolled up the American army. The colonials lost 500 dead and 1,500 prisoners of war. The remnants pulled behind earthworks at Brooklyn Heights. Howe ordered his engineers to build fortifications opposite the colonials. The British would approach the American army under cover along routes designated by British sappers. Washington was soon aware that the battle was lost, and he made plans to evacuate his army to Manhattan. On August 29, as night fell, a storm and fog blew in. Under cover of darkness and thanks to the rowing ability of Glover's Marbleheaders and Hutchinson's sailors from Salem, Massachusetts, the remains of the Brooklyn army were brought to safety in Manhattan. At this point, Washington should have given up Manhattan and moved his army to Westchester. However, he tried to defend Manhattan Island with a dispirited army. Nathaniel Greene wanted to burn the city and move upstate. Congress finally gave Washington permission to give up Manhattan. The general lacked transportation to move his army, and his army was again split. The main part of the army was pulled to Harlem Heights (125th Street), and another 4,000 men with artillery and stores remained at the Battery. On September 15, the

British and Hessians landed on what would be East 34th Street from Long Island and gradually took over Manhattan. The colonials rested on Harlem Heights and were joined by the men from the Battery who were led around the British by Aaron Burr, thus allowing the Americans to score a temporary victory in the hollow below Harlem Heights. There was considerable delay in further movement by the opposing armies as September slid into October. Washington left Manhattan covered by a guard under Glover. He reached White Plains on October 28. Manhattan was lost and with it Fort Washington with 2,000 prisoners of war.[4]

Before we leave the debacle at New York, let us return to the period when the colonials dug fortifications in New York. The civilian population was not particularly friendly, but the prostitutes in this seaport community were distinctly friendly. Syphilis, a major problem in Europe, was not a serious problem in the colonies. There were certainly pockets of venereal disease in the areas that immediately surrounded the harbors of Boston, New York, Philadelphia, and Charleston. The disease was probably reintroduced to the eastern seaboard by European sailors. Infected men passed the disease on to the friendly women and the "business" women in the seaport, who in turn passed it on to some of the locals. The majority of the population, however, had little or no experience with the disease. It was not that the people in the hinterland were chaste, it was simply a matter of the isolation of most farming communities. The men in the colonial army were brought to a "foreign" city away from their wives and family restraints. With time on their hands and money in their pockets, they fell into the vice of "sin city." This continues to be a problem for the military, especially in foreign ports.

Theories of the Syphilis Epidemic in Europe

FROM THE NEW WORLD TO THE OLD?

There were two theories to explain the emergence of syphilis in the western world. The first was that Columbus's sailors brought it back with them from their first visit to Hispaniola. The second was that it had been present in the Old World for many centuries and became virulent perhaps due to a mutation. The first theory was the most widely held. The trail of devastation wrought by syphilis in Europe could be traced to the period after the discovery of the New World.

Ruy Diaz de Isla was a physician from Baeza near Palos. He was the first western physician to see and treat the new disease. He examined the literature of Europe as well as that of the Arabs to find a hint about what he saw, but none of the past experts could help him. Forty years after his investigation and observations, he wrote a book about the disease. Columbus's three-ship armada reached Hispaniola, and the men naturally found relief with the aboriginal females. The disease in Hispaniola must have been present for generations, and the populace had a considerable level of immunity, so they were not covered with skin lesions, deformed, or disfigured. Certainly a woman with active secondary disease would cause the men to stay "buttoned up." (The primary chancre in women is not obvious and the tertiary disease is not infectious.) The *Nina* and *Pinta* with their complement of sailors returned home (the *Santa Maria* was destroyed). It was conceivable that the men suffered the chancre in the harbor or on board ship, and they may have reached home port before or with waning secondary lesions. The ships arrived at Palos on March 15, 1493. Shortly thereafter, Columbus, with some Indians and crewmen, set off for Barcelona, where the monarchs were visiting, to regale them with his discoveries. The trip was over land, with stops along the way. Palos and the places along the way were full of "groupies" who were willing to give their favors to these great explorers with exciting stories to tell. A line of syphilis followed the initial course taken. The men left behind by Columbus then followed their leader to Barcelona via Seville with further dissemination of this "present" from the New World.[5]

FROM THE OLD WORLD TO THE NEW?

The alternative theory did not accept Hispaniola as the source. It claimed that the treponeme started as a saprophyte living on dead organic matter, then became a commensal living in harmony with an animal host, and finally became a parasite of man with variable virulence. The earliest example of this mild relationship between the spirochete and the human host was the disease "pinta." Pinta was a rather mild illness affecting the inhabitants of the Caribbean littoral. It was predominantly a skin disease with a rash that healed with depigmented or hyperpigmented areas on the skin. Pinta meant painted. It may have been brought to the New World over the land bridge between Alaska and Siberia. The next and more potent spirochetal parasitic relationship was frambesia or yaws. Frambesia was derived from the French word meaning raspberry, which described the skin lesions. This was a non-venereal disease seen in warm, moist climates such as Equatorial Africa. It was probably brought to America with the slave trade. It was seen where very little clothing was worn due to climatic conditions. The lesion occurred primarily on the skin, but it could be followed by ulcers with deeper involvement as well as bony disease. Bejel or endemic non-venereal syphilis was the third rung. This disease was seen in hot, dry areas where people were covered. The lesion was spread from the mouth and lips of the victim usually to the hands of others. All of these illnesses occurred in young children who then built up an immunity to the spirochete. Supposedly, the advance of bejel to true venereal syphilis followed the development of cities with close living and dressing and where the only contact between humans was sexual. (Here the theory, like the treponeme, seems too fragile to survive.) The sudden widespread epidemic seen in Europe at the beginning of the sixteenth century was blamed on pockets of the disease throughout Europe that suddenly flared up as a result of a mutant strain of the treponeme. Further proof that the diseases were due to gradual evolution of the treponeme was that the different treponemal organisms could not be differentiated from each other. None of them were able to be cultured. They appeared the same in a dark field examination and all gave the same results in the V.D.R.L. and FTA-ABS tests used to diagnose syphilis. (A weak argument at best. The smegma bacillus and the tuberculosis bacillus are first cousins, but the problems they produce are poles apart.)

Both camps of theorists pointed to the Bible to support their beliefs. The "Hispaniola group" believed the epidemic that killed thousands of Jews in Gaza could not be syphilis, because it did not kill that rapidly. It was probably bubonic plague. The concept of the sins of the father visited upon the sons to the third generation, mentioned in the Old Testament, could have been a description of congenital syphilis. This could not be syphilis, however, because lues did not extend beyond the second generation. Descriptions of men with running sores in the groin were not applicable, because glands rarely break down in syphilis. This usually occurred in lymphopathia venereum.

The group that favored the belief that syphilis existed first in the Old World advanced other arguments from the Bible, citing descriptions of a disease mentioned in Genesis, Leviticus, Deuteronomy, and Proverbs that could be interpreted as secondary syphilis. It was felt that David developed syphilis from Bathsheba and that Lot's affliction was syphilis. In addition to the Bible, they also pointed to Roman literature where there were descriptions of ulcers in a disease caught from prostitutes. They also claim there were no bony pathological findings of syphilis in the pre–Columbian mummies of Peru. The bony lesion found in the South American disease was not luetic. They claimed this was "espundia," a disease of South America. This was countered by the "Hispaniola group," because there were no bony lesions of syphilis in Europe before 1495. However, some bony lesions of leprosy could resemble syphilis. Furthermore, when the Spaniards reintroduced it to the mainland of North and South America, it acted like a virulent new epidemic among the Indians. The "Old World" believers felt that Spain's expulsion of its Jews in 1492 helped spread syphilis to Asia and Africa, where they were accepted by the local population.

HISTORICAL TREATMENT

In his book, *Tractado Contra el Mal Serpentino*, de Isla called it the serpentine disease, because the eruptions and disease were as hideous, loathsome, feared, and ugly as the serpent. It was originally thought to come from the air, and the "science of astrology" was used to explain its presence. Similarly, God's anger at the sin of lust and its gratification were cited. However, physicians early recognized that it came from sexual intercourse. The term venereal is derived from Venus, goddess of love. However, they had to find other ways to catch the horror in order to explain why priests and nuns developed syphilis. Drinking and eating utensils were blamed by physicians who believed in the precepts of the Catholic church. (Actually, the treponema is a very fragile organism that dies almost immediately after leaving the moisture and warmth of the human body.) De Isla believed the disease was in the same class as leprosy. He described three stages. The first was the skin eruption on the genital organ and the presence of buboes (nodes) in the groin. He also described a purulent discharge from the penis and pain in the groin (his patients obviously had gonorrhea as well, and they may have had chancroid). The chancre was on the prepuce or corona. It was not painful and healed by itself in two to four months. The second stage came on with rheumatic pains followed by skin lesions. This could occur months to years after the chancre healed. He believed this stage was not contagious (actually, it is wildly contagious, particularly from the condylomata in warm wet areas of the body). There were buboes over the body with lesions in the throat, lips, and eyes. The third stage followed very soon if not treated. The patient developed fever, swelling, and bone disease and then died in horrible pain. (This was probably a description of the late second stage, because these writers were not aware of the central nervous system, cardiovascular, and other systemic symptoms of the third stage.) To prevent the disease, de Isla urged his reader to wash the penis with water or urine after intercourse. The author urged doctors to examine prostitutes regularly. If infected, they should be put out of business for one year. They could work if they had ulcers (wrong). He also urged that maids be examined frequently, particularly those employed by women in love. (He probably alluded to their swains relieving their urges with the woman's maid.)

He advised the following treatment if the patient had the disease: no sex, no fatigue, no alcohol. A healthy diet of meat, vegetables, and fruit was prescribed. The patient ate fish once a week (preferably on Friday), and meals generally were kept light. The patient arose early, took mild exercise in the morning, and went to bed early. A physic for constipation was prescribed. De Isla recommended a mercurial ointment to the chancre if it did not disappear spontaneously. The patient was bled for congestion. If the patient developed balanitis (again, probably gonorrhea), the chancre was cut out. If the patient was otherwise in good health, the area was cauterized. For the second stage, the sufferer was treated before skin lesions occurred with a mercurial unction started with a half ounce. This was increased by half ounces daily for nine days. The head of the penis was washed with lye once weekly until cured. If scalp lesions developed, the scalp scabs were not washed if a purulent drainage was present. If a discharge was present, the hair was shaved and the head washed with lye or wine in manchined (a poisonous fruit from America) every three days. This was followed by the application of mercury powder or silver sublimate ointment. For ulcers of the face, mercury was rubbed in, followed by silver and cow's fat. For mouth ulcers, mercury gargles were given as well as goat's milk. For eruptions on hands and feet, physics, goat ointment, and cloves were used. De Isla observed that when the patient developed an additional disease with fever, such as malaria, this would arrest the disease. This observation was forgotten for centuries until malaria was injected to treat paresis in this century. The patient had to stay indoors for 30 days while on mercury. He did not wash with water. He rubbed the mercury into his wrists, elbows, shoulders, sternum, knees, ankles, abdomen and spine until salivation started. This was repeated for five nights. It was rubbed in 18 times and required a total of 15 ounces of mercurial ointment. The salivation indicated absorption of the mercury with a systemic effect.[6]

Berenger de Corpi was the first physician credited with the use of mercury to treat syphilis. He kept it a secret and became wealthy. Vegas and Fallopius introduced the treatment to the public. Mercury was used for many years for skin eruptions. Arabs used it as a plaster or ointment and Vegas and Fallopius initially used it this way. Vegas, perhaps recognizing its systemic nature, also used mercury internally. They used red oxide of mercury and oxygenated muriate of mercury applied to the parts affected. Forty years after syphilis appeared, mercury pills were sold publicly. They were called pills of Barbarosa and came from Turkey. They contained mercury, rhubarb, scammony, musk, amber, and honey well triturated and formed into a mass with lemon syrup. Doctors were initially afraid to prescribe it because it was a poison. They tried sudorifics for years. Guaiacum officinale was used. It was a tree from Santo Domingo introduced to Europe in 1517. Sassafras and sarsaparilla, used by the American Indians, were also brought to Europe to be tried.

Eigteenth-Century Theory and Therapy

Gonorrhea has been known far and wide for millennia, and no group can take "credit" for its introduction to the human race. There are suggestive writings from Ancient Egypt, China, Japan, the Old Testament, and Assyria. Hippocrates described strangury (blockage and pain of the urethra). Rhazes and Avicenna described urethral strictures and the use of a catheter to relieve them. William of Saliceto, in the thirteenth century, described the disease well enough to make the diagnosis. Despite the existence of this disease for millennia and the comparatively recent appearance of syphilis, many physicians felt gonorrhea and syphilis were manifestations of the same disease.[7]

Dr. John Hunter, of anatomy and surgery fame, set the clock back on the study of venereal disease by his experiment on himself in 1767. He injected into his own urethra some material taken from the genitals of a patient with a discharge. He later developed a mucous drip and the onset of a chancre. He therefore assumed that gonorrhea and syphilis were different manifestations of the same disease. Obviously, the discharge was contaminated with the treponema. Most medical writers prior to Hunter agreed with this belief and were "vindicated" by his experiment.[8] It took ninety years before the two were separated after studies in France by Philippe Record.

Dr. F. Swediaur of London, a physician in the late eighteenth century, discussed what we would call syphilis. Syphilitic ulcers on the genitals (chancre) developed the third or fourth day after an "impure connection." (This is a little early.) The obstetrician could get a similar lesion on his fingers from delivery. In the treatment of this ulcer, the physician was admonished to make sure it was from syphilis. Mercury was given internally and red oxide of mercury in lard was applied topically, or muriate of mercury as a powder was applied. It could also be applied by mixing it with the patient's saliva. Treatment was continued until the ulcer healed, and all hardness of the skin disappeared. The patient was given mercury internally, or buboes developed. The chancre usually healed by itself in a few weeks, but the use of mercury internally and externally prevented the generalized buboes, which were part of the secondary stage of syphilis. Mercury was a reasonable specific for syphilis. If the ulcer did not respond to mercury, it was treated with a saturated decoction of guaiacum or sarsaparilla. Sometimes opium taken internally and by application helped. At other times a lotion of zinc with camphor or copper sulfate could be applied.[9]

Dr. Buchan talked about gonorrhea, and his initial treatment was sensible for the time. However, he also resorted to mercury. (Perhaps he used mercury as an eighteenth-century penicillin to treat all manner of venereal infections.) For gonorrhea he advised a cooling diet made up of vegetables and milk broth. The patient refrained from "heating" foods, such as alcohol and spices. It was recommended that there should be no heavy exercise or sex. The part was bathed in warm milk and water. (There must have been something in milk, particularly when added to bread, because this was used frequently in many poultices. Perhaps we have lost something in modern emollient therapy that they used.) Sweet oil or linseed tea was injected into the urethra to relieve symptoms. To cure, astringent injections were given—white vitriol in rose water three times a day. Gentle purges were prescribed. Bleeding was necessary for severe inflammation. Nitre and gum arabic were used orally to increase urine flow; or gum arabic and cream of tartar, which was a milder diuretic, was recommended. An emollient clyster acted as a fomentation for inflamed parts. A poultice was applied to the part made of wheat bread and milk, with fresh butter or sweet oil or warm water. The testicles were supported in a truss. After inflammation subsided, mercury was started. Mercury pills were given three or more a day until the mouth hurt. Calomel or corrosive sublimate might be used instead. The patient was advised not to take so much as to cause salivation. If mercury caused griping, it was counteracted with senna. If the patient could not take mercury orally, a preparation of blue ointment (prepared with quicksilver and hog's lard) was rubbed into the thighs at bedtime while the patient stood before a fire, then the area was covered with flannel. This was done nightly unless it caused mouth symptoms. After the inflammation subsided, gonorrhea was at a final stage—the gleet. To treat gleet, the debilitated blood vessels were braced. There was a need for strong astringents. These included bark, alum, vitriol, galls, and tincture of gum kino. These were injected into the urethra. A cold bath as a bracer was taken every morning for four weeks. If this did not cure gleet, mercury and medicines to treat the acrimony (sarsaparilla or sassafras) were suggested. If not healed, it was due to ulcers in the urethra. Medicated bougies were inserted for as long as the patient would tolerate them.[10]

Present day medical practice will look with horror at the treatment prescribed. We use a few shots of penicillin or qther antibiotics to cure this problem. However, think back to the early thirties in this century before sulfa came into use. The urologist used similar treatments and injections to cure this social disease. With the development of antibiotics, the urologist had to turn to another source of remuneration. Fortunately, men lived longer, and removal of their prostates replaced the treatment of gonorrhea to finance houses and automobiles.

Syphilis and armies were like Hansel and Gretel. They went into the unknown hand-in-hand. Baron Von Swieten in his *Medicine in the Armies* spent considerable time with lues venera. As mentioned, his work reached the English army through Dr. Pringle. Von Swieten felt syphilis consisted of many different disorders, subject to the part affected. He knew ulcers of the penis were chancres, warts on the genitals were venereal verrucae, and swellings in the groin were buboes. He knew that lues venera inside the urethra was different from the other forms. The soldier here had difficulty passing urine and had a discharge. He pointed out that syphilis could "get into the blood" (which, of course, it does very early in its course). It could spread over the entire body, and where it grasped a foothold, it created the problem seen. In the skin it formed a rash, and then pustules formed and broke down to produce ulcers and crusts. It could affect the fatty tissue and led to ulcers that burrowed and caused terrible scars. It could involve the throat and roof of the mouth. This resulted in spots, then hoarseness, followed by pain when the sufferer swallowed. The lesions, wherever they were seen, destroyed the soft parts and then attacked the contiguous bone. In the mouth, there was destruction of the bones of the palate. The bones developed localized swellings. The soft bumps were gummy, the hard ones were exostoses. The end result was caries, with bone pain worse at night. If the bones were "corroded," cure was difficult, and the problems would recur.[11]

The writings of eighteenth-century army surgeons were brief and to the point. They did not spend time with thoughts about the nature of the disease, as was common among the learned medical scholars who preceded them. Instead, they were excellent observers and observed what seemed to work. They discarded what did not work.

Conclusion

I have not seen any reports of the treatment of venereal disease by the American Revolutionary surgeons. That it was a problem can be deduced from the short-lived congressional law to fine officers $10 and enlisted men $4 if they developed venereal disease. They hoped to harvest enough money from this source to supply blankets and bed clothing for the sick in hospitals. Certainly, men like Cochran knew the treatment of venereal disease in the English army from their experience with British surgeons during the French and Indian War. This knowledge must have been conveyed to the surgeons from rural communities who joined their regiments. The university-trained physicians who gravitated to the upper echelons of the medical department had studied syphilis in their courses in "Physick."

Was syphilis a serious problem in the short New York occupation? I believe it was, because a "foreign" army always attracts the prostitutes of the community. During his stay in New York City, Washington commented on the number of his troops unfit for duty because of venereal disease. Whereas the civilian population remained aloof, the *filles de joie* were more than friendly to the men with money in their pockets. The short encounter with Venus frequently resulted in a long encounter with Mercury. Were syphilis and gonorrhea as destructive as the enteric fevers that broke out in New York as a result of the breakdown of the sanitation system in that city? Of course not! However, a soldier who could not urinate because of pain, had painful swollen testicles and joints, who developed urinary obstruction, or whose mouth was so sore from mercury that he could not eat, was hardly fit for duty.

— 6 —

Dysentery and the
Prisoners of War

Recently, the federal government struck a medal that was awarded to all service people who were prisoners of war. It was the last of a series of acts taken to recognize the hardships endured at the hands of a foreign enemy. I worked in a veterans' hospital for a time, and I am aware of the special treatment afforded these veterans. There was a special section for POWs, and they usually received complete postwar care if they wished to have it. Except for the destruction of allied prisoners in Japanese hands (including the Death March) and the wholesale death of Russian prisoners held by the Nazis, prisoners could hope to be exchanged sometime during their captivity. They might return physically and emotionally impaired, but they could look forward to seeing home and family sometime in the future.

In the history of warfare, this was a new development. In antiquity, war was fought to take another's territory. The enemy had to be destroyed. The aboriginal inhabitants were kept from the reproduction of their kind to make way for the new conquering inhabitants. Consequently, male prisoners were killed, and their women and children were taken into the tribes of the victors. Here they were raised in the tradition of the new masters. The next level up after annihilation of the enemy was slavery. The vanquished who were injured were killed outright. The uninjured might be taken to the victor's homeland to become slaves, particularly if they had a skill that was useful. Greek slaves were taken to Rome as teachers, physicians, etc. Others could be used as household or farm help. Those who could not be used were sold. If a prisoner could be sold at auction, he could buy his own freedom. This self-purchase from slavery led to the concept of ransom. Ransom could be paid by the soldier, his family, or his nation. In warfare in the Middle Ages, common people put their lives at risk, not for patriotism or fealty to an overlord, but rather to plunder and hopefully to catch someone of high station for ransom. A "king's ransom" could make a common soldier comfortable for life. It could purchase land to be passed on to his children.[1] This was nicely described by Paré. During one of the constant wars between France and the Austrian-Spanish-Netherlands empire, a group of Spanish soldiers captured Monsieur de Bauge. They did not know his worth, but a leader of the emperor's forces recognized him as a gentleman because his shoes and feet were clean, and his socks were white and thin. He gave thirty écus for him, enough for a night of drinking. The new captor wanted 15,000 crowns to be paid to two merchants who would act as intermediaries. The story ended unhappily for the second captor. The Duc de Savoi and the Queen of Hungary took the prisoner because he was "too large a morsel" for his captor. He received nothing for his prize. (Some businesses turn a profit, some do not.)

The concept of ransom did not stop brutality toward prisoners. Paré described the siege of the Château of Hesden in 1553. The army of Charles V gave terms to the French defenders. All of the nobility and officers would be taken for ransom. The common soldiers would give up their arms and leave. However, when the Emperor's forces entered the fortress, his Spanish troops killed prisoners savagely. Those saved for ransom had their genitals bound with arquebus cord tied to a pike. They yanked the cord with great violence and derision "as if they wished to sound a chime." The prisoners were asked to what family they belonged. If they showed no hope for profit, they were killed cruelly. If not, "their genitalia would have fallen into gangrene and mortification." Generally, their throats were cut.[2]

The custom of slavery for prisoners of war persisted until the eighteenth century in parts of Europe, as is verified by the writings of Rousseau and Montesquieu who deplored the poor treatment of the prisoners and slavery of belligerents. However, it was gradually becoming customary to deprive prisoners of their freedom during the war, but to restore it once hostilities had ceased.[3] (This is the concept followed in "modern" warfare.) There was one shining spot in the total picture of inhumanity of captor to prisoners that has been relegated to the sidelines in the recent past. This was the concept of parole. The prisoner of war gave his word to his captor that he would obey all the stipulations exacted by the victor in return for freedom of movement. This was a common practice in the American Revolution. The early days of the American invasion of Canada were crowned with success, and several forts along the water route between New York and Canada were easily taken by the Americans. The British officers were freed after they accepted the following:

> That the commissioned officers taken in the forts of Chambly and St. John be put on their parole of honor that they will not go into or near any seaport town, nor further than six miles from the respective places of residence, without leave of the Continental Congress and that they will carry on no political correspondence whatsoever, on the subject of the dispute between Great Britain and these colonies, as long as they remained prisoners. By order of Congress, John Hancock, President November 17, 1775.[4]

The benefit to the captors was the savings of resources needed to feed and guard the prisoners. Interestingly, the enlisted men frequently had no "parole of honor" to give.

The best thing a nation could do for its soldiers taken by the enemy was to trade them for the prisoners it held. This was not done frequently in our war with England. Early in the hostilities England considered any captured soldiers traitors rather than prisoners of war and thus not eligible for exchange. When Americans were released, they were often so debilitated as a result of the poor treatment at British hands that they died shortly after exchange, or they were sent home and spread their infectious diseases to their families and communities. Furthermore, Washington did not favor exchange because he believed that the British would return their exchanged prisoners back to the ranks to avoid the need to replace them with men sent 3,000 miles on a destructive sea voyage. However, there was an exchange of prisoners on the battlefield without government knowledge or interference. The commanders of the opposing armies carried out the exchange on their own authority.[5]

It has been said that "history is written by the victors." We were taught that the colonials treated our prisoners well. This is probably true, although they did have prison ships off New London.[6] The copper mine that served as a prison at East Granby, Connecticut, was dark, dank, and stayed at a constant cool 56 degrees Fahrenheit. More American Tories were kept in the mine than British soldiers. Unlike the British, the colonials had "back country" where prisoners could be kept safely without fear of escape through a hostile population. The first major group of prisoners was taken after the British withdrew from Boston. British ships, unaware of a change of status of the port of Boston, were seized, and their soldiers and sailors were taken prisoner. Similarly, in the early days of the invasion of Canada, British soldiers were taken. The greatest haul in the war came from the defeat of Burgoyne at Saratoga. The victors could not handle the mass of prisoners taken and signed a "convention" with the vanquished. (Gates gave this convention without consulting Congress.) The prisoners were to be marched to Cambridge, there to board English ships bound for England. They gave their parole not to take up arms during the remainder of the war. Congress initially approved the convention but later repudiated it. The British and Hessians were marched to Rutland, Massachusetts. The Hessians were detached at Rutland, and the British were marched to Virginia, and then to Pennsylvania where they remained until the end of hostilities.

The Hessians fared rather well in Rutland. The officers were quartered in private homes and the enlisted men lived in barracks and were free to walk about town. They could also hire themselves out to local farmers. The Hessian soldiers were under the medical care of Julius Friedrich Wasmus, a squadron surgeon, who kept a journal. This position was third in rank among surgeons of the line and was subordinate to the regimental surgeon and the company surgeon. He was probably the equivalent of a surgeon's mate in the

British or American armies. One of the surgeon's duties in the Hessian army was a throwback to medieval times—he was also a barber and had to shave the officers daily.

The Hessian medical service was set up for 17,000 Hessian troops. There was a hospital with physicians and surgeons as well as a staff in the field. The hospital table of organization listed four physicians, two surgeons general, eight surgeons, four apothecaries, two purveyors, three clerks, four commissioners, and two cooks. The field staff had 45 regimental surgeons. Under them there was one surgeon per company. Under the company surgeon was the squadron surgeon. The surgeon of the German armies was held in low esteem by the Americans as well as by his own troops.

Wasmus carried out routine medical care of the soldiers around him. Food was scarce for the prisoner of war. Homesickness was severe, and a few were reported to have died of it, but the more likely explanation was the presence of a fatal disease, and the patient probably expressed anxiety about his return home before he died. Scurvy was a serious problem in camp. Dysentery developed among the prisoners of war living with the farmers but not among those in the barracks. There were no deaths reported from that disease. The men also required treatment for chest diseases, such as tuberculosis as well as venereal disease. (Presumably they fraternized with the locals.) Despite all these hazards, only ten Hessians died during captivity from sickness and injury. Many Hessian troops died on the trip over to America, and when it was time for repatriation, several preferred to stay on this continent. Several surgeons remained in Canada. Some were given permission to stay and others took "French leave."[7]

Between Saratoga and Yorktown a few British army prisoners were taken. The British taken at Yorktown were marched to Winchester, Virginia, and then to Frederick, Maryland, for internment until the war was formally ended two years later.

British mariners fared considerably better than did any other group. Most were taken by American privateers and brought to the home port of the American ship. Once on shore, no specific action was taken. It was too expensive to keep them in prisons.

Neither the central government nor the state governments were willing or able to support them. Consequently, these men were turned loose and could fend for themselves. Many probably blended into the English-speaking community and became inhabitants. Many had been impressed into the British navy and had to undergo the harsh treatment meted out to able seamen by ships' officers. Therefore, few tried to return to active British duty. Very few of them were exchanged for American seamen.

Some signed on as privateers on American vessels or joined the Continental navy.[8] This was an extremely dangerous decision for them. If retaken by the British, they were tried as deserters and hanged. One prisoner described the ghastly hanging of a deserter. He was placed on a floating platform in a river with the noose in place attached to a stable gibbet. As the tide went out, the platform dropped and the victim slowly strangled. This might require four hours to complete the deadly task.[9]

One group needed special consideration: those injured in battle and their caregivers. Prior to the War of the Austrian Succession, no specific treaties had been signed concerning military hospitals overrun by the opposing army. An agreement signed by the French and English at that time proclaimed that military hospitals were neutral and neither medical staff nor patients were subject to capture, retention, or exchange as prisoners of war. The Continental Congress was happy to abide by that treaty's concept. However, early in the war, the British government did not consider the Continental Congress a government, and the Revolution was not an authentic war. This was borne out by the situation that developed after the capture of the fort at Chambly. Dr. Huddleston, surgeon of the Royal Fusiliers, was taken prisoner. He requested his release and transfer to Quebec on the basis of this treaty. Congress responded positively and set him free with a letter to General Carlton to release all American physicians and surgeons held captive. Further, it specified that if a hospital was captured, patients should receive the same food and care as the enemy sick. Patients and attendants were not to be considered as prisoners of war. If Carlton did not agree, Dr. Huddleston, on parole, had to return to captivity. The accord was refused by Carlton. Huddleston returned and went into captivity.

Later in the war, the British Parliament relented and allowed medical people of the belligerent army to cross battle lines and treat their nationals. The Americans reciprocated.[10] During the war, Dr. Rush was able to cross the lines to care for Americans in British hospitals. He was properly impressed with the conduct of the British hospitals and strongly criticized the American ones.[11] Another group allowed to cross lines under a flag of truce were the wives of officers who were casualties. Wives and families of British and Hessian officers crossed the ocean with their husbands and were permitted into American hospitals to nurse their spouses.[12]

The British faced a serious problem when they had to feed and house large numbers of prisoners of war taken at one time. This situation occurred after the battles for New York City, which were described earlier in the text. Many Americans were taken at Fort Washington and Fort Lee along with those picked up in the retreat from Brooklyn, Manhattan, White Plains, and New Jersey. The British, like every invading army before and after them, controlled only what their troops occupied. They controlled only New York, which suffered a devastating fire in the middle of September 1776 and lost a third of its buildings. There was no hinterland to which they could farm out the prisoners. In addition to their own troops, as well as the largely Tory New York civilians, the

British had 4,000 to 5,000 prisoners of war taken in the fighting. The American officer prisoners signed a parole and were billeted with private families who received the equivalent of two dollars per week per officer for food and lodging. The American officers could receive money from friends and relatives for clothing and shoes and were permitted to exercise and move about the city. The enlisted men were packed into churches, sugar warehouses, King's College, and the hospital. Some were hanged without trial. This, however, was not official policy.

The crowding was most notorious in the sugar warehouses where typhus and smallpox broke out. Twenty men at a time were allowed in the courtyard for thirty minutes of exercise in the open air. Six at a time were allowed at the windows for fresh air. The men had no seats or beds and had to sleep on filthy straw. Deaths reached about 12 per night. Fires for cooking were allowed only one day in three. The staple of their diet was wormy ship's biscuit. Anything the prisoners could catch was eaten with relish. The sick were not separated from the well. The "healthy" could choose to be inoculated when the British doctor visited. Many preferred to inoculate themselves. The men also developed diarrhea and dysentery and were not able to reach the privies. Excrement covered the floor where they sat and slept. There were no lights at night. The sick tried to reach the "tubs" made available for their use and stepped on their fellows who tried to rest on the floor. Churches were converted to hospitals for the sick prisoners, but the men refused to go because no one returned from there. Mortality was estimated at one percent per day. The dead were stacked until they were carted off for burial outside the city limits. The defensive forts and trenches these men had dug several months earlier became their own mass graves.[13]

Prisoners from the Battle of Long Island had earlier been kept in cattle transport ships until New York was taken. Then they were imprisoned on shore. Food was scarce and they were forced to eat insects and rodents. William Cunningham was appointed provost marshal by General Gage. He sold the prisoners the food they were entitled to receive. British rations for a prisoner were one pound of meat, three biscuits, and a quart of water every three days. Cunningham substituted spoiled for fresh food, and he was accused of poisoning prisoners. He hanged prisoners at the slightest provocation. The hanging stopped only when the women of New York petitioned the commanding general to stop the indiscriminate hanging. It seems the screams of the dying men disturbed the civilian population. Complaints about the poor treatment reached General Washington. He contacted the British and sent an investigator under a flag of truce. The complaints against Cunningham were verified; he readily admitted to his activities and was transferred to Philadelphia where he perpetrated the same offenses on American prisoners held there. The provost was then transferred back to New York. It was only after the capture of Burgoyne's army at Saratoga that treatment of American prisoners improved. A British physician, Dr. Debuke, was commissioned by the British to care for the American sick. The Americans claimed that he poisoned and otherwise killed many of his charges. The commissary for prisoners was a lucrative position for any self-serving Briton. He received rations for himself and family plus one guinea per day for provisions for his prisoners. He frequently sold the prisoners their rations and pocketed the money.

Ethan Allen, of Ticonderoga fame, was an officer prisoner of war in New York. He was on parole and was allowed to visit the enlisted men. He saw the starvation and inhumane treatment and believed it was an attempt to destroy the youth of America and to force their enlistment in the British army. Few did! After Princeton and Trenton, the Americans had some British prisoners, and some exchange could take place. The British prisoners were healthy. The American prisoners, some of them imprisoned for six months or more, were ghosts of their former selves. They were diseased scarecrows who died shortly after exchange or spread typhus wherever they went. Ethan Allen estimated that 2,000 died in captivity during this period.[14]

The first British prison ship, the *Whitby*, was anchored in Wallabout Bay, off Brooklyn, October 20, 1776. In addition, the British used the *Prince of Wales* and the *Good Hope*. The inmates on the *Good Hope* burned it to the water line. Some prisoners were shipped to Africa and India to work for the British East India Company. Few returned. One prisoner was able to escape, and he described conditions as well as his mode of escape. The British authorities did not hang prisoners taken on Long Island, but they harassed them on the way to prison. Prisoners were made to sit on coffins with nooses around their necks while being moved.

The terrible treatment meted out to the captured American soldiers in New York prisons cannot be compared to the utter disdain for human life perpetrated on the men on board prison ships. The men captured in land warfare were considered combatants. The privateers taken at sea were treasonous pirates and handled accordingly. Many of the survivors of the horrors left documents for posterity. One of them was Christopher Hawkins, who left a description of prison life aboard the *Jersey*.[15] The *Jersey* started out as a warship, but because of its age and rot, armaments were removed, and it was made into a hospital ship. It was sent to America on May 6, 1776 and became a storeship in New York Harbor. Then it became a hospital ship once more. In the winter of 1779–80, it became the prison ship of horrors. The ship was originally anchored in the East River and was then moved to Wallabout Bay. Sails and rigging were removed. Portholes were closed, and twenty-inch square holes were cut in the sides. These were covered by crossed iron bars to allow in light and air.

Prisoners on board were starved in order to force them to enlist in the British navy. Food meant for the prisoners was stolen by the guards and then sold to the intended recipients. Prisoners were formed into messes of six men.

One of the group would go to the steward to get the daily rations for his mess. If a prisoner stole food from his mess mates, he was punished by them under British supervision. He often died from the punishment. The allowance per man was two-thirds that of a British seaman. Naturally, the bread was moldy and full of worms. Pork was discolored, beef was old and hard, and peas were badly cooked and largely indigestible. The food given the prisoners was very likely condemned for use by the British navy. The meat was cooked in sea water taken from the side of the ship into which had been dumped the daily wastes of a thousand men. The food on the prison ship was never cooked adequately, because firewood was limited. There were no vegetables available except for peas. Water was scarce, full of sediment, and foul-smelling.

At sunset the men were sent below decks where they remained until morning. Only two at a time were allowed on deck after sunset for bowel movements. Practically everyone had diarrhea or dysentery, so many dirtied themselves before they were allowed topside. The holds were hot and stank from the wastes.

In addition to American prisoners of war, the *Jersey* also housed French and Spanish prisoners, who were treated even worse than the Americans, and were kept in the lowest reaches of the ship. These prisoners were more likely to enlist in the British army and navy as a means of escape than were the Americans.

A working party of prisoners, under a prisoner officer, cleaned, removed tubs of feces, and brought up the dead. Those who worked received extra rations plus a little rum. They were allowed on deck before the rest of the prisoners were allowed up each morning. Treachery of a prisoner against his mates, such as leaking an escape plan, resulted in killing of the traitor by the others. If a prisoner was caught in the act of escaping, he was executed summarily. In winter the prisoners did not have enough clothes to keep warm, and had to keep moving or pack together for mutual warmth. Water was shipped to them from Manhattan. As a result of the distance from its source, water was limited. Hawkins pointed out that fresh water flowed in abundance from streams and rivers on Long Island into the Sound. Water buckets were watched on deck by British marines. Prisoners could drink as much as they wished from the buckets, but they could take only one pint back with them for cooking. Pigs were kept on board to provide meat for the crew. The bran used to feed them was frequently stolen by the prisoners.

The more difficult prisoners on the *Jersey* were sent to the prison ship *John*, where conditions were worse. The *Strombolo*, the *Hunter*, and the *Scorpion* were hospital ships anchored along side the *Jersey*. All three could not handle the sick from the *Jersey*, and part of the *Jersey* was used as a hospital deck. The *Hunter* was basically a storeship for medical supplies and quarters for the surgeon's mate and crew. Most patients sent to the hospital ships died. They were not as crowded as the *Jersey*, and they had awnings on deck as well as wind sails at the hatchways to conduct fresh air between decks. Hatchways were left open at night, because the patients were too weak to attempt flight. Several patients occupied one bunk on the hospital ship. When a patient died, his clothes were appropriated by the "nurses." His hair was shaved off for future sale. Many of the nurses on board were thieves, frequently taken from British jails. The patients received a gill of rum and twelve ounces of bread or flour per day. They could pay the nurses to buy more food on shore.

The *Jersey* was visited daily by an army surgeon who made only cursory rounds because of his fear of contagion. Physician prisoners were also brought on board, but they frequently obtained parole and left. Tory physicians and clergy from New York refused to come on board. Mortality rates were appalling; generally only five of thirteen survived. About 11,500 died on board the *Jersey* and the hospital ships in Wallabout Bay. Most deaths were due to typhus, smallpox, or dysentery. The causes were filth, crowding, poor ventilation, limited supplies of contaminated water, a deficiency of protein and vitamins, poor medical care, and lack of sanitation. Mops and buckets were available to the prisoners, but they were too weak and depressed to use them, and the guards took no interest in helping. Finally, the ship was moored in a low, swampy area prone to "miasmas" and associated malaria. The ship was old and decayed with the decomposed remains of marine life in the bilge water.

Men volunteered for the burial detail because they were taken to shore where they dug trenches in the sand. The bodies were laid in these shallow graves covered with a few shovelfuls of sand. No burial ceremony was recited. Anything that could be sold was carried back to the ship by the burial detail. Tides and wind removed the sand covering the older bodies. The exposed bodies and the bones bleached in the sun. After the war Amos Chaney collected over 600 pounds of bones for which he received one cent per pound. They were reburied in 1808 by the Tammany Society in a vault donated by John Jacobson. In 1832 the land was put up for taxes. It was purchased by Benjamin Romaine who built a sepulcher over the vault, which eventually fell into decay.

The British crew of the *Jersey* included a commander, two mates, a steward, a cook, twelve sailors, twelve invalid marines, plus soldiers detailed from their regiments on Long Island. The soldiers were changed every week. Hessians were reasonable guards, English were fair, but the Tories were the worst. On April 19, 1783, all prisoners were released, and the ship was set adrift in deep waters where it sank.

Several thousand American soldiers were taken in the capture of Charleston, South Carolina, and the battle of Camden. They were placed on the prison ship *Concord* in the harbor. Eight hundred died in thirteen months, 530 enlisted with the British army in order to get out of prison, and 740 were exchanged in June 1780. Dr. Hays, the British physician general, refused to help them in any way and was probably responsible for the high death toll. However, the Tory women of Charleston brought food and clothing to the sick Americans on board.[16]

Privateersmen taken in the West Indies were placed on prison ships off Antigua. Heat and yellow fever killed most of them. They were hired off the ships with the promise of garrison duty in Jamaica. Some signed up but escaped to fight again.

If a privateersman was caught by the British, the best situation for him occurred when the ship sailed toward a British port. The prisons in England were far superior to those on the American side of the ocean. However, the trip could be devastating. The treatment the prisoners received on board the ship varied with the captain. Many officers, both in the army and navy, were sympathetic to the colonial cause (less so after independence was declared). Many felt the colonists were Englishmen fighting for the rights of all Englishmen and not the treasonous pirates that Parliament branded them. The problem again was space and provisions. A ship that left a port bound for home was packed to the gunwales. The capture of one or two privateersmen with a complement of about 100 men each created a severe problem for the captain. Some officers encouraged the prisoners to help the crew run the ship in return for extra rations.

Occasionally, there was a British dignitary on board who had suffered at the hands of the revolutionaries, and he could vent his vindictiveness on the prisoners. One such case was described in Fanning's narrative. Fanning's ship, the *Angelica*, was taken by the British ship *Andromeda*. The men were asked to enlist in the Royal Navy, but they all refused and were threatened with execution when they reached England. Their baggage was taken. Any ornaments and clothing desired by the British seamen were stripped from the captives. All other clothing was removed, and they were given a "frock and trousers" and placed in the hold. The *Angelica* was set afire because the British did not have a prize crew to put on board. The prisoners received two-thirds the rations normally given to prisoners of war. They were placed in the hold of the *Andromeda*, which was as hot as an oven. The men stripped naked. They were allowed on deck once a day, one man at a time. The British seamen were severely affected by scurvy, and it was felt they could not put down an uprising in their weakened state. The prisoners thought about this constantly. General Howe, on his way home on the ship, ordered that the prisoners' provisions be cut. They were to receive enough food to keep them alive plus half a pint of water per day per man. However, their prison was near the general's private supplies and just above the water supply of the ship. With Yankee ingenuity, they were able to satisfy their needs. Several British seamen died of scurvy on the trip to England, but the prisoners came out of the hold hale and hearty. The ship docked in Portsmouth, and the prisoners were removed for questioning by an admiralty commission. They were treated properly, then sent to Fortin prison for piracy and high treason.[17]

Israel R. Potter, a patriot who was wounded at Bunker Hill, told a similar story. He was fortunate to be evacuated to a hospital in Cambridge where he recovered. Potter then volunteered for the ship *Washington*, part of George Washington's navy whose purpose it was to interdict the flow of goods to British Tories quartered in Boston. His ship was taken, and Potter was sent as a prisoner of war to England. He and the other prisoners were placed in irons because they had attempted to take the ship. He developed smallpox and was hospitalized at the Marine Hospital at Portsmouth. Potter was then returned to prison from which he escaped and made his way to freedom with the help of British civilians.[18]

Charles Herbert's *Relic of the Revolution* described a situation similar to Fanning's. The ship *Dalton* was taken, and the crew was taken prisoner. The men crossed the ocean in the cable room of their captor. Their clothing was stolen by the British seamen. The prisoners developed scabies and were infested by other vermin. They had no bedding, and there was no room for all to lie down so that even the crew had to sleep in shifts. When the ship arrived in port, conditions improved generally. The sick were taken off and placed in hospitals. Herbert developed smallpox by self-inoculation, because he was reasonably fit and fed and could tolerate it. He was placed in a pox ward of the Royal hospital, which could accommodate 1,500 patients. His diet in the hospital was one pound of beef, one pound of potatoes and three pints of beer daily. Herbert was bathed and given new clothes. The nurses and doctors were kind, and the nurses shared their stores of tea with the patients. After his recovery, he appeared before judges who found him guilty of high treason and sent him to jail. His daily ration in the prison was one pound of bread, one-quarter pound of beef, one pound of greens, one quart of beer, and the soup in which the beef had been boiled. The provisions supplied were not enough for the vigorous seamen, and they were forced to cook grass, snails, hooves found lying around, as well as the refuse from the prison kitchen. The men sometimes sold their clothing for food with serious complications as winter approached. British civilians were able to come and observe them, and many were surprised that the prisoners resembled themselves and spoke English. The prisoners made small objects to sell to the visitors. The money was used to purchase food. If a prisoner was caught attempting to escape, he was placed in the "Black Hole" for 40 days with half rations. In the hole he slept on the bare ground without cover.

Fortin prison was originally built as a hospital for seamen. There were two large spacious buildings separated by a large yard. One building held officers, the other was for able seamen. The prisoners slept in a room 200 by 40 feet in hammocks that were folded away in the daytime, leaving them room for exercise. Next to the buildings there was a level yard three-quarters of an acre in size. In its center was an open shed, which was airy and had seats for the prisoners. They could congregate there when it was very hot. The entire yard was surrounded by an eight-foot-high wall. There was a second wall 20 feet away. Each had a gate. The outer gate was open during the day for communication with the town. The prisoners were confined to the inner court. Outside the fence were civilians armed with clubs and dogs. They received five pounds for every prisoner they caught (one-half guinea per Frenchman). Many guards told the prisoners they would allow them to escape only to pick them up for the reward. Those who attempted escape and were caught would be designated as the last to be exchanged. Those who did escape frequently did so with the help of civilians. They were transported to the coast and placed on small boats called "wherries" to sail to France.

The prisoners tried to run their own affairs. Thieves among them were punished by running the gauntlet. When an infraction had been committed against their guards and all were to be punished, they chose one of their number to admit to the crime and take the punishment for all. He would be paid by his fellows for the ordeal. Traitors of escape plans were whipped mercilessly if caught. The sailors even started schools in prison where they were taught reading, writing, and arithmetic as well as navigation. Men who were captured as ordinary seamen advanced to the rank of masters of vessels as a result of this education. Others who were illiterate learned to read and write. The prisoners could write to other prisoners and even send mail overseas. The prisoners started a "sick fund" from the money they received or could earn. This was used to purchase necessities and drugs for those who were sick among them. There were few deaths from sickness among the prisoners after they settled into their routine. However, with the arrival of a new batch of prisoners, illness broke out again. A shipment of French prisoners brought "spotted fever" (typhus), others brought consumption, smallpox, and other diseases. The prison was "smoked" frequently to prevent epidemics. Mortality overall ran about five to seven percent. The crew of the *Dalton*, 120 strong, spent three years in prison. Of this group, nine men died of illness in prison. As on board ship, treatment on land could be bad depending upon the individual in charge of prisoners. Fanning described an incident of one such captain of the guards. The prisoners used the wall to hang their shirts for drying. This captain started to burn the clothing. When the prisoners tried to grab them to put out the fire, he ordered his men to shoot those prisoners who touched the wall. One prisoner was killed, and several were wounded. Some of the men who became sick in jail under "mysterious" circumstances felt they were being poisoned by their British guards. Some claimed they found ground glass in their bread. Their claims were investigated by the British authorities, but no decision was ever handed down.

Mr. Wren, pastor of a congregation next to the prison, collected money from his parishioners for the prisoners. He was able to give each man 25 pence per week for a period of two months. His activities were not isolated. Prior to the Declaration of Independence, British civilians subscribed

8,000 to 10,000 pounds for prisoners of war relief. The queen was believed to have donated 1,000 guineas of her own money toward this fund. This charity ended with the news of the separation. Benjamin Franklin, among his other duties, raised money to help feed the prisoners in England. Most of the money raised went to purchase additional rations from the civilians. Formal rations were supplied once a day at noon. The hungry men frequently consumed the entire amount at that time.

Prior to the French participation as active combatants, British seamen could not be held prisoner if brought to France. However, this changed after Saratoga and the formal declaration of war. British prisoners who landed in France could be used for exchange. Ben Franklin was active here as well. He corresponded with Britain in an attempt to set up such an exchange. The British initially were not interested, but as the war progressed, they did agree. Fanning's narrative described an exchange, because he was one of the early lucky ones. The exchanged prisoners were lined up and marched through town with a British escort that played "Yankee Doodle." Along the road of march the local inhabitants lined the streets. Some wished them well; others damned them for taking up arms against the king. They were placed on a ship and sent to France. The French called all Americans "Bostonians," welcomed them warmly, and raised money to provide clothes for them. As a sidelight to this tale, Fanning signed on again as a privateer. He was again captured and thrown into another jail. This was filthy with bed bugs, lice, and fleas. He referred to them as "Dutch lice," because he was confined with Dutch prisoners who, he felt, were unusually dirty. Fanning was allowed out of jail during the day after he gave his parole. He spent his days visiting with the young Cornish women, who must have been sympathetic. Fanning was again exchanged and again taken prisoner and again exchanged. The war's end found him on a French ship.[19]

When I read accounts of the kindness of British civilians toward the prisoners, I wondered why they were willing to help these "treasonous rebels." I believe the answer involved the media. The English did not have television or radio, but they had newspapers, which they read avidly. Those who could not read or afford a regular newspaper could listen to someone read it aloud. Seventeen newspapers were published in London at that time, and most were shipped to all parts of the islands. The papers were largely Whiggish in attitude and therefore supported the colonists, and swayed public opinion in their favor. The Tory government realized this power and subsidized writers and newspapers to print the Tory point of view (*London Gazette* and *General Evening Post*). Prior to the outbreak of hostilities, Ben Franklin, colonial agent, bombarded the newspapers with letters and articles to explain the colonists' stand and attitude. He frequently succeeded despite the excesses of Sam Adams and John Hancock. An equally important factor that swayed public opinion was Thomas Paine's *Common Sense*. This was published in England and sold thousands of copies. Despite the outbreak of hostilities and the loss of English lives, the colonials still had their supporters in England. There was a violent uproar when North's government turned to Germany to lease foreign soldiers to fight in America. The powerful merchant class felt the war in its pockets and wanted it stopped. Just as Americans two centuries later became conscientious objectors to our involvement in Vietnam, many British refused to fight colonists in America. British officers tried to sell their commissions when they learned they were being shipped to America. Several general officers refused to take commands in America.[20]

Most deaths among prisoners of war, particularly on the prison ships, were due to smallpox and typhus with yellow fever added in the West Indies. However, dysentery was a "handmaiden" to these frequently fatal illnesses. Men of robust constitution could be shrunken to skin and bones by dysentery, and it could turn morbidity into mortality. Similarly, men with serious diseases could be tipped over by dysentery. We have no statistics for the mortality associated with dysentery in the Revolution. However, statistics kept in London between 1667 and 1720 show that one-fifth to one-third of all deaths were due to intestinal infections. Of course, this included the old and sick and the young without resistance. The deaths among newborns heavily skewed the statistics.

Wherever a large group of people was crowded in a small area under less than clean conditions, there was fertile ground for dysentery. The pathogenic organism was introduced to a group by food, water, and probably flies and improper disposal of human waste. Groups of soldiers away from the routine restrictions of normal life were notoriously susceptible. This applied to the army of Xerxes in 480 B.C. as well as to Theodobert's invasion force in Italy in 538 A.D. Civilians who lived under adverse conditions were not exempt. It was described in epidemic form in all of the English colonies. Dysentery took the old, the young, and the infirm. It weakened the robust so their productiveness was destroyed.[21] Washington was afflicted with dysentery several times. On one occasion, he traveled to Williamsburg to see a specialist for relief.

We know dysentery affected the troops camped around Boston in 1775. It was also a severe disease in Pennsylvania and New Jersey in the summer of 1777 where it was called "putrid diarrhea."[22] Dr. Ebenezer Beardsley described an epidemic in a regiment of Continental troops. The men were quartered in a house. One hundred of the regiment fell sick. The rest of the army and the civilians in the city of New York were free of disease. He believed the disease resulted from quartering the men in low underground rooms or garrets that did not allow free circulation of air. The rooms were small, and the epidemic resulted from the putrid atmosphere. Upon removal to larger airy places, the men recovered, and only two died. Dr. Beardsley used this knowledge in the care of the sick in the army in future campaigns. The doctor found that even in large rooms, those stuck in the corners did poorly. He concluded that people in large airy rooms were less likely to develop putrid fevers. Those who were sick were moved into airy rooms or out in the open. He believed that feather beds and warm close rooms were the principal causes of fatalities.[23]

As mentioned earlier, dysentery was a problem faced by civilian and military populations alike. What did they think about its causes, and how did they try to treat it? Buchan devoted a chapter to the problem in his textbook of medicine. He observed that it was a disease of the spring and autumn. It seemed worse in marshy areas after a hot dry summer. The disease attacked people exposed to night air, or where air was confined and unwholesome. Dysentery was fatal in camps, ships, jails, and hospitals. The disease was brought on by anything that obstructed perspiration or rendered humors putrid, for example, poor diet, bad air or wet clothes. Dysentery was most frequently communicated by infection. Even just the smelling a patient's stool could communicate the infection. Miasmas and odors spread disease. Protection was afforded by smelling something stronger, such as vinegar-soaked pledgets in the "gold headed cane," the symbol of the physician. This concept of the connection between smell and disease survived into the present century. I can remember summers when polio epidemics developed. We wore "amulets" with garlic or other strong smelling material to keep the disease at bay.

Like most medical writers of the time, Buchan was an excellent observer, but he often reached the wrong conclusions from his observations. His description of the symptoms bore this out.

> There is flux of the belly, violent pains of the bowel, blood in the stool with a constant desire to go to stool. The illness starts with a chilliness, a loss of strength, a quick pulse, great thirst, and a desire to vomit. Stools are at first greasy and frothy, then blood streaked, then almost pure blood with small filaments like bits of skin. Worms may be passed up [vomited] or down during the course of the disease.... The patient may push out part of his bowel. Gas is troublesome. Pain and blood separate it from simple diarrhea.... It can be differentiated from cholera morbus, because there is no violent vomiting. It is fatal to the young, the old and the sick. Vomiting and hiccoughing are a bad prognostic sign as are a green stool [rapid passage] or black stool [bleeding in the tract]. This indicates that the disease is putrid. Additional bad prognostic signs are a weak pulse, cold extremities, difficulty swallowing and convulsions, as well as inability to insert a clyster.[24]

Buchan believed that the best therapy was cleanliness. This protected the patient and his attendants. The patient's clothes were changed frequently. Stool had to be removed and buried immediately. Fresh air was allowed into the patient's room, which was also sprinkled with vinegar or lemon juice. He urged the doctor to keep the patient's spirits up. The victim was not to wear a flannel waistcoat next to his skin, because that would cause sweating without overheating. The patient was to abstain from flesh, fish, or anything that could turn rancid or putrid in the stomach. Buchan preferred a diet of apples boiled in milk, light pudding, and broth from the gelatinous part of animals. A gelatinous broth could cure the disease if it had not turned putrid. The attendant was advised to boil flour until it was as hard as starch. The patient received two to three tablespoons in milk and water well sweetened. In putrid dysentery, he urged a free intake of ripe, fresh fruit and raw or boiled milk. This counteracted putrefaction. Whey was taken orally or by clyster. If whey was not available, barley water with cream of tartar or barley and tamarinds was substituted. Efficacious too was warm water, water gruel, or water into which a hot iron was plunged several times. Camomile tea prevented mortification of the bowels. Buchan advised the following course of therapy: First, a cleansing of the passages with a vomit of ipecacuanha, then weak camomile tea. A day after the vomit, rhubarb or Epson salt every other day for three doses was given. This was followed with frequent small doses of ipecac mixed with syrup of opium. If this was not effective, a clyster of starch or fat mutton broth with laudanum twice a day was prescribed. By mouth, the patient took gum arabic and gum tragacanth in barley water hourly. If these did not help, Japonicum confection followed by a decoction of logwood four times a day was tried. To prevent a relapse, the patient was not allowed liquor, fish, or meat but could have only milk and vegetables. The patient was told to go to the country for clean air and exercise on horseback or in a carriage. The patient was advised to drink lime water and fresh milk, as well as bitters in wine or brandy. The patient had to avoid night air, the sick, the smell of putrid animal material, and he was advised to stay away from privies used by the sick.[25]

Dysentry defied all therapy, and because of this many treatments were advanced. Duffy, in *Epidemics in Colonial America*, offered the following treatment: Bleed the patient, prepare pills of grated pepper, turpentine, and flour to be used as directed. Give the patient a drink of butter or oil to which has been added beer and molasses. Insert hot lard and boiled eggs with the shell into the buttocks.[26] Dr. Rush, in a compendium of common diseases, discussed his therapy of dysentery. "Bleed if the pulse be full or tense and give a half an ounce or six drams of salt or two or three tablespoons of castor oil every morning or every other morning or forty drops of laudanum every night. Let your patient drink plentifully of weak fresh broth or ran or flax seed tea."[27]

The therapy mentioned that seemed most effective was sending the patient home or to the country. (This suggests that the disease was probably self-limiting, and if the patient went "to the country," he would be removed from the source and stop his own reinfection.)

In *Principles and Practice of Infectious Disease*, the authors discuss dysentery for the physician today. There are two types of dysentery: bacillary due to shigella, and amebic. The bacillary type does not produce liver complications and is six times more common. Shiga described gram negative rods in the stool and showed agglutinins to them in the plasma. It takes an inoculum of less than 200 viable bacteria to cause the disease in a healthy adult.

This explains its easy spread in families, institutions, and camps. The bacteria invade the intestinal mucosa and destroy it. Generally, they do not invade below the mucosa nor invade the blood stream. The organism causes a fever and toxemia. Bacteria multiply in the small intestine and then spread to the colon, resulting in lower abdominal pain, urgency, tenesmus and bloody mucus. Micro abscesses develop that coalesce to form large abscesses that cause the mucosa to slough.

The disease today is most common in infants and preschoolers because of a lack of hygienic habits. The severity and mortality of the disease are proportional to the degree of malnutrition. The treatment is basically fluid replacement and cleanliness. Antibiotics are of questionable benefit, although ampicillin and trimethopium-sulfamethoxazole in good doses may shorten the course of the illness. Antidiarrheal drugs, such as anticholinergics and opiates, should not be used because they increase the duration of the disease and its infectivity.[28]

— 7 —

Typhus and the
Army Hospitals

Typhus followed armies like a shadow. The massive destruction of soldiers from this disease shaped the history of mankind. If the conditions present in an army were reproduced in civilian life, typhus became an equally destructive force. In farming communities where the population was spread out, there was minimal personal contact and the disease, if present, was rare. However, in cities where people were packed together and cleanliness and sanitation were not controlled, the stage was set. All that was needed was the principal actor, the louse. Such was the situation in the army hospitals of New Jersey and Pennsylvania in 1777 and 1778, and it almost destroyed Washington's army.

Typhus is a rickettsial disease due to R. prowazecki. The organism is an intermediate form between bacteria and viruses and will grow only intracellularly. It is believed that rickettsia started as parasites in insects. Its most ancient host was probably the tick. The organism can live in ticks from generation to generation without any harm to the parasite or its host. A more recent association with the flea is suggested by the flea's ability to survive infection, and its ability to rid itself of the parasite in about a month. The infection of lice is relatively recent, because the louse is killed by the parasite as is its newest host—man.

There are two forms of typhus: the murine or endemic form and the epidemic form. The murine form is a disease of rats and mice caused by R. typhi. It infects the rat flea when the flea takes a blood meal from an infected rat. It is spread from rat to rat by the feces of the flea rubbed into the bite. If the rat dies, the flea requires an emergency host and will attack man for its next meal, and thus the organism arrives inside its new host. The epidemic form is caused by R. prowazecki. The natural host is the louse. The human louse's optimum habitat is in the clothes next to the skin and hair. This provides the proper temperature and humidity. The female lays about 60 eggs every six days. The eggs or nits are laid in clusters and protected by a chitinous material and attached by cement to clothing and hair. The egg can hatch in five to six days if the temperature and humidity are right. The hatching process is slowed at lower temperatures, and the process will stop if the temperature gets too low. If the host dies of the disease and his body temperature drops, or his temperature becomes too high as a result of the disease, the louse will leave and look for another human and thus spread the disease. The louse is a bloodsucking insect and will consume about one c.c. (about 1/28 of an ounce) of blood with each meal, during which it will defecate five to six times. The causative organism is taken in with the blood meal, and it invades the lining cells of the louse's stomach where it proliferates. It bursts out of the cells and passes with the feces onto the skin of the next human. Four to five days of incubation are required before a person shows evidence of the disease. The patient recovers when the rickettsial organisms are destroyed by his immune mechanism. In rare cases, the rickettsia invades the reticulo-endothelial system of the liver, spleen, bone marrow, and nodes and becomes dormant. Years later, perhaps due to a lapse in resistance of the host, the rickettsia can reactivate. This results in the milder Brill's disease, and an epidemic of typhus can follow. Brill's disease seems to affect mostly people from Russia and other parts of eastern Europe.[1]

Typhus was described by Hippocrates in the first book of Epidemion. His patient, Selenius, developed fever, soreness in the back and neck, and headache. For several days he had fever, intestinal symptoms, pressure in the abdomen, insomnia, and delirium. On the seventh and eighth days he developed severe sweats. On the eighth day an eruption of red spherical spots without suppuration appeared. He died on the eleventh day. Typhus (as well as other epidemic diseases) was claimed by some to be the plague that destroyed Athenian power in the Peloponnesian Wars. This series of events was described in the second book of the History of Thucydides. The disease spread from Ethiopia to Egypt, then Libya, then Piraeus and on to Athens. (An interesting side-light in history described smallpox in an almost similar progression.) In the summer of 430 B.C., large armies plus the civilian population around Athens took refuge within the walls of the city. Many of them developed the illness very suddenly. The patients had headache, red eyes, inflamed throat and tongue, sneezing, hoarseness, and cough. (These early symptoms resemble the start of typhoid fever and many other infectious diseases.) This was followed by vomiting, diarrhea, thirst, and delirium. Patients died on the seventh to ninth day. Survivors were weak and suffered persistent diarrhea. When the fever was at its peak, red spots appeared on the skin. In severe cases, where the victim recovered, he developed necrosis of his fingers, toes, and genitalia. Others lost eyesight and memory. This epidemic started in the summer, but most typhus epidemics occurred in the winter.[2]

Apparently Europe enjoyed a hiatus from typhus for at least 1500 years. At least the medical writers in the first millennium did not describe the disease. In 1083, a "spotted fever" epidemic affected a monastery in Salerno. It is possible that typhus existed in endemic form in Europe in the twelfth century. The definitive host of endemic typhus was the rat. The black rat was brought to Europe by the Crusaders. It lived in prehistoric Europe for centuries but had died out for unknown reasons until its reintroduction early in the second millenium. The brown rat came later from Mongolia and overwhelmed its black cousin to become the serious source of typhus in Europe. Epidemic typhus probably came from Asia or Africa via Cyprus to Spain. The army of Don Fernando, the Catholic, hired Cypriot mercenaries to dislodge the Saracens from Granada (1489 to 1490). It was claimed that typhus destroyed 17,000 Spanish troops, while the Saracens destroyed only 3,000. From Granada, typhus spread over the Iberian Peninsula and into Europe in the sixteenth century. The Spaniards probably carried it to Mexico in 1545. Authorities believed the New World was free of typhus prior to the Spanish conquest. However, archeologists found a pre–Columbian Mayan hieroglyph that pictured a man covered with spots, with his head in his hands, and bleeding from his nose. This could have been a related rickettsial disease. In Peru, pre–Columbian mummies had nits. This at least suggested a lice-infested society. Most societies had to bear the cross of the louse. However, the Hottentots and Syctheans ate theirs, and early English physicians prescribed them to treat jaundice.[3]

In 1528 a French army of 28,000 encircled Naples and tried to starve the city into submission. Typhus struck, and half the army and its general, Lantrec were dead in 30 days. The French retreated, and the defenders of the besieged city broke out and attacked and destroyed the remnants of the French army. As a result, southern Italy fell into the camp of Spain. Spain was united with the Austrian Hapsburgs to produce a huge empire in Europe under Charles V, the Holy Roman Emperor. In turn, Charles V lost 10,000 troops at the siege of Metz from typhus. In 1566 a German army of 80,000 under Maximillian II faced the troops of Sultan Suleiman of Turkey in Hungary. Typhus caused such destruction among the German troops that the fight against the Turks was given up. In 1632 during the Thirty Years War, Gustavus Adolphus's Swedish army faced Wallenstein at Nuremburg. Typhus killed 18,000 of the combatants and the armies separated. Typhus spread from Europe proper to the British Isles, and the armies of Cromwell and Charles I were decimated at Reading in 1643. The eighteenth century produced a change in alliances and combatants, but this did not affect the impartial louse and its rickettsial parasite. The wars of the Spanish and Austrian succession were accompanied by typhus, as was the American Revolution. In the early nineteenth century, Napoleon's Grand Army, in its invasion of Russia, was struck down. Certainly respiratory and enteric fevers took their share of French soldiers, but it was typhus predominantly that turned the army of 500,000 into 20,000 stragglers who were able to reach the safety of the French border. World War I brought with it many typhus deaths in the Middle East and on the eastern front among Russian soldiers. In World War II a serious epidemic was staved off in Italy with massive use of DDT on the Italian population.

In the American Revolution, typhus was second to smallpox in the destruction of American troops. It developed in the hospitals of New Jersey and Pennsylvania in 1777 and 1778, a time of very low morale in Washington's army after a series of defeats in New York, New Jersey, and Pennsylvania. However, let us start at the beginning and trace the colonial army from its early success to the debacles in the middle colonies, and the crowded hospitals set up at a safe distance from the British advance.

The number of casualties from illness without a shot fired in anger in the Boston campaign prophesied the problems to be seen in an undisciplined army of civilian soldiers. Of an army of 19,365 men, 2,817 were unable to perform their military duties. It should be remembered that these "soldiers" were New Englanders with the same backgrounds, exposure to the same illnesses from infancy to adulthood, and treatment by the same level of physicians. The army was surrounded by a sympathetic civilian population that supplied its needs. Their new leader, General Washington, described them as the dirtiest group he had ever seen. Washington's earliest general orders concerned hygiene and sanitation.

The army from New England was joined by regiments from the middle states and the south to form the army in New York, which contained representatives of seven colonies. These included mountain people from the south as well as lowland farmers.[4] They brought malaria, probably typhoid and/or typhus as well as smallpox. Discipline in the American army was lax, and general knowledge of disease was limited. General Washington again ordered latrines to be dug deep and covered after three days. Each day fresh dirt was to be thrown into the latrines. All wastes around camp were to be burned daily. In the summer of 1776 Washington prepared the defense of Manhattan. The men worked with pickaxes and shovels during an unusually hot summer. Poor sanitation resulted in polluted water supplies. By late August, the army was debilitated by illness. General hospitals were set up at King's College Hospital as well as in private homes and churches.[5] John Warren set up a general hospital in Long Island with three surgeons and three mates. Warren also set up a line of medical command. He set regimental surgeons and mates 300 to 500 yards behind their infantry. He wanted them behind a hill if possible. They were to dress the wounded on or near the field of battle. If the regiment was within a fort or on a defensive line, that was where the surgeon and mate were to be. If the regiment was broken up, the surgeon reported to the commander for a new assignment. The surgeon's prime duty was to the men of his regiment and brigade. He was to stop the flow of blood from a wound by tourniquet, ligature, lint, and compress, and remove all extraneous bodies from a wound, reduce fractures, and dress wounds. Warren instructed the surgeons in the proper use of tourniquets. They were not to fasten them so tightly that circulation would be stopped for a prolonged period as this would increase inflammation and excite a fever, nor so loose as to allow rebleeding. The wounded were then to be removed to a brigade or general hospital. If the general hospital was overwhelmed by sick and wounded, the hospital surgeon would apply to the brigade commander or division commander for more regimental surgeons. The regimental surgeons who were assigned to the general hospitals were to check with the hospital surgeon for orders about their duties. The regimental surgeon, with the regimental commander's concurrence, was to appoint certain infantrymen as bearers of the wounded. The surgeon had to have available wheelbarrows and other means to carry the wounded.

The Battle of Long Island and Manhattan was a complete, one-sided victory for the British. Washington's casualties were sent to hospitals in Hackensack, Hoboken, Weehawken, and Newark, New Jersey, as well as to Fishkill and Peekskill, New York. The Battle of White Plains resulted in more casualties, and Dr. Morgan set up and worked in a hospital in North Castle. Sick and wounded from White Plains were also sent to Norwich and Stanford, Connecticut. As Washington continued his retreat across New Jersey, the sick and wounded were transported from the hospitals of eastern New Jersey to Morristown, New Jersey. They were then moved to Bethlehem, Pennsylvania.[6] Bethlehem at this time was a community of about 300. It was home to the Moravian sect. Washington sent a letter to the Reverend Ettwein, head of the community, and requested the use of their facilities for 250 casualties. This was granted, and Reverend Ettwein moved the single brothers out of their quarters in order to accept the American casualties. The brothers' house was a stone structure three stories high; 50 by 80 feet. It was first used as a hospital from December 1776 to March 1777. During the first month of occupation 62 casualties died, mainly from exposure. This was a result of transfer of patients from other hospitals in open conveyances. A total of 110 died that winter. Other hospitals were opened in Philadelphia, Easton, Allentown, Princeton, and Wilmington.[7] The mortality in these areas was extreme. In Philadelphia alone 2,000 troops died in the fall and winter of 1776 to 1777. The coffins had to be stacked in graves in Potter's field.[8]

Following the American defeat at Brandywine Creek in September 1777, the sick and wounded were sent to Ephrata, the home of the Dunkards, another monastic community. They received 500 sick and wounded. The community acted as a hospital in the winter of 1777–78. The Dunkard brothers acted as nurses and paid with their lives when typhus broke out. As a result of the loss of Philadelphia, the sick and wounded of that city were moved to Bethlehem, and the single brethren's house was again occupied. Those casualties were joined by the casualties of Germantown, raising the population to 450. By Christmas of 1777, there were over 700 patients in a house considered crowded with 400 occupants. The men were packed in with inadequate ventilation. They were filthy, but many stayed because they had no clothes to wear back to duty. Typhus fever visited, and 300 died in the last three months of 1777. Of eleven surgeons and mates, ten caught typhus, and one died. All three hospital stewards caught typhus, and two died. Every orderly and nurse developed typhus. The disease spread to the civilian population and caused the death of seven brethren. The hospital was occupied until June 1778. Of the 1,500 soldiers treated during this period, 500 died. Many had been admitted with only minor wounds and illnesses. Two hundred troops from North Carolina died at Bethlehem. This represented half of the total casualties of the state during the entire war. Of 40 patients from a Virginia regiment, only three were to return to duty.[9] The soldiers came to the hospital in a weakened condition due to dysentery and respiratory illnesses, and typhus supplied the coup de grace. Those casualties lucky enough to be cared for in the regimental hospitals frequently survived.

In April 1778 General Washington sent an inspector to check the percent of fatalities per hospital admission. He reported back that in Cambridge in 1775 about six percent died. In the battle for New York City in 1776 ten percent of hospital admissions perished. In Pennsylvania and New Jersey in the winter of 1777–78, twenty percent died. In the Bethlehem hospital during this period, thirty-five percent were lost. Dr. Rush visited the hospital at Bethlehem, and blamed the deaths on overcrowding and unclean air. Rush was a prolific letter writer, and he used his pen to attack Dr. Shippen, director general of the medical department. In his defense, Dr. Shippen claimed the high mortality rate was due to the lack of clothing and bed coverings to keep the men warm and clean. In addition, he put the blame on the casualties themselves. They were raw, undisciplined men, unused to camp life and exposure to hardship. He also attributed the high mortality rates to the movement of casualties in open wagons in winter.[10]

Benjamin Rush wrote extensively about typhus from first hand observation of the disease at Bethlehem. He believed typhus was caused by perspiration and respirations of human bodies kept confined where the air could not be diluted and rendered inert by mixing with the atmosphere. Rush believed the principal diseases of hospitals were typhus gravior and mitior. Typhus mitior was the most common, particularly in the winter. Breezes mitigated it. Cold weather made typhus active. If patients were moved in winter, half of them became sick with typhus. Drunken patients were most subject to the disease. If a typhus patient developed large ulcers on his back or legs, his prognosis was much better. Rush advised doctors that throat ulcers and buboes due to typhus should not be mistaken for signs of venereal disease. Rush believed the disease could be spread by clothes and blankets. It was a disease poorly tolerated by blacks. He also advised that treatment be started with vomits produced by tartar emetic. This was followed by laxatives, bark, wine, opium, and blisters. An emetic would check the fever in the early state. His ideas on causation included lack of cleanliness, fatigue, poor diet and accommodations, as well as the use of linen clothes instead of woolens in the summer. Like most observers he abhorred crowding, and the presence together of large numbers of men of different "manners and habits." Rush believed the best and quickest treatment was to get the soldiers out of hospitals and into private homes.[11]

The Moravian community at Lititz, Pennsylvania, was also used as a hospital for eight months and ten days in 1777 and 1778, and 120 deaths were reported during that time. There were similar hospitals with similar mortality figures at Warwick, Mendham, Allentown, Reamstown, Schafferstown, and Buckingham. Hospitals were opened in barns, factories, private homes, churches, taverns, and schools in eastern Pennsylvania. Despite a devastating experience with spotted fever with high mortality, nineteen years earlier,[12] the Moravian communities saw the need and accepted the danger.

The destruction of personnel in the hospitals of eastern Pennsylvania was repeated at Princeton, where a hospital was opened after the defeats at Brandywine and Red Bank, New Jersey. The Princeton hospital was under the supervision of Dr. Tilton of Delaware, a graduate of the College of Medicine in Philadelphia. Tilton was a good observer and a well-trained physician. However, his description of typhus at his hospital differed from the descriptions of the others. Dr. Tilton was himself a victim and nearly died of the hospital fever. Upon recovery he described the illness but never mentioned the skin rash so typical of typhus and other rickettsial diseases. His description ran as follows:

> The disease gave notice of its approach by a languor of the whole body and the head felt it was compressed as in a hoop. The symptoms were treated by blood letting and an antiphlogistic course. After some days, the pulse begins to sink, a dry tongue develops, followed by delirium and the whole train of putrid symptoms supervenes. At this point, blood letting must be used with caution whereas it was helpful at the onset of the disease. A vomit was deemed excellent as it opened and squeezed all the glands, thus shaking from the nervous system all the contaminating poisons before their impressions are fixed. However, when the fever is fixed, mercury is of the greatest importance. This remedy has the power of subduing all manner of contagion and all infections with which we are acquainted. Thus, besides syphilis, itch, etc. without fever, it is regarded as a specific in smallpox, measles, scarlatina, yellow fever, etc. Mercury set secretions afloat.[13]

Tilton's treatment of typhus was two drams of calomel, one dram of opium, and fifteen grains of tartar emetic all added to syrup to produce 60 pills. These were taken one or two daily. If the pulse fell, accompanied by a dry tongue and delirium, patients were to be treated with stimulants such as bark, wine, volatile salts, and blisters. Tilton had to convalesce for eight months after his illness before his old strength returned. Consequently, he believed the soldier could not be fit for duty after a case of typhus. The prolonged convalescence after the disease suggests typhoid fever. A clear distinction between the two diseases was not made until the nineteenth century. In any case, Tilton commented that the hospitals "swallowed up half the army of 1777–78."

As described earlier, Tilton and Rush wrote extensively about typhus, and it was also described in Buchan's medical textbook. Buchan called it malignant, putrid, or spotted fever and attributed it to foul air and poor ventilation as developed in camps, hospitals, and jails. Other factors included the ingestion of too much animal food and spoiled corn. The patient developed sudden weakness, nausea, vomiting, violent headache, and throbbing arteries in his head. His eyes became red, inflamed, and a painful and ringing noise developed in his ears. He developed pain in the stomach, loins, and back. His tongue and teeth developed a black crust. According to Buchan, the patients frequently passed worms. Black spots developed on the patient's skin, followed by bleeding from all orifices. Buchan's treatment included placing the patient in a cool room with fresh air, where vinegar and lemon or orange juice were evaporated in the air and the skin of a lemon was held near the nose. Patients were to drink orange and lemon juice as well as Rhenish and Madeira wine. To open the bowels, the doctor prescribed cream of tartar or tamarinds. The patient consumed a light diet of fruit and vegetables. Medication included a vomit and clysters. The patient was not bled. Peruvian bark was employed in serious cases. If the glands became swollen, the physician promoted suppuration with poultices and then drained them.[14]

Baron Von Swieten of the Austrian army called typhus "continued fever." When a fever of this kind produced an inflammation, the disease took the name from the part affected, e.g., pleurisy, peripneumony, "quinzy," but since this was not localized, it was called continued fever. Von Swieten believed it was caused by fatigue and lassitude, excessive exertion, or too much alcohol. The disease caused a loss of fluid, leaving the blood thick and acrid. His therapy included frequent large bleedings early in the disease. It also included barley water drinks of honey and wine vinegar as well as emollient decoction, oxymel, and nitre. If the patient improved, the surgeon switched to an anti-febrile decoction. A continued fever due to putrid dissolution of humors was very dangerous. It occurred when soldiers were encamped in marshy areas or packed too closely together, which prevented air from renewing itself. This was a common problem in ships and hospitals. When the air could not be changed, it became corrupted from the effluvia of bodies as well as the stink of excrement and putridness of gangrenous parts. This led to putrid fever, which was contagious. The patient had alternating shivering and heat, frontal headache, loss of appetite, and a crusted dry tongue. There was gradual loss of vision and hearing, and he became languid. Purple spots of irregular shape developed on his skin. If the patient developed black stools, which indicated bleeding, and livid stripes as though from a beating, his outlook was grave. A good prognostic sign was an easy sweat, black sediment in the urine, and easy expectoration. Other good signs were parotid swelling and white aphthae on the tongue. Von Swieten was against bleeding later in the course of the disease because it decreased the strength and brought on delirium, and he advised instead that the air around the patient was to be changed. The fear of army hospitals was shared by soldier and physician alike.[15]

In proportional terms, more surgeons died in military hospitals than line officers.

Ship's fever, jail fever, camp fever, hospital fever, and continued fever, were all terms used for the same disease, typhus. Ship's fever was not a common problem in American ships, because seamen joined willingly and came from sparsely settled areas where typhus was uncommon. The situation in England was considerably different. Sailors came from crowded hovels in filthy cities. Some were impressed from jails where the disease was rampant because prisoners remained in jail with the same clothing without any opportunity to wash. This plus poor nutrition made them ideal candidates for typhus in jail and on board ship. Typhus was the second most serious disease after scurvy faced by the surgeon and crew. Doctors Lind, Trotter, and Blaine of the British navy related the disease to filthy rags impressed prisoners wore on board. They urged that a new recruit be quarantined before he was permitted to board a fleet ship. His clothing was removed, and he was given a clean set. He was taught to use soap and his clothing was fumigated with brimstone. Lind urged that able seamen be given a uniform and their rags be discarded. The uniform served two purposes. It seemed to prevent the spread of disease, and the men could not safely sell it for liquor money.[16]

Civilian populations did not escape typhus, and there were many epidemics of "spotted fever" in Europe. Among them, Salerno 1083, Bohemia 1085, Germany and Tabardillo in Spain 1480–1490, France 1528, Hungary 1542 and 1566. The epidemic in Hungary was so bad that spotted fever and morbus hungaricus became synonymous. They were all probably typhus, because the population was "lousy."[17] An observer described the body of Thomas à Becket, killed in 1170: "As his body cooled the lice flowed from the seven layers of clothing surrounding his chilling body like water boiling over a simmering cauldron."[18] Pepys, years later, described his visits to the barber where his wig was cleaned of nits.

Typhus reached epidemic proportions at the end of the fifteenth century in England. There were sporadic outbreaks among jurists, the so-called "black assizes" in Cambridge in 1522, Oxford 1577 and Exeter 1586. Prisoners taken from jail for their day in court passed lice containing typhus to court officials who were too close to them. From them, the disease spread to the population at large. Bad harvests were also a cause of spread. Farmers, displaced from their land, took to begging and went from town to town with "hitchhikers" in the seams of their rags. In the countryside typhus was known as "famine fever." Typhus became endemic in England in the mid-seventeenth century where it destroyed ten percent of the people who caught it, but it could flare up into epidemics as well. In 1750 there was a repetition of the "black assizes" in London when typhus broke out at the "Old Bailey." It killed two judges, the lord mayor, an alderman, a barrister, several law students, court officials, jurors, and idle onlookers at court.[19]

The English inhabitants in America believed typhus was brought here by the German immigrants who left Europe to escape the destruction of the Thirty Years War, which ravaged Germany.[20] They also accused the Scotch-Irish when their migration seemed to overwhelm the "Native Americans."[21] Typhus was never a major problem in Colonial America, which was an agricultural society spread over a large area with limited person-to-person contact. However, the Revolution ended that idyllic condition.

— 8 —

Valley Forge and Scabies

In the spring of 1777 General Howe was preparing to sail up the Hudson River to join in the three-pronged attack on northern New York when a change in plans from London authorized him to go after the main prize—Philadelphia. On July 23, 1777, he embarked with 15,000 men and materiel on the trip to Chesapeake Bay. The Hudson River plan was turned over to Sir Henry Clinton. Clinton sailed up the Hudson and captured a few forts, but gave up his expedition after General Howe ordered him to send troops to reinforce his attack on Philadelphia. Howe's fleet landed at Head of Elk, Maryland, approximately 60 miles south of Philadelphia. His troops had to remain below decks on the long sea voyage, so they were sick and dispirited when they disembarked. His horses, kept under the same conditions, sickened and died. Howe was able to purchase replacements, and the rest on dry land reinvigorated his troops. Finally, he was able to start his march north to gain his prize.

Meanwhile, Washington moved his army south through Philadelphia to meet the British threat to the capital of the colonies. The two forces met at Brandywine Creek, a beautiful area in southeastern Pennsylvania. The British had better intelligence than Washington from local Tories. On September 11, 1777, Washington's armies were rolled back. The American army, still a fighting unit, retreated through Chester to Philadelphia. Congress moved to Lancaster and then York, Pennsylvania. Howe sent a foraging party west around Philadelphia to replenish his supplies. Those men came upon Valley Forge and occupied it temporarily. In Valley Forge, they found large quantities of food, horseshoes, and entrenching tools. They confiscated what they needed, and they burned the grist mill and forge before they left on September 23, 1777.

Washington sent Mad Anthony Wayne with a detachment of troops to fall on Howe's baggage train and destroy it. Instead, Wayne's forces were surprised by the British and almost annihilated at Paoli. In addition, Howe outsmarted Washington with a feint toward Reading, a major American depot. In his attempt to counterattack, Washington left Philadelphia undefended, and British troops under Cornwallis were able to cross the Schuylkill River and enter Philadelphia on September 26, 1777. The remainder of the English troops under Howe occupied Germantown. Washington tried to hit the British army at Germantown with a two-pronged attack that would have been difficult with a well-trained, cohesive army, let alone a green group of men. The attack was initially successful, but it failed miserably, causing 1,000 American casualties.

With his army still intact, Washington represented a threat to the over-land supply of Howe's forces in Philadelphia. Howe stormed and captured Fort Miflen and Fort Mercer on November 22, 1777, and opened the Delaware River. He could now supply his men by ship. Washington received reinforce-ments from Gates's army after its stupendous victory over Burgoyne, and he fought the British at Whitemarsh in December without any significant results. Howe withdrew his army to Philadelphia to winter in the city, and Washing-ton turned west to Valley Forge.[1]

Washington chose Valley Forge because of its good defensive position. In addition, he received a warning from the Supreme Executive Council of Pennsylvania that it would withdraw his Pennsylvania troops if he did not camp within 25 miles of Philadelphia. The Pennsylvania troops represented a substantial percent of Washington's army. Therefore, Washington decided on Valley Forge, 18 miles west of Philadelphia. Valley Forge was an iron forge started earlier in the century by Evans, Walker, and Williams near the Mount Joy elevation. It became a complete iron manufacturing plant to which the own-ers added a grist mill and a saw mill. The surrounding area was fertile, and workers could be fed from the well-run farms. The surrounding forests were used to make charcoal for the forge. Two stone houses were built for the own-ers. Early in the war, the mill and forge were used to make flour and ordnance for the army.

Valley Forge was a desirable place for Washington's army. From there it could interdict British foraging parties in the countryside, and there was enough forest left to build huts for the army, and food was readily available in the neighborhood. The site was on a plateau 250 feet high, protected on two sides by the Schuylkill River and Valley Creek. It was also near Reading where the sick and wounded could be sent. Reading also served as a depot for sup-plies. Eleven thousand men left Guelph Mills for the march to Valley Forge. Prior to the march, Washington shipped his sick and wounded to neighboring hospitals. His remaining troops were reasonably healthy when they arrived at their destination on December 19, 1777. The frozen, rutted roads chewed up the men's shoes, and 2,000 troops arrived barefoot. There were no animals for butchering, and the army had only 75 barrels of flour to hold them until a sup-ply line could be established. Some rations and rum reached the army by New Year's Day.

Brigade areas were laid out, and shelters were thrown up. Washington and his generals rented the stone houses in the area for headquarters and accom-modations, and he assigned teams of twelve men each to build huts of logs chinked with clay for the enlisted men. The huts were to be six and a half feet high, fourteen feet wide, and sixteen feet long, and were to be lined up with doors that opened onto the company street. These streets were covered with boards to control the mud. A fireplace of clay and mud at the rear of the hut supplied heat. Behind these were to be similar huts to house six to eight company officers or three field grade officers or one general officer. By February 8, 1778, most of the men were in reasonable shelter. However, the occupants soon despoiled them by throwing uneaten food and bones into the corners, so they rapidly took on an odor of decay. Dr. Rush visited the camp in March 1778 and described it as dirty and stinking, with men barely covered with rags. General Wayne reported that the whole army was sick and crawling with vermin. The soldiers were farmers and backwoodsmen with no knowledge of sanitation. Washington had to order regimental officers to inspect the huts twice a day for cleanliness. The smell was finally dissipated in the spring when the clay was removed from between the logs, allowing fresh air to flow through. Also, tar or gun powder was burned in the cabins to neutralize the odor, much as an air freshener is used today.

Food was limited during the cold winter when it was needed most. Men could forage in the countryside, and supplies might be bought from neighboring farms. However, the farmers near Philadelphia were less than sympathetic to the cause. Tory purveyors could buy supplies for gold, but the soldiers had only paper money. Oxen were sent from around Philadelphia, but the roads were so bad that the men were left without meat for days at a time. Meat represented the basic part of their diet (about one pound per day). Fodder and protection from the weather for horses was limited or nonexistent. As many as 1,500 horses died during the encampment. The carcasses were frequently left where the animals fell.

By the middle of March, supplies started to reach them in greater amounts. In April, the shad were running in the Schuylkill River, and fishing parties supplemented their diet. Gradually, cabbage, potatoes, turnips, and onions became available. There were no eggs or coffee, and tea could be bought only with gold. Flour supplies were uncertain. Indian meal was available, but rice was reserved for the sick. Salt was rarely obtained. The men made "fire cakes" of flour and water baked on flat rocks near the open fire. Alcohol was limited, and a black market grew up for it. Men sold their clothing and equipment for the available spirits. Clean water was available from rivers, creeks, and wells. Horses, needed for the cavalry and to pull cannons and wagons, replaced those that died by May 1778.

Clothes were limited. Occasionally the men were ordered to seize clothing from civilians. Shoes were worn out by the long marches, and clothes fell to rags. Hides of cattle were bartered for shoes. Men would trade 30 pounds of rawhide for one pair of shoes. Washington offered a monetary prize for anyone who could think of a way to convert hide into serviceable shoes. The consequence of poor footwear was frostbite. This usually resulted in amputation followed by shock, sepsis, and even death. Once the huts were built, the tents the army carried were cut up to make clothing. An occasional prize such as the British sloop *Symmetry* supplied cloth, boots, stockings, and shoes. State legislatures sent supplies. Unhappily, they still had parochial attitudes about the army, and they designated the supplies for men from their state. The troops were not above stealing clothes from the sick or dead. By February 5, 3,989 soldiers were unfit for duty due to lack of uniforms. In March French ships made their way to American-held ports with supplies of wearing apparel. At the end of April, new shoes reached the men. On June 18, however, when the army left Valley Forge, approximately 100 of the men were without shoes. Food and clothing were available in centers of population, but the roads were so bad that they could not reach the army. The rivers froze, and the necessities could not be sent from the depot at Reading by boat. Teamsters demanded too high a pay scale to transport material on land. Those who did work had to contend with the breakdown of wagons on the rough, rutted roads. Contents were abandoned where they lay.[2]

It has been reported that 3,000 troops died that winter at Valley Forge or in the hospitals around the camp, but there are only 30 grave sites in Valley Forge proper. Respiratory disease carried off the largest number of poorly fed, poorly clothed and poorly housed soldiers. In the six months at the camp, snow fell or was on the ground for 29 days, sleet one day; there were seven days of rain and ten of severe cold. (A later encampment at Morristown existed through the coldest winter in memory, but deaths were fewer because of better conditions and training.) The army sickened shortly after its arrival at camp. As late as May 1778, 4,000 were sick at Valley Forge and its environs, predominantly soldiers recovering from smallpox inoculation, but the usual camp illnesses were represented too.[3] The regimental hospitals handled most of the sick in camp. The hospital was usually set up in an available hut in the company area. The individuals who were too sick for the limited supplies and abilities of the surgeons but not sick enough for the general hospital went to a "flying hospital." There were one or two of these intermediate hospitals with each brigade. They were built by the troops and were fifteen feet wide, twenty-five feet long and nine feet high, covered with boards or shingles rather than sod, so the earth could not fall in on the occupants. Windows were on two sides, with a chimney in the rear. The hospital was erected near the center of the brigade area about 100 yards to the rear. There was usually not enough straw, and patients slept on the cold ground. This led to greater mortality figures secondary to respiratory disease.

The general hospitals for the encampment were at Reading, Bethlehem, Easton, Lititz, and Yellow Springs. The hospital at Yellow Springs, ten miles from Valley Forge, was the first permanent army medical facility. It was a three-story frame building that measured 100 feet by 36 feet, with porches on three sides. The first floor had a kitchen, dining room, and utility rooms. The second floor had two wards, and the third floor was divided into small rooms. It housed 1,300 soldier patients during the Valley Forge period; most were victims of typhus fever. The institution was well run with a purveyor who was responsible for purchasing needed material for the hospital, such as equipment, bedding, straw, food for special diets, beds, clothing, candles, eating implements, and kitchen utensils. He also provided drugs, dressings, and medical equipment for the staff. The purveyor supervised clerks, teamsters, and storekeepers. One of his duties was to maintain meticulous records for a Congress suspicious of expenditures by the medical department.

Hospital duty was dangerous duty. Consequently, the worst men of the outfit were made orderlies. As a result, the care the patients received was less than optimal. Washington tried to get women to serve in the hospitals to relieve troops for active duty. Patients were crammed into the hospitals. Reading Hospital, with a capacity of 360, had 900 patients. Quaker meeting houses were confiscated to use as hospitals, despite the members' objections. (The Quakers were neutral or Tory in sentiment.) Churches and barns were also commandeered. There were little or no supplies for the sick. Straw and clothing were reissued to the new casualties after the death or return to duty of the previous user. In Bethlehem, a third of the patients died. The hospital at Lititz had a better record. Only 66 of the patients sent from the Valley Forge encampment died.

The general hospital was examined by the inspector general at regular intervals. His reports generally showed poor record keeping, poor care of the patient and many desertions by the sick to return home for better care. The patients were supposed to be visited by their company officers as well as by senior officers. This rule was based on a general order, but it was rarely obeyed. Patients had one set of clothes with which they entered the hospital, and they were not provided with an alternate set while the originals were being cleaned. Consequently, they refused to give up their clothing for cleaning. Therefore, vermin and scabies mites persisted in their garments.

Washington ordered parties to be appointed to bury dead horses every week. He also ordered garbage pits to be dug, and the use of latrines by his men (called "vaults" in his orders). The latrines were to be dug by the quartermaster, and they were placed where deemed necessary by that service group. Each morning, freshly passed wastes were covered with a fresh layer of earth. The vault was filled in when it approached ground level. The general ordered sentries to shoot at men who relieved themselves at places other than latrines. The miscreant also received five lashes for his offense. Offal from slaughter pens had to be buried daily. With the approach of warm weather, the stench at camp became so bad that it was moved one mile away by June 10, 1778.[4] In May, new clothing reached camp. The soldiers were given time to wash their old uniforms and to bathe in the river. Smallpox inoculation was carried out on reinforcements as well as on those veterans who had never had the disease. Of 4,000 troops inoculated, only ten died of the disease.

In his command at Valley Forge, Washington had 74 infantry regiments. Each regiment was composed of nine to thirteen companies; each with 77 officers and men. He also had a brigade of artillery and a corps of engineers. A brigade consisted of four battalions or regiments. Three brigades formed one division. During the six months at Valley Forge, five soldiers and two civilians were given the death sentence for desertion or spying for the enemy; but not all punishments were carried out. Other crimes were punished by whipping. Crimes reported included robbery, embezzlement, and attempted sodomy. Washington violently opposed gambling, but it was impossible to stop this among soldiers with time on their hands.[5]

The troops came from ten states. There were no levies from Delaware, South Carolina, or Georgia. Washington's army was predominantly of British extraction. About half of his Pennsylvanians were foreign-born (mostly German). There were about two percent blacks and a sprinkling of Indians. Generally, the men were dedicated to the effort and aware of the issues. They were confident of the war's successful outcome. The conversion of a ragged, despairing "army" into a trim, dedicated fighting force was largely due to the efforts of Von Steuben. He drilled the men relentlessly, but he also looked after their health and well-being. He developed rules of sanitation, which were incorporated into army regulations, and he made sure that they were observed. Among his changes was an insistence that the straw used for a soldier who died or recovered was to be burned. The bedding was washed prior to reissue. He also insisted that his troops washed, shaved, and kept their hair short. When the army left Valley Forge on June 19, 1778, the troops were ready to do the job for which they had enlisted. They left the encampment when they learned that the British were quitting Philadelphia.[6]

Sir Henry Clinton received orders from London that he had to evacuate Philadelphia because the American Revolution had become a broader European war. Some of Clinton's troops were sent to the West Indies to fight the French; others went to St. Augustine, Florida; and the remainder were to go to New York City. He used his ships to send the sick and wounded by sea. He also carried heavy baggage, as well as many Philadelphia Tories who feared retribution from the Patriots. His fit troops were to march across New Jersey to Sandy Hook. Washington saw this as an opportunity to smash the British forces, because they would be strung out over a long distance. He attacked the British at Monmouth Court House on June 28. The general would have had a resounding victory if General Charles Lee had attacked instead of ordering his men to retreat. Charles Lee was an officer in the British army before he joined the colonials, and was considered the military expert among Washington's officers, but he was always pessimistic about the ability of the green Americans to withstand the might of trained British troops. Washington relieved Lee of his command in the middle of the battle, and he ordered the troops to attack. However, the opportunity to smash Clinton's lines was lost. Charles Lee was court-martialed and cashiered from the service. Nightfall ended the fighting on that sweltering June day, and Clinton was able to continue to Sandy Hook and New York City with his army intact. The battle at Monmouth was the last major battle fought in the north. The work of Washington, Von Steuben, and other leaders to maintain some semblance of military order and sanitation in camp was finally effective.[7]

What of the individual soldier and his immediate superiors? How did he tolerate the biting cold and the snow and sleet in which he had to function day after day? How did he manage in his smoky, stinking hut with one side of his body cooked by the fireplace and the other side cold? How did he function on irregular rations poorly prepared, and how did he tolerate guard duty at night standing on a hat because he had no shoes? We can learn something of these problems from the diary of Albigence Waldo, a regimental surgeon from Connecticut. Waldo started as a surgeon's mate with the 8th Connecticut Regiment after Lexington and Concord. By the autumn of 1775, he was surgeon to the 11th Connecticut Regiment. Dr. Waldo completed his apprenticeship before he enlisted.[8] Waldo marched with his regiment to Valley Forge, and he saw the troops' health deteriorate due to fatigue and exposure. He commented on their "contentment and spirit of alacrity" despite the problems they faced. Like all soldiers, he complained about the civilians at home enjoying their wives and families while "we suffer for their benefit." The troops had "fire cakes" and water until cattle could be driven in. On Christmas, they were still in tents, and the sick did not have better protection from the elements than the fit. He complained that the enlisted men's families were cared for at public expense if articles they needed were above "common price." The officers' families were not that lucky. The money sent home by the officer purchased very little, and his family had to beg for the necessities. The officers received tearful letters from their loved ones, and many resigned their commissions to go home to care for them. In 1779 Waldo had to resign as well because his family was poverty stricken without him.[9]

Scabies infected the troops in epidemic proportions shortly after their arrival at Valley Forge. In Washington's General Order of January 8, 1778, he noted that too many men were unfit for duty due to "the itch." He ordered the regimental surgeons to examine the troops in their units. The infected soldiers were isolated in separate huts and treated with sulfur in hog's lard.[10] Thacher, in his *Military Journal of the Revolution*, described a visit by General Israel Putnam to a hospital whose occupants suffered with the "ground itch." He asked the physician why they were not cured. The physician replied that there was no lard to make the ointment. The general responded, "Haven't you ever cured the itch with tar and brimstone? No, then you are not fit for a doctor." Sulfur was in limited supply, and some troops approached their companions in the artillery to obtain the element. At this point, the need for treatment outweighed the need for artillery. Some soldiers tried their own treatment. One covered his entire body with mercury ointment, and he died the next morning. Another drank six gills of rum (about one and a half pints) to stop the itch. He too died.[11] The surgeons tried to obtain sulfur from Dr. Cochran, director general of the middle department, without much success. Drs. Shippen and Potts wrote letters to the president of the war board to make him aware of the troops' problem, and their need for sulfur—also without great success.[12] The association of scabies and lack of cleanliness was known. To produce soft soap, General Weedon ordered receptacles for dirty tallow and wood ashes left in all brigade areas. There was also an area set aside to boil the feet of cattle to extract the oil. Soap was made and rationed to the soldiers on a weekly basis. They received three ounces of soft soap or one ounce of hard cake per week.[13]

Scabies followed armies relentlessly. Baron Von Swieten, in his *Diseases Incident to Armies*, urged that soldiers infected with scabies be isolated from their fellows. He described the disease for regimental surgeons, pointing out that it occurred first between the fingers with vesicles of clear fluid that caused severe itching. The victim scratched and broke the vesicle, and it spread the disease to other parts of his body. The broken vesicle was followed by a crust. If not cared for, the crust was replaced by an ulcer that could burrow into the fat below the skin. He urged cleanliness with frequent changes of clothing and linen. Von Swieten was a practical observer of illness, but he was also a product of university training. As such, he believed in internal and external treatment of the disease. He advised that the patient be bathed in water to which sulfur had been added. The soldier's clothing was fumigated in the open air with brimstone. The skin was anointed with Ethiops mineral (a black amorphous mercury sulfide, with a large excess of sulfur, in hog's lard). He advised not to cover the entire body with one application. The arms were treated the first day, the legs the second day, the trunk the third day. The cycle was repeated until the crusts fell off, the ulcers healed, and the patient was cured. The internal treatment included a diet free from salt. The patient was purged every eight hours with Ethiops mineral and antimony. Between purges, the individual received flower of sulfur and Ethiops mineral orally.[14]

Buchan thought scabies could not occur in the presence of cleanliness, good diet, and fresh air. He knew it was rarely a fatal disease; however, if it lasted too long it would "vitiate the humors." If driven internally without proper evacuations, it produced fever and inflammation of the viscera. Sulfur was prescribed internally and externally. Buchan advised the application of a salve composed of flowers of sulfur plus sal ammoniac in hog's lard or butter. Essence of lemon was added to control the odor. This was rubbed into the body at bedtime three times a week. Like Von Swieten, he urged that not all pores be covered in one application. Before the salve was applied, the patient was bled or purged. To keep the body open, he received flowers of brimstone in cream of tartar dissolved in treacle each morning. (Treacle was a sweet, syrupy material used to convey medicine. In the armamentarium of the Middle Ages, treacle was a mixture of many materials, sometimes as many as sixty, including ground unicorn's horn. The horn was considered a universal panacea and antidote for poisons of all sorts.) Buchan urged that the patient remain in one set of clothes for the entire treatment. After the patient was cured, his clothing was thrown away, or fumigated with brimstone and then washed. Otherwise, the disease would recur. Buchan recognized the association of clothes with the disease, but he never thought of the vector in the clothing. He had a secondary treatment if the patient could not tolerate the smell of sulfur: powder of white hellebore root in an ointment. The lesions and distribution of scabies might resemble syphilis, and many used mercury. Buchan advised strongly against the use of mercury for this disease.[15]

Dr. Reuben Friedman produced the most extensive work on scabies, its history and therapy. He suggested that scabies may have been described in Hebrew scripture as "zaraath." The Greeks had also been aware of scabies. They called it psora. However, this included all cutaneous eruptions with itching. Quintus Curtius, in the *History of the Wars of Alexander*, described a skin condition among the soldiers. After they bathed in a salt lake, their bodies broke out in scabs, which they spread to their companions. The illness may have been scabies or impetigo. Hippocrates believed scabies was a cutaneous manifestation of an internal derangement of the humors. He advised treatment with blood diluents and drastic purges. It is believed that the ancient Greeks knew of the "itch mite," since acarus, the scientific name, is of Greek derivation.[16] Aristotle talked of "lice in the flesh" that produced vesicles. Celsus, in 25 A.D., suggested external treatment with ointments containing myrrh, saffron, copper, nitre, lead, sulfur, and pitch. He also advised the application of sulfur in pitch for any itch.[17] Galen felt it was a disease of the melancholy humor. The bad humors passing through the skin caused scaling in vesicles. He advised internal and external treatment; however, external treatment had to be limited in scope because this might drive the disease internally and cause dropsy. If the vesicles remained, the causative humors had a pathway to leave the body. Galen's beliefs were retained by the Arabs who passed them to Christian Europe. His principles of therapy for this disease persisted into the nineteenth century.[18] As late as 1867, sulfur was taken internally as part of the treatment of the disease. Peasants, quacks, and "old women healers" in Europe knew external treatment was adequate and safe.

The ancient Sumerians, perhaps in the time of Abraham, may have used sulfur in the treatment of skin disease. St. Hildegard, when she was abbess of the convent of Rupertsburg, wrote a treatise called "Physika" in 1150–60, in which she described the presence of a mite-related skin disease. The mite was also described by the Arabian physician Zohar in 1280; however, he did not associate it with scabies.[19] Bernard de Gordon (1307) described scabies as one of the communicable diseases that included plague, erysipelas, and anthrax.

Whole populations could be involved, and its incidence was inversely related to cleanliness and skin care.[20] In 1721, Johannes Schweibe felt the organisms were generated from sweet fruit, developed in the stomach, and crawled out to areas under the skin.[21] Dr. Sydenham originally, and Rush in 1815, prescribed various internal decoctions as well as bleeding and purging to cure this debilitating disease. One prescription consisted of Venice treacle, plus an electuary of egg, Virginia snakeroot, oriental bezoar, and syrup of candied citron. This was followed by a distillate of holy thistle, plague and treacle waters, and syrup of cloves. The patient was to drink warm posset (hot milk and liquor sweetened and spiced). If this did not help, Sydenham advised the application of a liniment of sharp powdered dock (a weed of the buckwheat family), pomatum, flowers of sulfur, and oil of rhodium. In Colonial America, there were patent drugs for the "itch." "Button's True and Genuine British Oil" was good for a multitude of illnesses in man and beast and for the "itch." Wharton's itch ointment was hawked as well.[22] In 1731 Benjamin Franklin's mother-in-law placed an advertisement in his *Pennsylvania Gazette* for a cure for the itch. It was a sulfur ointment, and it cured the disease without adding internal medications. She claimed it was also good for lice. It smelled good and was even safe for suckling children. The cost was two shillings per ounce.[23]

Sir John Pringle devoted one chapter of his book *Observations on the Diseases of the Army* to "the itch." He did not compare it to the fatal contagious diseases such as dysentery, hospital fever, smallpox, or measles. However, he felt it was in a class with syphilis in disability statistics among his troops. He described it as contagious and believed it was communicated from a "foul person" through his clothing and bedding. It was due to small insects found in the pustules. Pringle felt that Leeuwenhoek had described these animalcula from his work with the microscope. In the second edition of his book, he gave credit to Bonomo who had described the mite. Bonomo believed that external treatment was all that was necessary. Pringle denied that the "itch" was due to a change in the air or diet, but rather to individuals who had the disease originally. It was spread predominantly in hospitals, because all sorts of patients were admitted and packed together. Sulfur was the cure, usually with one application. However, more than one application was necessary in severely involved areas. He also gave sulfur internally to catch the mites too deep to be reached by the externally applied medication. He urged sulfur instead of mercury because of its safety.[24] Pringle observed that the treatment of officers was less effective than enlisted men, because enlisted men had no changes of clothing. He received treatment in his original clothing, and the organisms were killed in the treatment. The officer changed his clothes during the treatment, and he put the infected clothes back on after he was cured.[25]

In the Seven Years War, a Prussian physician, Dr. Ackermann, wrote that often half of a regiment had to be hospitalized for scabies. Dr. Baldinger, another Prussian doctor, described soldiers whose entire body from the neck down was covered with scabetic crusts. Schmucker, chief surgeon to Frederick the Great, described the contagion of scabies in field hospitals. He observed that those who washed daily with soap developed the disease less often. Prussia's enemy in the war, Austria, had similar problems described by Austrian surgeons.

In the eighteenth century, learned physicians agreed that scabies was an internal disorder due to body humors. Therefore, emetics, bleeding, purging, and blood-cleansing drugs were prescribed. They also advised treatment to prevent pushing the disease back into the body from the skin. Therapy included peppermint water, fennel water, corn poppy blossoms, and dilute sulfuric acid. This therapy took up to six months to effect a cure. Other physicians prescribed antimony and mercury. A pharmacist, Bonomo, believed it was due to an external parasite. In a letter written to the naturalist Francesco Redi he described the mite and explained that its burrows caused the itch. The pharmacist advised external treatment with mercury, sulfur, vitriol, and sublimate.[26] Bonomo also described how women inserted needles into the vesicles and withdrew the mite.[27] In folklore, the disease was treated by whirling a black cat with a spot of white around the patient's head three times. The charred remains of nine barley corns plus nine drops of blood from the cat's tail were then mixed and applied with a wedding ring while walking around the patient three times, invoking the name of the divinity.

We have no statistics about the incidence of scabies among soldiers in the American Revolution. However, letters home to their families described the infestation. Under orders of William Shippen, Jr., director general of the medical service, all poor sick in the Philadelphia almshouse were removed, and their places were taken by soldiers infected with scabies. In Philadelphia in 1776, Shippen said that of 440 sick in a hospital, 78 were hospitalized with the itch. *The Lititz Pharmacopoeia*, composed by William Brown, physician general of the middle department in 1778, called for lard ointment containing thirty-three percent sulfur for scabies. The scabies mite was neutral in its attacks on the contending armies of the Revolution. Both sides suffered. The British soldier may have suffered more than the American, because he had to take internal treatment as well as ointments. He received saline purges plus sulfur internally and externally. Mercury was tried for awhile, but it was dangerous and less effective. When sulfur was given internally, it was supplied with nitre and cream of tartar or molasses. Scabies traveled with the armies, and it was spread to civilian populations wherever the army camped. Scabetic soldiers sent home to convalesce spread the disease in their communities.

The disease is still reported in the military. In 1946 Walter Libmann, M.D., reported that 65 percent of the patients in the skin clinic presented with scabies or its complications (pyoderma and furunculosis). Sixteen percent of sick-call patients had scabies.[28] It affected all ages and ranks. The disease in the military was endemic in peacetime and epidemic in wartime due to the lack of cleaning material and sanitary facilities. Scabies accompanied venereal disease among service people.

Malaria and the Southern Campaign

The mosquito is ubiquitous throughout the world. It was present on earth long before man's appearance. There are mosquitoes embedded in amber from the period when reptiles were the dominant animal species.[1] Malaria was known and described from many areas in the ancient world. However, there is no evidence it existed in the Western Hemisphere. The vector of malaria, the anopheles mosquito, probably existed in America before Columbus, although it may have been carried here in the water storage casks on the three ships that left Palos in 1492. Certainly the plasmodium organism could easily have been brought to Hispaniola by the sailors on board. Spain, and much of Europe, suffered from malaria by this time. After the Spanish invasion and conquest of Mexico and South America, malaria became widespread in the Western Hemisphere. Malaria was well established on the eastern seaboard when the British, Dutch, and Swedes established their outposts in what would later become the thirteen American colonies.[2]

There was some suggestion that malaria was the "seasoning" disease of the early settlers on the east coast.[3] In fact, however, England and other colonial powers had malaria at home. It was more likely that typhoid fever was the "seasoning" disease, because the mortality rate from typhoid was more compatible with the decimation produced among the early colonists. Malaria rarely killed the victim in the first or in early repeated attacks. Duffy, in *Epidemics in Colonial America*, argued that it was one of the most fatal of all colonial illnesses in the long run. As with dysentery, repeated attacks of malaria weakened the patient's capacity to survive attacks of the devastating epidemics of smallpox and yellow fever, or the insidious presence of pneumonia and tuberculosis.

Malaria existed in all of the thirteen colonies in the seventeenth century. For some unknown reason it had disappeared from New England by the outbreak of the Revolution. Then, the furthest northern extension of the disease was probably New York City. The absence of malaria in New England was probably the explanation for the feeling that it was a healthy place compared to the more southern sites of habitation. The tidewater areas of Virginia and North and South Carolina were notorious for malaria as evidenced by the repeated attacks suffered by George Washington. The disease was endemic in the south, and it reached epidemic proportions in the summer and fall. The marshes in the south and the heavily irrigated fields of rice agriculture in South Carolina created an anopheline breeding paradise.[4] British medical officers commented on the severity of swamp fever around Charleston, South Carolina, and Savannah, Georgia.[5]

Cotton and tobacco cultivation in the south were labor intensive, high cash crops ideal for slavery. In addition, it was believed that the blacks were resistant to malaria, and they could work through the summer and autumn unlike their white masters. There was some basis for this belief. Blacks with the sickle cell trait were resistant to falciparum malaria, the most deadly form of the disease. The plasmodium organism that caused falciparum malaria could not digest sickle hemoglobin. It was the protection produced by this trait that resulted in the predominance of sickle-containing inhabitants in West Africa, the area where most American slaves were obtained. All other groups, aboriginal or slave traders, were forced out of this area or died. Thalassemia hemoglobin, a similar mutation, in the Mediterranean littoral, seemed equally effective against falciparum. Blacks were also relatively resistant to vivax due to the absence of the Duffy antigen on their red blood cells, which prevented invasion of the cell. In addition, a deficiency of the glucose-6-phosphate-dehydrogenase enzyme, more commonly described in blacks, interfered with the growth and development of the parasite in the host's blood.[6]

Malaria played a significant role in the war in the south. The morbidity in the contending armies was high. Fortunately, the mortality was low. In the north, the frigid winters were generally used for encampment, refitting, and retraining rather than for active hostilities. In the south the cold was not a major problem. However, the malarial season was a "time to find the high ground" as Nathaniel Greene did with his army in the summer of 1781. The Rhode Island general led his troops to the high hills of Santee while Lord Rawdon, his counterpart in the British army, brought his troops to Orangeburg.[7]

Following the "draw" in the battle of Monmouth in June 1778, the major field of war shifted to the south. Some battles of no major consequence, except to the combatants, were fought in the north. A fiasco for the Americans and their French allies played itself out at Newport, Rhode Island. In the spring of 1779 Anthony Wayne defeated the British and took Stony Point on the Hudson River. Light Horse Harry Lee on August 18, 1779, took Paulus Hook.[8] Benedict Arnold invaded Connecticut with a British force and burned New London. He massacred the garrison and then left. He achieved nothing except to increase the animosity toward him of all patriots in America.[9]

The strategy of the British was to split the southern states from the rest of the rebellious nation, much as they tried to split away New England earlier in the war. The British felt they had two groups in the south they could count upon to flock to their colors. These included the Scots who had supported "Bonnie Prince Charlie" and other leaders in the Jacobite uprisings of 1715 and 1745. For some reason, the Scots transferred their allegiance to the House of Hanover from the house of Stuart after the loss at Culloden in 1746. The second group were the small farmers in the highlands who hated the tidewater plantation owners more than they did the English.[10] The war in the south started in 1776 when Sir Henry Clinton tried to capture Charleston with a British fleet. The city was defended by Major General Lee and Colonel Moultrie. Access to the city was between James Island and Sullivan's Island, which was protected on its seaside with temporary fortifications. The British tried to get to the rear of these defenses, but they failed. Cannonballs thrown by the British fleet seemed to bounce off the palmetto logs used in the island's defenses. The fire delivered by the batteries in Charleston was enough to dissuade the British from pushing their attack any further. In the back country, battles between Whigs and Tories occurred with ferocity and brutality on both sides. Loyalist Scots were defeated by Patriots at Moore's Creek Bridge, North Carolina, on February 27, 1776. This battle ended all major Tory depredations against their neighbors until the successful invasion of the south late in 1778.[11] In December 1778 British Lieutenant Colonel Campbell landed below Savannah, Georgia. He was opposed by American troops under General Robert House. British troops were able to get behind the Americans and attack from front and rear. House withdrew to South Carolina. The British took Augusta and controlled all of Georgia. The opening success of British forces resulted in the vindication of British beliefs in potential allies. Loyalists flocked to their colors. General House was replaced by Major General Lincoln of Massachusetts who tried to retake Georgia with a combined force of Americans under General Ashe and French under Count D'Estaing. These troops were soundly defeated by General Prevost leading British troops. The Americans lost General Pulaski; the French fleet picked up its troops and departed in October 1779. The only benefit of the battle to the Americans was to impress on Sir Henry Clinton that he had to consolidate his troops. The British therefore vacated Newport, Rhode Island, and Rochambeau with 4,000 French troops marched in and occupied it in July 1780.

The next objective in the British southern strategy was to capture Charleston. In April 1780 British ships under Admiral Arbuthnot successfully crossed a sandbar in Charleston Harbor. The South Carolina "navy" under Whipple was pulled back, and ships were scuttled in the Ashley River to prevent passage of the British fleet. The British were able to pass Fort Moultrie, and Sir Henry Clinton invested Charleston, which was under the command of General Lincoln. Cornwallis commanded the British infantry and Lieutenant Colonel Banastre Tarleton the British cavalry. The British cavalry defeated its American opponents at Santee. The British now controlled the country between the Cooper and the Santee Rivers. The Americans in Charleston were surrounded. Lincoln capitulated on May 12, 1780. The British captured more than 5,000 troops as well as shipping and ordnance. They also captured intact the entire medical establishment of South Carolina. Of the prisoners, the militia units were disarmed and allowed to return to their homes. The continental troops were made prisoners of war on ships in Charleston Harbor. Cornwallis then took Augusta, North Carolina; Ninety-Six; and Camden. The American Colonel Buford retreated to North Carolina. His group was caught by Tarleton's cavalry at Waxhaus. Buford surrendered, but the prisoners were massacred by Tarleton's troops. After news of the massacre leaked out, the cry of "Tarleton's Quarter" was the rallying cry on American lips.

After he had secured South Carolina, Clinton took the majority of his troops back to New York. He left 6,500 troops under Cornwallis to "clean up the south." De Kalb with the Maryland and Delaware line (some of the bravest troops in the Continental army) moved south. General Gates, still fresh from his victory at Saratoga, was sent from Virginia to take command of the entire southern theater of war. He chose to march his army along a poorly settled route. This meant there was no adequate source of food available for his troops nor forage for his horses. His troops were forced to subsist on green corn, unripe fruit, molasses, improperly prepared meat, and cornmeal resulting in severe diarrhea. When the line of march passed through marshlands infested with mosquitoes, the men fell victim to malaria. With this poorly prepared army, Gates met Cornwallis at Camden. Gates's line broke when his militia panicked and fled. Cornwallis defeated Gates handily, and the latter took off for points north, probably ahead of the militia. Among the casualties was General De Kalb, who was killed on September 8, 1780.

Cornwallis then set out to conquer North Carolina. He suffered a serious setback at King's Mountain with the loss of a quarter of his troops, and he retreated back to Charlotte. This defeat at King's Mountain gave the North Carolina Tories second thoughts about enlistment in the British army. The rainy season set in, and the ground became marshy with an attendant overgrowth of mosquitoes. Troops sickened with malaria. Cornwallis developed a bilious fever (probably malaria) and turned his command over to Lord Rawdon. The British were pulled back to Winnsborough, near Camden. Behind the British troops, Marion, Sumter, and Pickens carried out a guerrilla war that destroyed troops, ordnance, and morale.

Nathaniel Greene replaced Gates on October 14, 1780. Clinton sent General Leslie to join Cornwallis. Leslie landed at Portsmouth, Virginia. Cornwallis sent Tarleton out to destroy Brigadier General Morgan, who, despite suffering from chronic rheumatism, fought Tarleton at the Cowpens on January 16, 1781. Cowpens was a resounding American victory. The British suffered 900 casualties. Greene pulled his army back to Virginia, and Cornwallis followed. The American general skillfully moved his green army across the

Catawba, Yadkin, and Deep Rivers with the British in pursuit. This retreat left North Carolina in British hands. Greene then recrossed the Dan back to North Carolina. He fought Cornwallis at Guilford Court House March 15, 1781. The Americans retreated from the field, but they inflicted severe losses on the British troops; about a third of the British were killed or wounded. The Americans lost 326 dead, wounded, and prisoners.[12] In the English Parliament, Fox said of the victory, "Another such victory would destroy the British Army."[13]

Now it was the turn of the British to pull back and Greene to follow. Loyalists refused to join Cornwallis who pulled back to Wilmington, North Carolina. At this point it should be noted that Benedict Arnold's attack on New London was an attempt to force the American command to pull some of its troops away from the southern theater of operations. After Arnold left Connecticut, he was sent to Virginia in January 1781 at the head of a large British force to try to subdue that important state. His troops marched to Richmond and destroyed it; he put his troops back on transports and proceeded to devastate settlements on the James River, and moved to Portsmouth to build up its defenses. General Arnold received reinforcements, but his command was taken over by General Philips who used it to capture Petersburg from Virginia militia under Baron Von Steuben. Philips destroyed Petersburg, and he devastated its environs. He then returned to Petersburg where he was to link up with Cornwallis who pushed north from Wilmington. Lafayette and his troops followed Philips while Greene invaded South Carolina. General Philips in Petersburg, Virginia, succumbed to bilious fever. Command of the British troops returned to Benedict Arnold, joined by Cornwallis. The British forces chased Lafayette around Virginia, but they failed to destroy Lafayette's troops who had marched to Virginia from Peekskill, New York. The British finally pulled back to Richmond, then to Portsmouth, by order of General Clinton. Clinton expected a major attack on New York, and he ordered some of Cornwallis's troops to be sent north. Cornwallis was to set up a defensive position on Chesapeake Bay so that the British fleet could winter there instead of in Halifax, Nova Scotia. Cornwallis initially tried old Point Comfort, but this was not defensible. He then chose Yorktown and Gloucester on either side of the York River. The British army pulled into these positions on August 1, 1781.

Meanwhile, Greene's plans for South Carolina involved a combined use of his regular forces with the guerrilla troops under Pickens, Marion, and Sumter, with added help from "Light Horse Harry" Lee. The guerrillas would disrupt supplies, and the troops under Greene would attack the strong points. The British defense of South Carolina was an inverted "T" from Charleston west to "96." The upright of the "T" ran from the Wateree River north to Camden. The battles for South Carolina started April 25, 1781, with the battle at Hobkirk's Hill. The Americans had to retreat from the field with about equal losses on both sides. However, Greene's army was still intact. Greene's greatest service to the war effort was to conserve his army and keep it intact much as Washington had done in the north earlier in the war. Greene won no victories, but he won the war. Although victorious, Rawdon, the British leader, had to abandon Camden and retreat south to the waterway, which formed the east-west defenses of the British line. Greene unsuccessfully tried to conquer "96" and move back to Charleston.

The hot, muggy summer weather of South Carolina put a stop to hostilities. Both armies suffered large losses from malaria. Greene took his troops to the high hills of Santee. Rawdon camped at Orangeburg. The guerrilla forces continued to attack British supply lines and outposts. Rawdon gave up his command to Lieutenant Colonel Alexander Stewart because of a combination of poor health and failure to destroy Greene's army. With the approach of August 1781, Greene's troops, recuperated from their labors and relatively free of the malaria they had suffered in the marshy areas of South Carolina, were ready to fight. Greene's army met Stewart at Eutaw Springs on September 8, 1781. Again the British retained the field, but Greene's army inflicted forty percent casualties on the British, causing them to retreat back to Charleston. Despite repeated victories in South Carolina, the British were finally left with Charleston alone.

Washington and his French allies were ready for a concerted effort to defeat the British. Rochambeau and his troops from Newport joined Washington in Westchester, New York, on July 5, 1781. They moved south on August 19, 1781. French Admiral Barras moved his fleet south. Washington wanted to capture New York City, but Admiral DeGrasse, with the main French fleet, sailed north from the West Indies to the Chesapeake. He advised the American general that he could remain in the area until October, but then he had to return to the West Indies. Washington with 19,000 men marched around New York and turned south. The British general, Clinton, was fooled. He believed that Washington was headed for Staten Island. DeGrasse reached Chesapeake Bay before the British Admirals Graves and Hood. The French had 28 ships of the line, as well as four frigates and 3,000 infantry. The French fleet fought the British fleet on September 5, 1781. With the additional forces supplied by Admiral Barras, De Grasse won a slight victory over the British. More significantly, the French closed Chesapeake Bay to the British fleet, which turned and sailed to New York. Washington's army arrived, and together with Lafayette's troops hemmed in Cornwallis. Cornwallis could not turn south because Greene's forces were there after the battle at Eutaw Springs. Cornwallis expected Clinton to sail down and evacuate his troops so he made an attempt to break out and failed. He then capitulated to Washington in October 1781, surrendering 7,500 troops. Across the river, Tarleton capitulated at Gloucester. Clinton dispatched a fleet to rescue Cornwallis, but it arrived too late, and the surrender was signed October 19, 1781.[14]

Half of Lafayette's troops were off the line because of malaria. The New England troops who accompanied Washington to Tidewater, Virginia, had had no previous exposure to malaria. They developed the disease shortly after their arrival. Malaria along with dysentery compromised the fighting strength of both adversaries. Of the 20,000 troops on both sides at Yorktown, 570 were killed. A far greater number were sick. Sixteen percent of Cornwallis's troops as well as the general himself were unfit for duty with malaria.[15] General Cornwallis was so sick that he turned his command over to Lord Rawdon, and he was unable to appear at the surrender ceremonies. At Yorktown, the majority of hospitalized patients were sick, not injured. There were 193 French and 107 American wounded casualties in the hospitals. Sick troops were also sent to hospitals in Williamsburg, Hampton, Portsmouth, Fredericksburg, and Charlotte. In September 1781 William and Mary College was turned over to the French to use as their hospital. In November 1781 a wing of the college used for an officer's hospital caught fire, and the patients had to be moved. French casualties were also housed in Elizabeth City.[16] The British had 1,500 sick in their hospitals at Yorktown. They were moved to Gloucester and cared for by their own doctors. They had practically no supplies to treat the sick. As soon as the surrender was completed, Washington pulled his troops out and marched them to the Hudson River encampment to prevent further decimation from malaria.[17] The American sick and wounded could be discharged from the service at their request and receive $5 a month until cured, or they could join the "Invalid Corps" at full pay to do garrison duty.

Further south, Greene awaited the cooler weather of November to continue fighting. The British withdrew from Wilmington and held only Charleston and Savannah. After Yorktown, British General Leslie proposed to Greene that they stop hostilities and await the impending truce. Greene refused, and a unit under American General Wayne tried to take Savannah and failed. However, by July 11, 1782, the British withdrew from Savannah, and Wayne entered the city. On December 14, 1782, the British evacuated Charleston and for all intents and purposes, major fighting in the war ended. In Great Britain, Lord North resigned in March 1782; Rockingham succeeded him, but he died on July 1, 1782.[18] Negotiations for peace crept along for a year. The American peace commissioners, who feared a French "double cross," signed a separate peace treaty without the French and Spanish. The war in America ended. British troops finally left New York at the end of November 1783, although the Treaty of Paris had been signed in January of that year.

There was no description of malaria by the American surgeons in the Revolution. However, the British regimental surgeon of Fraser's Highlanders, Robert Jackson, left a complete description of the disease in different parts of America. He observed languor, debility, flatulence, headache, and drowsiness. The patient's veins "subsided," his nails became pale, then blue, and the skin was dry and constricted. There was diminution of heat of the extremities, yawning, weariness, and a desire to stretch the limbs. He complained of a sensation of cold felt in the back, "as if water ran down." It came and went with aggravated violence. The whole body was involved with rigor or shaking and chattering teeth. The coldness was replaced by "glowings of heat," which grew stronger and lasted longer. All sensation of cold disappeared. The fever rose, the veins became full, the face flushed, and the body bore marks of distention. This phase lasted one to four hours. This was followed by a dampness of the forehead and breast, which extended to the extremities. The fever dropped, and the patient's body returned to near normal. Jackson believed that the cold fit might not occur in the summer. The tumult and weakness that terminated in the sweat went off in some patients in urine and stool. Rarely, the patient did not have the fever or sweat. These were replaced by local pain in the paroxysms and were often accompanied by a comatose state, convulsions, or tetanic affection. Vital and natural functions were variously affected in different people or in the same person at different stages of the paroxysm of fever. The pulse started slow, languid and weak, then more frequent, but small and contracted. Then it became strong, full and hard with the sweat; the hardness and frequency then abated and became normal. (The extent of physical diagnosis at this time was observation of the patient and taking his pulse. Many variations of the pulse could be detected by a competent examiner.) The patient developed nausea, retching, and vomiting until the body was in a sweat. The patient's respiration started slow with sighing. This was replaced by frequent laborious breathing. His mental faculties declined with fever, but they could become acute with continued fever. Excitement, delirium, and deranged intellect could continue throughout the course. The patient's urine was thin and pale at first, then high colored with heat. This was followed by a thick and turbid urine, with the sweat associated with a copious lateritious (brick-red colored) sediment. The observer believed that single tertians began between 10:00 A.M. and 2:00 P.M. and lasted one to two hours in America.

Dr. Jackson then made certain generalizations. He felt that single tertian was most usual in spring and summer. In June, July, and August double tertians developed. As the weather cooled, single tertians recurred. Dysentery and dropsy developed in August, September, and October. Jackson believed that intermittents were not dangerous if treated decisively at the start. He rarely saw fatalities in a paroxysm, but rather with deterioration to dropsy and dysentery. Danger signs in the patient included a flushed face that was dark and overcast and appeared greasy and dusky. In addition, despondence and a stern look in the eyes were prognostic signs. A white glutinous covering of the tongue was also dangerous. When these signs appeared, the doctor had no time to prepare the patient with cathartics and emetics. He had to start bark immediately. He believed those preparations prior to bark were generally useless. He also did not believe that bleeding the patient helped in hot climates. Tartar emetic did not shorten the disease, but antimonial emetics made the bark work better, which was the chief remedy. The French used it cautiously, and the Germans rarely. The bark imported into England was probably adulterated or inferior, because it required a larger dose to do the job. He prescribed two drams every two hours during the afebrile period. Sometimes the patient required massive doses. Sometimes, the stomach rejected it, and stools came rapidly. Occasionally bark did not work, and the doctor resorted to blisters on the back of the neck and head to make the bark work better. Sometimes aromatics, chalybeates (medication impregnated with iron salts), and snake root helped. If snake root was given with bark, there were no relapses, and the improvements developed more rapidly. Jackson believed that if he returned his patients to duty rapidly, their health was preserved.

Finally, he compared mortality in the different armies. The Hessians did not use bark and lost a third of their troops stationed in Georgia in one year. Some British surgeons, who used it timidly, lost a fourth of their troops. Those using it in good doses lost only one-twentieth of the troops. Bark did not help in dysentery. Here, Jackson used the usual blistering, cathartics, opium, ipecachuana, snake root, camomile flowers, and wine. To treat dropsy, he advised exercise, wine, stimulating liquors, highly seasoned food, friction to the body (usually with flannel), and blisters. Cantharides in a tincture was the best diuretic. Other diuretics were chalybeates and colombo root.[19]

The History of Malaria

Malaria is an ancient and widespread infection affecting mankind. Intermittent fevers were frequently described in Babylonian-Assyrian writings. The god of pestilence of Babylon, Nergal, was depicted as a flying insect. Malarial fevers were probably described in the Old Testament (Leviticus described a burning ague, and Deuteronomy talked about an inflammation). It was probably recognized 3,000 years ago in China by the writer Huang Ti. Old Indian literature described a fever with splenic enlargement. In a Sanskrit reference from 600 B.C. (the *Susruta*), the mosquito was described as the cause of the disease. Malaria was probably introduced into Japan by Chinese invaders, as Japanese writings alluded to the disease only after these invasions.[20]

Malaria probably was a significant cause of the downfall of Greece from its heights in the classical world. Ancient Greece was free of the plasmodium. Its citizens were vigorous, patriotic, religious, and active members of their societies. The Athenians reached great heights in art, science, and philosophy. There are no writings to suggest the presence of malaria in Greece before the middle of the fifth century B.C. It was probably introduced into the Greek peninsula when Greek warriors invaded Asia and Africa, particularly the invasion of Egypt in 456 B.C. The soldiers and their foreign slaves returned with a stowaway in their bloodstreams.

The geography of Greece may be responsible for malaria's widespread decimation of its population. There are mountains separated by valleys where the majority of the population lived and farmed. The runoff of the mountains created pools in the valleys, which frequently became stagnant. The mosquito was present and available to receive the plasmodium. It required about fifty years to spread throughout the population. This resulted in a withering of the nation's intellectual growth. Unlike most infectious diseases, malaria did not weed out the unfit. It simply lowered the vitality of the general population. By 300 B.C., Greece was easy prey for the invasion by its neighbor to the west.[21]

Hippocrates recognized the association of fevers with marshes and described patients with large spleens and fleshless bodies. He was also aware of a "cold" stage characterized by weariness, headache, nausea, vomiting, and shivering. The pulse was quick, small, and hard. Urine output increased. This was followed by the "hot" stage seen as heat and red skin. The pulse was full and bounding associated with delirium and thirst. The final stage was the sweat with a drop of fever, and the patient fell into a deep fatigued sleep. Hippocrates distinguished the quotidian fever, which lasted six to twelve hours each day, from the mild tertian which lasted about nine hours every two days, from the malignant tertian which lasted up to forty hours out of the forty-eight, and from the quartan, which lasted nine hours every three days. He described the chronic sufferer as one with a large spleen, evil complexion, ulcerous and emaciated, who suffered foul breath and constipation. The physician described malarial cachexia characterized by fear, depression, and melancholy. The overall loss of health and vigor probably resulted in decreased morale, conscience, duty, patriotism, and brilliance, which indeed occurred about 300 B.C. It was also associated with increased pessimism in philosophy, sentimentalism in literature, and an increase in morbid brooding about death.[22]

The spread of malaria into Italy is difficult to date. Some trace the fall of the Etruscan culture to malaria, but this is unlikely. The Etruscans dug irrigation tunnels below the ground to drain the marshlands and reclaim the land for farming. Whether it was used as a tool against malaria is conjectural. The Romans who followed the Etruscans extended their work to increase productivity of the soil. Malaria may have been introduced into the Italian peninsula in approximately 200 B.C..[23] The Romans were never prize winners in medicine or medical writing, but one can infer malaria's presence from plays and speeches that have come down to us. It is believed that malaria was introduced from Africa by Hannibal's mercenaries.[24] The devastation of the Punic Wars converted normal farmland into marshy areas, which were excellent breeding places for the mosquitoes. The peasants, long the backbone of Rome and its armies, became unproductive due to physical decay and the associated moral decay. They left the land and flocked to the city, which resulted in increased congestion and left the farmland to return to marshes. Added to this was the period of civil wars in the first century B.C. Farmers left their land in wartime, because they feared isolation and death at the enemy's hands. This swelled the mobs and forced Rome to import its food from the conquered provinces. It is claimed that malaria turned the stern Roman character into the dissolute, bloodthirsty, immoral spirit depicted in current movies and books.[25] The autumn rains in the Italian peninsula created the necessary pools for the larvae to mature. The widespread prevalence of malaria in Italy is attested to by the three ancient temples to the goddess Febris whose help was sought to relieve the supplicants of this debilitating disease. The presence of the temples, perhaps dating to the fourth century B.C., negates the theory of the Punic Wars as the period of introduction of malaria to Italy.[26] In Italian, "bad air" is mala aria, and the name of the disease is derived from this term. The etiological agent, plasmodium, was not identified until 1880 when Alphonse Laveran, a French medical officer in the Constantine Hospital in Algiers, discovered it and determined the vector to be the mosquito.

Malaria spread from Greece and Rome to the rest of Europe except to the Scandinavian countries and northern Russia. The Dutch used windmills to drain marshy areas to increase their productivity. However, a land full of canals with slowly moving water was a fine breeding ground for the mosquito. The introduction of the parasite resulted in great morbidity and mortality among the population. Sir John Pringle mentioned the "intermittents" in the low countries in his book. Sir Gilbert Blane described the destruction of British troops in the Walcheran expedition of 1809. In four months, 4,000 of a garrison of 18,000 were dead of the fever. Repeated attempts of the North Sea to take back the land from the Dutch resulted in outbreaks of malaria.[27]

In England, the disease was called ague from the Latin, *acuta* (sharp). The enlarged spleen was called an "ague cake." Malaria may have been introduced into the British Isles during the Roman occupation. It is claimed that the Romans lost an army in Scotland due to malaria. The Thames estuary around London, as well as Kent, Bridgewater, and Lancashire were notorious for their marshy areas. In Kent, the disease was so common that malaria was known as the "Kentish Disease."[28] In parts of England, marshy areas with their associated malaria were so bad that the overall life expectancy was 14 years. In the town of Wrangle, sixty percent of the population died before their 21st birthday. There is the story of one old farmer who lived at a higher elevation but whose wives were from the "lowlands." He went through five wives, all of whom died before the age of 20.[29] The term "malaria" was introduced into England in the correspondence of Horace Walpole to H. S. Conway dated July 15, 1740. He described "the horrid thing called the mal'aria that comes to Rome every summer and kills one."[30] It was not until 1850 that England became relatively free of malaria. This followed the successful drainage of the fens and marshes with tiles used to build drains. In the process 680,000 acres were reclaimed for agriculture.[31]

Early Treatments

Before the discovery of bark, various medications were tried to treat the illness. Herbs mixed with evil-tasting materials were compounded to drive out the invader. This technique was not specific for malaria, but it was a general concept of therapy to drive out the demons. The Indians and Chinese used arsenic to treat the disease. Some herbs used in China were later found to contain antiplasmodial chemicals. Hippocrates prescribed rest, massage, hydrotherapy, diet, change of residence, purges, trefoil, asafoetida, and wine. He restricted food during the paroxysms of fever. The physician pushed barley gruel as well as honey in water or honey in wine. After the paroxysm ended, he prescribed mistletoe for the enlarged spleen. Of all the therapies he advised, the idea of a change of residence was obviously the best. Pliny the Elder in *Natural History* advised garlic in sour wine for quartan fevers. Pepper and verbena root were also prescribed in Greece. Galen called for emetics, purges, sudorifics as sweat inducers, cholagogues to carry off bile, and venesection. Galen's medical concepts were followed in Byzantium as well as among Arabian and Persian physicians. Avicenna used cool drinks and fruits, such as plums, pomegranates, and watermelon. The public put its faith in amulets that held hair from a goat's chin as well as dung and beetles in a red bag. Spiders were a specific for the disease, because they drew the poisons into themselves. Spiders could be taken internally or worn on the body. The disease could also be transferred to another person, animal, or object.

The specific therapy for malaria comes from the bark of a tree in South America. There are forty species of evergreen trees grown in the western Andean slopes of Venezuela, Bolivia, and Peru. The bark of these trees contains cinchona from which quinine is produced.[32] There are many stories told about the introduction of cinchona to western medicine. The most commonly told tale is that of Ana de Osorio, the Countess de Cinchon, who was cured of malaria in 1638 in Peru with bark. The Countess was the wife of the viceroy.[33] Another story described a soldier in South America left to die by his comrades because he was so weak with malaria. He drank the bitter water from a pool in which a log had been soaking, and he was cured.[34] One tale I find difficult to believe is that concerning the Jesuit missionary Juan Lopez who observed the Indian tribes using the bark in 1600. Malaria was probably introduced into South America in the middle of the sixteenth century. It is hard for me to accept the Indian use of this specific so soon after the introduction of the disease.[35]

The introduction of bark to Europe has many fathers as well. One story concerns the Jesuit missionary, Tafur, who returned to Europe with the Count and Countess de Cinchon. Tafur carried the bark to Rome where it was ground into powder in a Jesuit pharmacy and distributed throughout Europe by followers of Loyola. The name "Jesuit's Bark" for the remedy lends credence to this theory. Another contender is Juan DeVega, the physician to the Count de Cinchon. He is supposed to have brought it to Europe in 1641 and sold it in Seville for 100 reales per pound.[36] Then, there is Calancha of Lima, Peru, a monk who authored a book in 1633, which was printed in Spain in 1639 and in which he described the process of pounding the bark into powder. The natives then added it to a beverage to cure fevers.

The bark was not immediately accepted by the European conservative medical groups and the professors at the universities because it could not be reconciled with Galen's teachings. Others in Protestant Europe refused to accept it because the Jesuits controlled its distribution. Nevertheless, the drug found its way into use by the charlatans who dispensed it as part of a secret remedy to treat "the fever." One quack, Robert Tabor, was made rich and enno-bled after he cured the royalty of England and France.[37] Eventually, the trained physicians of Europe recognized the benefits of bark in ague, but they still did not accept its specificity in the treatment of disease without the addition of other medications.

Sydenham was completely aware of the specificity of bark in malaria in the seventeenth century. In 1740 Dr. Lind, of scurvy fame, prescribed large doses of the powder as soon as he made the diagnosis. He went one step fur-ther and urged its use in prophylaxis against the disease. Lind advised inhab-itants of malarial regions to take the remedy daily in alcohol.[38] In view of the proven effectiveness of bark in malaria, one wonders why so many additional treatments were given for the disease well into the nineteenth century. Charles Ledger, an Englishman, obtained seeds from the trees that grew on the west-ern slopes of the Andes Mountains and sold them to the Dutch. The Dutch planted them in Java, their colony in the East Indies. The area seemed to be made for their cultivation, and Java soon passed South America in its pro-duction of the bark. Java today supplies most of the natural quinine used in the world. The active product of the bark, quinine, was isolated by two French chemists, Pelletier and Caventou in 1820.[39] Quinine is known now to act as a protoplasmic poison. It destroys the organisms as well as the host's cells. It can damage white blood cells, decrease reflexes, and irritate the gut. Most of it is degraded in the liver; approximately a third is excreted unchanged through the kidneys. Excessive doses cause ringing in the ears, constrictions in the head, headaches, and vertigo. It is also recognized as one of the causes of sec-ondary thrombocytopenic purpura.[40] Two hundred years ago, Dr. Robert Jack-son knew that Peruvian bark was a specific for ague. According to Jackson, it worked by giving tone and vigor to the powers of life, and often communi-cated with the sanguiferous system. If strength, fullness, and vigor of the pulse followed bark, the fever disappeared. Basically it worked by changing the state of the body. The intermittents arose from an atonic state of the system. It did not prevent relapses, but they were milder.[41]

Malaria cannot be said to have played a vital role in the outcome of the war in the south, but it put large numbers of combatants out of action in both armies. Except for falciparum malaria, the disease usually did not kill its victims in the first or after several attacks. Unlike the other plasmodia, falciparum could invade the cerebral vasculature with coma and death. It also affected the kidneys and caused black water fever, renal failure, and death. It was probably the cause of death of British general Philips who was reported to have died of bilious fever. The recurrent attacks of fever followed by anemia and a swollen spleen left the soldier at less than combat readiness. Like most chronic debilitating diseases, it weakened the host and increased the mortality rate caused by other acute diseases.

Appendix:
The Health of
George Washington
and King George III

George Washington

EARLY YEARS

Like every other school child in America, I was brought up to believe in the honesty, integrity, and strength of the father of our country. After all, he admitted that he chopped down his father's cherry tree, and he was strong enough to throw a silver dollar across the Rappahanock River. When I reached my cynical twenties and thirties, I doubted everything. After all, Washington was a slaveholder. Although he took no salary as commander-in-chief of the Continental troops, he submitted an enormous, possibly padded, expense account. He executed a few mutineers during the war. With age and mellowing, the pendulum of my opinion stopped somewhere between the two extremes. In Washington's case, I am happy to believe that the pendulum leans toward the positive side.

During the many crises in our national history, we have almost always been blessed with a leader to help us overcome our dark days. Washington was one of several who came to the top like cream in a bottle of milk. He was a general, but he could not hold a candle to General Jackson or General Lee in the Civil War. I believe his real claim to fame was his ability to hold an army together in the face of the best trained, best equipped army in Europe. His "army" was a mass of poorly supplied, poorly trained farmers who believed in what they were doing, and who had real faith in their general. He was a brave leader and led his men from the front much as do the modern-day Israeli battle leaders. He placed himself in "harm's way" repeatedly. In leading Braddock's defeated troops from Fort Duquesne, he had two horses shot from under him and four bullet holes in his clothes.[1] In Princeton he rallied his troops when he rode his white horse between the two firing lines to within 30 paces of the enemy. He urged his men to victory and gave the new nation another lease on life.[2] The victory led many of his troops to extend their enlistment. In my eyes, his greatest contribution as a general was that he respected civilian authority. He accepted the supremacy of Congress over the military. He reported his actions and plans to Congress and accepted its judgment. He was a politician, but not as good a cajoler as Franklin, nor as wise or gifted with words as Jefferson. His formal education had stopped at the age of 14. He preferred hunting, fox-chasing, card playing, the theater and business to literary pursuits. While he is reported to have had a private library of 900 books, his own diary failed to mention any major periods of reading.[3] He was elected to the Virginia House of Burgesses several times and to the First and Second Continental Congress as well as to the Constitutional Convention. I am sure his wealth and major landholdings were responsible for his first two positions, and the successful outcome of the Revolution for the last position. His success as a general led to his unanimous election to the presidency.

What contributed to the makeup of this man? What was his genetic makeup, his health, his emotional state? On his father's side, longevity was not extended. Tuberculosis was a common problem throughout the family's history. Throughout his life, George Washington was frequently ill, and he thought he was near death repeatedly. Surprisingly, however, during the Revolution, he only suffered a sore throat while he wintered at Morristown. Emotionally, he was depressed too often, and he was ready to die when he was seriously ill. There also was a period of a persecution complex during the French and Indian War.

John Washington, George's great-grandfather, came to Virginia from England in 1657 with his two sons, Lawrence and John. Lawrence, George's grandfather, died at the age of 37 probably of lung disease, leaving two sons, Lawrence and Augustine. Augustine, George's father, lived to the age of 48 and died of respiratory disease. Augustine was married twice. His first wife, Jane Butler, died in 1726, after bearing four children, two of whom died in infancy. His second wife was Mary Ball, George's mother, who died of breast cancer at the age of 81. This union produced six children, of whom George was the oldest. Mildred was the youngest and died in infancy. When his father died, George went to live with his half-brother, Lawrence, at Mount Vernon. Lawrence married Anne Fairfax and had four children, all of whom died in infancy or childhood. Lawrence died of tuberculosis in 1752 at the age of 34. George's other half-brother, Augustine, died before age 40. Mary Ball must have introduced better DNA to the genetic pool. Of George's full siblings, Betty died at 64, Samuel at 47, John at 51, and Charles at 64. His nephew, George Augustine, died of tuberculosis. George Washington had no children of his own. It was not his wife's "fault." In her first marriage, she had four children, two of whom lived beyond infancy.[4] It is an accepted fact that the father of our country could not father children, perhaps because of his early case of smallpox and/or tuberculosis, either of which can affect the testicles and the conducting tubules from the testicles (vas deferens).

George Washington also developed severe depression in the face of chronic debilitating diseases. In his writings he mentioned being ready to die, and during his last illness, he told his doctors he was ready to die and to let him die peacefully. He may have been very suggestible as well. In 1758 he believed he was dying of the flux and pleurisy with fever. He was sick for four months and traveled to Williamsburg to see Dr. Anson who told him he would recover. And so he did a few days after the consultation.[5] Perhaps his depression in the face of illness was due to deficient or improper balance of the neurotransmitters in his central nervous system. On the other hand, he had a poor early life. His father died when he was only eleven, and he was unable to obtain the schooling in England that the sons of the first marriage received. His father figure was his half-brother, Lawrence, who was chronically ill and died at a young age. His mother was egocentric and resented his achievements, because they detracted from his attention to her. She also dissipated the inheritance he received from his father.

Early in life, he had an unrequited love for a married woman. Despite his marriage to the wealthy widow Custis, he loved Sally Cary Fairfax all of his life. The Fairfax family owned vast acreage in Virginia, and a cousin, also a Fairfax, managed the estates while the owner lived in England. The manager's daughter married Lawrence. When George went to live with his brother and sister-in-law, he was introduced into the higher strata of Virginia society. George became a surveyor at the age of sixteen with a license from William and Mary College, and he went to work for the Fairfaxes and spent a fair amount of time with them. George loved Sally Cary who married George William Fairfax in 1749 and admitted his love for her all of his life. He described a feeling of loneliness during his married life at Mount Vernon. However, perhaps because he was employed by the Fairfaxes, or perhaps because well brought up men in the colonies did not dally with married women, he never made overt advances to this lady.

The "persecution complex" developed around 1757. After the Braddock debacle, he again was dispatched to the "frontier" with France. He developed severe dysentery and fever. Washington gave up his command and left the army to return to Mount Vernon to regain his health. The illness persisted for months. At this period there was unrest in Virginia, and he felt he was the butt of false accusations. He felt personally humiliated and became more disturbed, more depressed, and developed a "persecution complex." He believed his friends were traitors to him. This in turn caused a flare-up of his dysentery, and his health grew worse. He corresponded with Lieutenant Governor Dinwiddie of Virginia and complained of remarks by other officers. He was rebuffed by Dinwiddie. His bloody flux continued for three more months.[6] It is an interesting sidelight that the Lieutenant Governor was suffering from the same problem at this time, and he went to England to heal himself. However, he died there.

George was born in Virginia in 1732 into a family of comfortable circumstances. Early in life he probably had measles and diphtheria. The case of measles could be assumed, because Martha developed measles during their life together, and he did not develop it despite his proximity. He had "black canker" of the throat which was believed to be diphtheria.[7] (It was not until 1821 that the Frenchman, Bretonneau, fully described this disease.) However, the assumption of diphtheria at this age was presented to rule out this disease as the cause of his terminal event since one attack produces life-long immunity. He grew up in the lowlands of Virginia, and his job as a surveyor forced him to spend many nights in the marshes of the Fairfax property. He developed malaria early in life, and he suffered repeated bouts of the "ague." At seventeen he became seriously ill with malaria and exhaustion.[8] After his first severe attack of malaria, he went on a surveying project across the Blue Ridge Mountains into the Shenandoah Valley. He returned in time to take his brother Lawrence across the Blue Ridge to try the healing waters of "Warm Springs." His brother, seriously ill with consumption, experienced some improvement. In September 1751 George accompanied Lawrence on a trip to Barbados to try to restore his health. At a dinner party, one of the household staff had smallpox, and George developed that disease. Those who believed it was a mild disease with minimal pitting postulated that he may have been inoculated with smallpox before he left Virginia. This is doubtful, because an inoculation that "took" gave lifelong immunity similar to the "natural way." A more likely explanation was that it was a milder variant of the virus. Other authorities believed it was a more serious case and left his face badly pitted. He lay ill until December 12, 1751, with Dr. Lanahan in almost constant attendance for 26 days. Lawrence then sailed to Bermuda in hopes of further improvement, but George returned to Virginia and arrived in January 1752.[9] That spring George developed a violent pleurisy. For this diagnosis, we must depend upon his physicians. The extent of most evaluations was to obtain a history, observe the patient, and feel his pulse. All chest pain was called pleurisy. In view of his family history, it probably was tuberculous pleurisy. During his period of recovery, he suffered repeated bouts of ague and was unable to work for extended periods.[10]

Lawrence returned to Virginia during this recuperative period, and he died of consumption on July 26, 1752. George lost a second and beloved father. Washington's life in Lawrence's home had been a happy period for the young man. He heard exciting tales of English wars, and this probably stimulated him to desire a military career. Lawrence was a member of the colonial forces sent to take Cartagena in Colombia in the War of Jenkin's Ear.[11] The Spaniards controlled the Caribbean basin and determined to keep all trade within their hands.

Masters of foreign ships, if caught, were mutilated. One such unfortunate sea captain was Jenkins, commanding a British merchantman. The Spaniards caught his ship and cut off his ear. Jenkins retrieved his ear, placed it in a bed of cotton in a small box, and set out for London. When he arrived, he went to Parliament and opened his box before the entire house. England declared war on Spain. In fact, the name of the "homestead," Mount Vernon, came from Lawrence's military exploits in Colombia. The leader of the force, greatly respected by Lawrence, was Admiral Edward Vernon.

Lawrence had achieved the position of adjutant general of the Virginia militia, a position George coveted. After Lawrence's premature death, George was made adjutant general of the southern district of Virginia, the smallest of four districts. He was made a major of the Virginia militia at 21 and received 100 pounds a year from the Virginia treasury. At this time trouble was brewing in the Ohio Valley, an area that attracted British and French explorers in the seventeenth and eighteenth centuries. Ownership was not contested until the mid-eighteenth century. Its value was in Indian trade, and it was a gate to the west and the south. The British looked at it as a natural expansion west of their colonies, which hugged the Atlantic Ocean. Many in Pennsylvania and Virginia saw the vast territory as a site for speculation. The British staked their claim to the area based on a treaty they had signed with the Iroquois Confederacy in Lancaster, Pennsylvania in 1744. The French looked at it as a bridge between Canada and their posts on the Mississippi River. France claimed control because of LaSalle's exploration in 1669–70. The Iroquois recognized British control over the Valley. In Virginia, the Ohio Company was formed and requested a grant of more than one half million acres from the King of England. This was granted, and the company rapidly started to settle the area. The Iroquois, frightened by the extensive incursion of white settlers, went to the French and denied the treaty. The French sent De Blauinville down the Ohio River to forbid further British advance. Governor Duquesne of Canada sent an army down and built forts in the contested area. The governor of Virginia requested from his king the right to intervene. This too was granted, and the governor was advised to tell the French to leave in a peaceful manner. If not, the British were to resort to arms. Dinwiddie appointed George Washington the messenger with a note to the French. He set out on October 31, 1753. He carried out his appointed task and delivered his note at Fort LeBoeuf just south of Lake Erie. Washington returned to Williamsburg to see the governor on January 16, 1754. The French took the note but disregarded its contents. Dinwiddie appealed to the other colonial governors to help him repel the French. George Washington was told to raise 100 men and go to the fork of the Ohio River to complete a fort started by the Ohio Company. Washington was unable to raise the "army," so Dinwiddie used assembly funds to raise a force of 300. Washington was now a lieutenant-colonel and second in command to Colonel Joshua Fry. The force left

Alexandria on March 21, 1754. Fry was killed when he fell off a horse, leaving Washington in command. On May 28, 1754, Washington had his baptism of fire when he led an expedition of 40 men who blundered into a French scouting party at the fork of the Monongahela and Allegheny Rivers. The Virginians killed 12, including their leader, De Villiers, Sieur de Jumonville, and captured the remaining 21. Washington's forces suffered one dead and two or three wounded. The captives claimed they were ambassadors with a note to the English, and they demanded immunity. Washington set them free, returned to Great Meadows, and built Fort Necessity. He received 400 reinforcements under Captain Mackey and set out to clear the Ohio Valley. The French sent a force of 700 from Fort Duquesne, and Washington retreated to the small palisaded fort at Great Meadows. On July 3, 1754, the French attacked the fort from cover, and the colonials lost one-third of the garrison. Washington was forced to surrender the fort. He signed a capitulation treaty in which he was forced to say that de Jumonville had been assassinated in the battle fought on May 28. This was a serious mistake by Washington, because the French could use this confession as proof of their moral right to be in the Valley. Washington brought the survivors of his defeat back to Virginia. In the eyes of the local population, he was a hero. However, the English and the governor of Virginia had a more jaundiced view of his diplomatic breach. The governor reorganized the Virginia regiment and broke it into separate companies with no rank higher than captain. Rather than accept this demotion, Washington resigned his commission. He returned to Mount Vernon and rented the plantation from his sister-in-law to take up his duties as a plantation manager.[12]

The French strengthened Fort Duquesne (later Fort Pitt; then Pittsburgh). The English had to dislodge the French from the valley, and they sent Major General Braddock with an army of British regulars to oust the enemy. Washington volunteered for service, and he was placed on Braddock's staff as an aide-de-camp.[13] In this army, he met Captain Horatio Gates, later to be his adversary in the Conway Cabal, as well as Thomas Gage who would command the British army during the American Revolution. The army left Cumberland on June 7, 1755, ready to meet and destroy the French. General Braddock had been trained on the open fields of Europe, and he could not handle the forests of America. Washington advised the general to pick 1,200 lightly supplied men who could move more rapidly than the full column and so could reach the fort quicker. The rest of the army could follow at a slower pace. This advice was accepted, and Washington accompanied Braddock with the forward echelon. Unhappily, Washington fell sick with the first of his five bouts of the "bloody flux." He was left behind, to be picked up by Colonel Dunbar's rear echelon.[14] On Braddock's order, Washington was treated with "Dr. James's Powders." This remedy contained antimony salt plus mercury and bark. It had emetic, cathartic, and diaphoretic properties. The powder was popular in England at the time, and Braddock carried it in his medicine chest. The patient seemed better after four days, but he could not mount a horse. The future general had to be carried in a cart with Dunbar's troops.[15] On July 12, they reached Braddock twelve miles from Fort Duquesne. Washington was still in pain, and he was forced to put pillows on his saddle in order to mount up for the attack. (It is probably irreverent to postulate that the future father of our country probably suffered thrombosed hemorrhoids from the frequent bowel movements caused by the flux.) The British forces were badly defeated by the French and Indians. The French force of 300, fighting from cover, vanquished the British force of 1,300 who tried to fight as though they were on the open fields of Europe. General Braddock and most of his staff were killed or seriously wounded. Washington was miraculously spared, and he sent back a courier to bring up reinforcements from the rear, but it was useless. The British had to leave the field to the French, and Washington led the retreat back to Virginia. The British lost about 300 wounded and 300 killed in their first experience with this different form of warfare.[16]

Washington, still too weak from dysentery, returned to Mount Vernon to gain his strength. This required five weeks of almost complete rest. During this period, there was considerable backbiting in Virginia. The colonials damned the British regulars and accused them of cowardice. They felt their own militia had behaved admirably under fire, and they heaped praise and adulation upon the "local boy" who led the retreat. According to the civilian population, Washington was the star of the whole wretched affair, and he became the best known soldier in the colonies. On August 14, 1755, he was made colonel of the reformed Virginia regiment and commander-in-chief of all Virginia forces, then composed of 16 companies. Washington tightened his command and laid down new rules for the recruitment of soldiers. No man would be taken if he was younger than 16 nor older than 50. No soldier would be less than five feet four inches unless he was strong and active. No man with old sores on his legs or subject to fits was accepted. The new recruits were examined by a regimental surgeon before they settled into quarters.

George Washington wanted to return and attack Fort Duquesne with his regiment, but Dinwiddie refused. Dinwiddie was replaced by John, Earl of Loudoun, commander-in-chief of British forces in North America, as governor of Virginia. The earl did not support Washington's plans either,[17] and George developed his second bout of dysentery and fever in August. He was ordered back to Mount Vernon by Dr. Craik, and he turned over his command at Winchester. It required many months of rest before Washington returned to good health. During this period he feared consumption, because he developed pleuritic pain. He was bled by Dr. Craik on November 8 without benefit. Dr. Craik admitted to being stumped by his patient's illness. "What's good for him in one respect, hurts him in another."[18] He called the Reverend Charles Green of Alexandria who doubled as a doctor. He prescribed jellies and a change in diet.

Washington was given hartshorn shavings and hyssop tea and canary wine. He was to have one to two glasses of wine daily with water of gum arabic. This brought no relief, and he told Dr. Craik he was getting worse. Craik advised complete bed rest on fear of death. That winter, Washington became seriously depressed. In January, he set out for Williamsburg for medical help, but he was forced back by the illness. In February, his fever increased, and his coughing became severe. His thoughts must have turned to Lawrence in his final months. He finally reached Williamsburg to see Dr. George Anson. He paid the doctor three pounds two shillings six pence. The doctor told him he would get well. This seemed to turn him around. In March of 1758, he went to woo Martha Custis whom he had met on the way to Williamsburg. She was a wealthy widow with 24,000 pounds from her previous marriage. Washington was an attractive swain (except for the scars). He was six feet two inches tall and weighed about 175 pounds. He had well-developed muscles and great strength. His bones and joints were large as were his hands and feet. Washington had broad shoulders. His chest was not deep or round. (This latter is questionable. Other observers claimed his chest was concave probably from infantile rickets.) He was thin-waisted and broad across the hips with long arms and legs. The future general had a well-shaped head gracefully poised on a superb neck. Featuring a large straight nose, blue-gray penetrating eyes, widely separated, and overhung by a heavy brow, his face was long, not broad, with high, round cheek bones and a firm chin. He had clear, pale skin, which sunburned easily. Washington had a pleasing and benevolent though commanding countenance with dark brown hair worn in a queue. His mouth was large and kept closed because of defective teeth. His features were regular and expressive of deep feelings. His demeanor was composed and dignified. Washington's movements and gestures were graceful and his walk majestic. He was also a splendid horseman.[19]

Washington reached a reasonable state of health in time for a new attack on Fort Duquesne in the summer of 1758. The army was to be led by General John Forbes with George Washington in command of Virginia troops. Forbes had 6,000 to 7,000 troops made up of Virginia and Pennsylvania militia plus British regulars. Washington suffered a recurrence of dysentery and body aching and again feared tuberculosis. However, he stayed with his command in the march to Fort Duquesne. The French were intimidated by the British forces. They burned Fort Duquesne and retreated to Canada without a fight. The British took the fort, rebuilt it, and named it Fort Pitt after Pitt the Elder, later to be raised to Earl of Chatham. Following the capture of the Fort, Washington arrived in Winchester in December 1758 in poor health, and he resigned from the army due to his health. He feared consumption and that he would die before he reached his home. After five years of soldiering, he returned to civilian life in January 1759.[20]

Meanwhile, the French and Indian War was drawing to a close. The British took Montreal and Quebec. The war in America ended, but the world war continued two more years, and in 1763 the Paris Peace Treaty was signed with Britain the uncontested winner. The victor received Canada and Florida, and the lands east of the Mississippi were free of the French and the Spanish. India came under British control as did much of the West Indies.

LIFE AS A VIRGINIA ARISTOCRAT

Washington married Martha on January 6, 1759. She was the daughter of Colonel Dandridge and the widow of Daniel Parke Custis who had died of bilious fever (possibly typhoid) at age 45. With her came her money, estates, and two difficult children; two of her children had died in infancy. The older child, George Parke Custis, was indolent and lacked stability. Patsy developed seizures at age twelve. In the four years before she died, Patsy saw a multitude of doctors and many remedies were tried without success. In his diaries, Washington listed the visits and treatments. Dr. Rumney was called frequently. Most times he stayed overnight, sometimes for several days. He saw Patsy from March 4 to March 17, 1768. He tried valerian for the seizures. This was a plant derivative with stimulant and antispasmodic properties. Dr. Rumney called in Dr. Mercer in consultation. Dr. Mercer prescribed mercury pills, purging pills, and other decoctions. Washington paid Mercer six pounds for his attendance on February 1, 1769. On February 16, Joshua Evans, a blacksmith, put an iron ring on Patsy's wrist to prevent "fits." English folk medicine of the fourteenth century described "cramp rings" to relieve or cure epilepsy when placed on the finger. They varied in design and composition, and they depended on a blessing, inscription, or the material itself for their efficacy. (This is not absurd in the light of modern man wearing copper bracelets to treat arthritis.) Several other doctors were called in at great expense, but none of their so-called remedies could prevent the inevitable. On June 19, 1773, Patsy died during a seizure. The Reverend Lee Massey performed the funeral services. During Patsy's life, Washington was quite wealthy, and the money expended was not of major consequence. He would have paid it gladly for Patsy's recovery. There is certainly evidence that he loved the child. When he left home on necessary business trips, he usually brought trinkets home for Patsy's pleasure.[21]

His relationship with his stepson, "Jackie," was less loving and more formal. Jackie at best was a difficult person without real ambition.[22] He was sent to a boarding school for one year, and Washington also paid for music lessons for Jackie without any obvious results. Before sending Jackie on a tour of Europe, Washington wanted him inoculated for smallpox, even though this was illegal in Virginia at the time. Washington opposed this law and wrote to the government about his feelings. He planned to send the boy to Dr. Henry Stevenson's inoculation clinic in Maryland. Martha refused permission, and this trip was canceled. The boy was finally successfully inoculated for small-pox on April 18, 1771. The operation was performed in Baltimore without Martha's knowledge or acceptance. That Washington was frustrated with the boy's behavior is evident when he finally turned to Dr. Stuart, a confidant, for help in handling the boy. The last straw was when Jackie married and rapidly proceeded to have four children. He was still very young, with no real educa-tion, and no training or land he could call his own. During the Revolution, Washington made Jackie his aide-de-camp. In 1781 Jackie developed "camp fever" and died, leaving a widow and children. His stepfather adopted the two younger children. The adopted son, George Washington Custis, would later become the father of Robert E. Lee's wife.[23]

In addition to Martha's estates, Washington inherited Mount Vernon. Lawrence's will specified that the estate would go to his wife. If she had no living children at the time of her death, the property would then go to brother George. All children of that union succumbed before their mother's death. Washington was now a wealthy landowner with parcels in several counties. From his writings, we can perceive that he was a good administrator and busi-nessman, and he enjoyed the lifestyle of the aristocratic landowner. He bought land with a fishery on it, and he signed a contract to sell the fish that were caught. The fish were salted, barreled and used for local slaves and for ship-ment to the West Indies to feed their slaves. He owned a brig, *The Farmer*, that he used for international trading. Washington also planned a commercial mill on his property with plans to buy wheat produced by the neighboring farms. The grain would be ground, and he would sell the flour. He paid Joseph Gort three pounds for one month's salary to cut stone in a quarry. He paid John Ball thirty-one pounds two shillings six pence wages for himself and five workers to build his stone mill.[24]

As the administrator of large estates, he had to be a veterinarian and a doctor. He described his invention of a sling to support a horse whose broken leg he set. The horse fell free, injured himself, and he was put away. During an epidemic of smallpox in Frederick County, some of his slaves developed the disease. He isolated the sick to prevent its spread. He believed in bleed-ing, and he used the terms of the "wise physicians" that disease was caused by peccant and morbific matter that had to be evacuated by phlebotomy. The landowner had slaves bled and had himself bled when he thought it necessary. Washington bled ten slaves sick with "rain and lightning" (fear), and they recovered. The "doctor" used bark on the slaves and on himself. He believed worms were the cause of most children's bellyaches. Washington believed in smallpox inoculation, and, as we saw, he had Jackie inoculated as well as his wife Martha and the slaves in the various plantations. He kept them on a "low diet and cool surroundings" during the eruptive stage. The slaveholder did not allow malingering among the help. If you are sick you should have a fever, and the fever will wear you down before long. Those who were truly sick got the best medical care available. He sent one slave to the best surgeon in Virginia for cataract surgery, and another to Pennsylvania to get therapy for a mad dog bite. He used a paid midwife for slave deliveries. Washington employed "Negro doctors" for minor illnesses. Dr. Rumney, who treated Patsy, was on retainer to look after his slaves (at fifteen pounds per year). He kept a medicine chest available for early treatment of illness. It contained mustard, bark, camphor, sulphur, antimony, cream of tartar, Glauber's salts, calomel, rhubarb, and jalap.[25]

The aristocratic planter still had time for the pleasures of life. He was an avid duck and fox hunter and fisherman. Washington reportedly paid six pounds ten shillings Maryland currency for a rifle and one pound sixteen shillings for a spaniel dog. This may be compared to thirty-one pounds he paid for a male slave and fifty-five pounds for a boy slave. The future president enjoyed card playing, billiards, and horse racing, and he gambled frequently. The ladies said he was "the best dancer in Virginia." An important social function of the time was a visit to neighboring plantations for several days and a return of the courtesy. Dr. Rumney was a frequent house guest both on medical visits and social visits. He visited with the Washingtons frequently after Patsy's death. Dr. George Craik, who later became Washington's physician, was a friend and frequent visitor before and after the Revolution.[26]

Washington was a strict nutritionist throughout his adult life. As commander-in-chief he insisted that his troops be fed vegetables with limited animal food. The general believed excessive amounts of animal food led to putrid fever. At his home, his eating times were absolutely regular whether guests were present or not. Breakfast was at 7:00 A.M. and consisted of eggs, corn cakes and molasses; dinner was at 3:00; tea at 6:00; supper was served between 8:00 and 9:00 and included fruits, cream, and cakes. He had household rules for civility at the table: do not appear angry at the table; do not eat with greediness; do not put food into your mouth until the last bite is finished. He did not smoke tobacco but did indulge in snuff. Washington enjoyed wine and drank two to three glasses of Madeira at dinner. When friends visited him at dinner, he toasted each with a glass of wine, and he had a few more after dinner. After supper, he excused himself from his company and retired for the night.[27]

Washington still had time and energy for politicking. He was elected to the House of Burgesses on December 1, 1768. He was a delegate to the First Continental Congress from Virginia. Washington's first night in Philadelphia was at the home of William Shippen, Jr. While in Philadelphia he visited the Pennsylvania Hospital and attended an anatomy lecture by his host. Washington also dined with Doctors Cadwalader, Bond, Morgan, and Rush. He was a delegate to the Second Continental Congress where he was named commander-in-chief.[28]

His life as a married man who supervised plantations was marred by recurrent illness. In 1761 he became severely ill. This may have been a recurrence of the malaria he suffered earlier in life. This is unlikely, because he knew about bark, which was a specific. More likely it was typhoid fever because of its longevity and the severity of his illness. He tried the waters at Warm Springs with some improvement, only to relapse on his return to Mount Vernon in September 1761. Washington felt he was going to die and did not fear the end. (This from his letter of October 1761.) He then went north to the mountains for the air. The persistence of the illness caused a severe bout of depression that made his symptoms worse. He was advised to seek medical help in Philadelphia, and he entertained a trip to England to get the best medical attention available. Gradually, however, he showed improvement. Washington spent about eight months in 1761 a victim of this illness.[29]

On March 3, 1768, near home after a fox hunt, Washington developed diarrhea with griping and straining. Perhaps it was another bout of dysentery. This persisted for one week, and then he "rid out" (took up his regular activities). The failure to mention bleeding, and the short duration of illness suggests food poisoning or a viral or bacterial diarrhea. In September and December of that year, he had recurrences of the same problem. Washington was under the care of Dr. Rumney, then of Dr. William Pasteur. In addition to these frequent bouts of diarrhea, he suffered numerous attacks of documented malaria. They started at age 17 with a recurrence at 29, three at 36, two at 54, and three during the last three years of his life. In the later attacks, Dr. Craik prescribed cathartics followed by bark, which provided prompt relief of the attack. Bark was one of the essentials in Washington's medical chest. He dosed himself, his family, and his slaves with the drug. It was a panacea for many diseases as well as a specific for ague. It is believed that the frequent doses of quinine, probably in near toxic amounts, were responsible for his loss of hearing later in life. He claimed to be deaf at 57. The attacks of malaria in his 29th year must have been debilitating, because he felt he was "near death" that year. Dysentery and malaria were recurrent enervating diseases during the colonial period; particularly in the south. While they did not usually kill by themselves, they lowered resistance enough to leave the major killers (pneumonia, smallpox, yellow fever, and tuberculosis) an easier target.

During the Revolution Washington made no entries in his diary. He had one bout of tonsillitis in 1777 while wintering in Morristown. This was treated with molasses and onions. At age 46, he developed a problem common to us all, presbyopia or "old sightedness," at the time his army encamped at Newburgh. He tried the glasses of all his officers until he found one that improved his vision. These were sent to David Rittenhouse in Philadelphia who duplicated the lenses and returned them to him without an examination.[30] Washington claimed to be almost blind at 51. (I am reminded of my grandfather who lived with us when I was growing up. When his eyesight became poor, he took a streetcar over the bridge to Orchard Street on the east side of Manhattan. A pushcart full of spectacles was his destination. Like Washington, he tried on glasses until one corrected his vision. I was amazed that he would endanger his vision in this way. I duplicated his actions when my time came, only I tried the glasses on in a drugstore.)

Washington probably started losing teeth at age 22 (other records say 40). By 28, he had many defective teeth, and he did not smile. It is reported that Paul Revere made his first set of dentures, but there is no corroboration. The famous rider silversmith is supposed to have made a set during the Revolution.

Washington's poor dentition and improper closure of his mouth are also claimed as a cause of his poor hearing. The combination of poor hearing and failure to smile were probably responsible for his "aloofness" described by his contemporaries. His poor mastication is blamed for his frequent abdominal pains.

Washington consulted many dentists for relief (John Baker, Joseph Le Maire, and Dr. Fendall among others). Dr. Le Maire or Dr. Le Mayeur was a French dentist who worked on Washington on July 16, 1783, on a visit to Mount Vernon. He later opened his office in Richmond, the new capital of Virginia. The good doctor placed ads in the local paper that boasted "operations on the teeth performed only in Europe such as transplanting." He offered to pay three guineas for good front teeth to anyone except slaves. John Greenwood, a Continental soldier from Connecticut, made several sets of teeth for "his General" later in life. At one point, Washington had one tooth in his lower jaw, and a plate was anchored to this tooth. It had eight human teeth pinned with gold into a plate of elephant or hippopotamus ivory. Later Greenwood carved dentures out of walrus tusks.

The artist Charles Wilson Peale made full dentures for him out of cows' teeth set in plates of lead alloy and pressed against the gums by springs. In 1796 James Gaudette made another set. By 1796 (some reports say as early as 1789), his last tooth was pulled, and in January 1797 Greenwood carved his last set. The teeth were made of hippopotamus or elephant ivory set in plates that had gold plate. The "Gaudette teeth" are probably responsible for the appearance of his mouth in Gilbert Stuart's familiar painting done when he was 64. The family claimed that the painting so distorted his face that they refused to accept or pay for it. Stuart's widow later sold it to the Athenaeum Society of Boston.[31]

THE PRESIDENCY

Between the time he relinquished his command of the troops of the Revolution and his inauguration as the first president, Washington returned to his home in Mount Vernon and resumed his responsibilities as landowner. He made a trip with Dr. Craik over the Appalachian Mountains to inspect land they owned jointly. They remained away from the tidewater for one month. In May 1787 he went to Philadelphia as a delegate to the Constitutional Convention.[32] It is there that he first came across the activities of the abolitionists. They "rented" slaves from visitors, then smuggled them to freedom. Washington, the owner of 216 slaves on his six plantations, claimed he deplored the institution of slavery, but he felt the abolitionists were wrong. In a letter to Robert Morris on April 12, 1786, he said that abolition must come through legislative activity, with probable payment to the owners. He left his slaves to his wife in his will with the proviso they were to be freed upon her death.[33]

The period before assuming the presidency was another time of poor health. There was the usual malaria. In 1787 he had an attack of "rheumatism." He could not raise his arm or turn in bed. He was sick for six months. It never recurred except for a sore arm (possibly tendinitis) in 1789. This may have been a bout of rheumatoid arthritis. This disease is associated with young people, mostly women, but there is an additional peak of recurrence at about age 55. In 1789 he had a mild attack of pneumonia.

Six weeks into his presidency, Washington developed a carbuncle of the thigh. The doctors thought it might be a malignant tumor or "anthrax of the hip." He was seen by Doctors Samuel Bard and John Bard. Washington again talked of dying to his doctors. The problem lasted 12 weeks, and he could not walk or sit. The surgeons finally performed an incision and drainage that brought about a drop in his fever and gradual return of health. After his recovery, he made a state visit to New England. In Boston, he was exposed to unusually bad weather, and he developed a respiratory illness with conjunctivitis. The disease also affected many other residents of Boston. The Loyalists in the area christened it "The Washington Influenza." Actually, it was part of an influenza epidemic that had started in the south and spread up the middle states and into New England. Despite the illness, Washington continued his visit. He inspected factories and met with persons of high position in the community. Upon his return to the capital in New York City, he recovered his health and resumed his activities as well as his exercises. He was an avid horseback rider, and he took walks around the battery as well as coach rides as a form of exercise. (This type of exercise was not exclusive to the colonies. In England, it was prescribed for King George III as well. It is difficult to see this as exercise, unless the exertion came from holding on while bouncing around in the coach.)[34]

The most serious illness of Washington's term in office occurred on May 9, 1790. It started with a cold and progressed to a very serious pneumonia. His physicians included Doctors Samuel Bard, Charles McKnight, and John Chaselton. Dr. John Jones of Philadelphia was called in "quietly" to check the illustrious patient three days later. There was great fear for Washington's life. On May 15, he went through a crisis with copious sweating. His expectoration went from "thin and ichorous" to well-digested. His articulation became distinct, and he proceeded to mend. During this attack, he felt another attack will "put me to sleep with my fathers." This time his premonition of death was almost true. He required several weeks of convalescence in Newport, Rhode Island, but by June 24 he was back to horseback riding. After his recovery, he toured the southern states and took along Dr. Craik's youngest son, George Washington Craik, who later became his secretary.[35]

Later that year the capital was moved from New York to Philadelphia. The yellow fever epidemic struck Philadelphia in 1793, but there is no evidence that Washington contracted the disease. The federal, state, and city governments were in Philadelphia at the time, and most lawmakers left town until the epidemic subsided. During that year, Washington developed recurrent fevers that persisted for seven to ten days. The diagnosis was not guessed at, but Jefferson in a letter remarked at how worn out he looked. (I wonder if he had the relapsing fever of brucellosis, because of his work around animals on the plantation.) In 1794 Dr. Tate of Philadelphia cured a "cancer of the right cheek." (It is doubtful this was cancer. Any hardened tissue on the skin like a fibroma, large scar, or exuberance of tissue was called cancer.) He returned to Mount Vernon to recover from the two months of therapy only to fall prey to another attack of malaria with a rapid weight loss of 20 pounds. It was about this time that he developed a tremor, which affected his handwriting. I would guess this was just a tremor of old age rather than Parkinson's disease.

While in Philadelphia, he met Dr. Hugh Martin, who claimed to have a secret cure for cancer. The basic ingredient was arsenic. He asked Washington for a testimonial, but the President refused on the grounds that medical cures should not be kept secret; certainly a proper attitude toward quackery. However, in 1796 Washington bought a set of Dr. Elisha Perkins's "tractors," one of brass and one of iron. They were drawn one at a time from the point afflicted to a point on the body as far away from the painful area as possible. This treatment was supposed to remove pains and inflammations from the body when it attracted the surcharge of the "electric fluid" that caused the inflammation.[36] Perkins was thrown out of the Connecticut Medical Society, not because of quackery, but because he patented the tractors and thereby obtained a monopoly. After duping the gullible of this country, he went to England and made another small fortune from the arthritics of that country.

RETURN TO MOUNT VERNON

In 1794 George Washington injured his back while horseback riding. This required no great treatment except bed rest. The remainder of his presidency was uneventful, and in the spring of 1797 he returned to his beloved, mosquito-infested Mount Vernon. In 1798 he had a serious bout with malaria again associated with excessive weight loss. It is said that George Washington weighed about 230 pounds when he returned to Mount Vernon.[37] During his short and final sojourn in Mount Vernon, there was an interesting incident with a rabid dog bite. The care the patient received gives us insight into therapy for this dreaded disease. Washington's body servant, Christopher, was bitten by a dog owned by a lady visitor. Shortly thereafter, the dog died in a state of madness. Christopher was sent to a physician in Alexandria who cut out the area, applied an ointment to keep it open and gave him a course of mercury. He was then sent to Dr. William Henry Etoy of Lebanon, Pennsylvania. Etoy said no further therapy was needed, although Dr. Etoy had a prescription for rabies that included an ounce of chickweed and four ounces of theriac plus one quart of beer. The dose was one wine glass full. Christopher did not die. The dog may have had distemper, or he may not have inoculated the rabid saliva, if he was rabid, into the bite.[38]

On December 12, 1799, Washington rode around the plantation at Mount Vernon from 10:00 A.M. to 3:00 P.M. in rain, snow, and hail alternating with a cold wind. His neck and hair were wet, and he did not change his wet clothes before dinner. The following morning, he awakened with a sore throat and remained indoors until afternoon when he went out into the snow to mark some trees to be chopped down. He was hoarse that evening but refused to take medicine for the "cold." On December 14, he awakened at 3:00 A.M. with a fever. He refused to disturb Martha or anyone else at this hour. By daybreak the patient was breathless and could not speak. He was given molasses, vinegar, and butter, which he could not swallow, and he almost suffocated from it. At his orders, he was bled one pint. Washington ordered flannel in a solution of hartshorn ammonia wrapped around his neck. His feet were bathed in warm water. At 8:00 A.M. he left his bed for a sitting position, but this did not improve his breathing. Dr. Craik was called, and raised a blister on Washington's throat with cantharides and bled his patient. Washington then gargled with vinegar and sage tea, which again almost suffocated him. Craik called for consultants. Dr. G. R. Brown from Maryland (author of the *Lititz Pharmacopoeia*) and Dr. E. C. Dick of Virginia responded to his call. The consultants arrived in midafternoon, and a fourth bleeding was completed, all in less than twelve hours. Calomel and tartar emetic were given. At 4:30 P.M. Washington gave instructions about his will. At 8:00 P.M. more blisters were raised and a poultice of wheat bran was applied to his feet and legs. He received an enema and inhaled a solution of vinegar and water. Blisters were raised on his extremities to draw the poisons away from his throat. Another poultice of bran and vinegar was applied. Washington told his physicians he was not afraid to die, and he thanked them for their attentions. "Doctor I die hard, but I am not afraid to go. I believed from my first attack that I should not survive; my breath cannot last long."[39] As a last effort, Dr. Dick suggested a tracheotomy. This was refused by Craik and Brown.

Tracheotomy was not an unknown operation. A manuscript written by

Matthew Wilson (1734–90), who was a preacher and a doctor, described the "bronchotomy" operation to be used in angina (sore throat), diphtheria, or if the throat is enlarged by a tumor of the thyroid. An incision was made in the "cuspera anterior" to admit air to the lungs to preserve life in a violent compression of the larynx or other process. To avoid the recurrent nerves and great blood vessels, the skin below the tumor was picked up and incised three-quarters of an inch long above the third or fourth ring of the trachea. The lips of the wound were parted, and a small transverse incision into the windpipe was performed. A silver cannula, one-half inch long, with a couple of little rings at the top of it, through which a ribbon was passed was inserted. The ribbon went around the neck and kept it fast in the wound. After cure, the tube was removed. This left a simple wound and required only a superficial application to close.[40]

There was a storm of criticism after Washington's death. His doctors were castigated as well as the medical profession in general. Doctors Craik and Dick published a description of his illness in the *Times* of Alexandria. The cause of death was listed as "cynanche trachealis," a term that had been used by Cullen, professor of Medicine at Edinburgh, in 1778. He described an inflammation of the glottis, larynx, or upper part of the trachea that produced a peculiar croaking sound in the voice with difficult respiration, and a "sense of straightening about the larynx." This was associated with fever, and it frequently obstructed the airway and resulted in suffocation and sudden death. The attending physicians further described the illness as starting with an ague (here a shaking chill, not malaria), pain in the upper front part of the throat, a feeling of stricture, cough, difficult but not painful swallowing, fever, and rapid laborious breathing. They did all the right things as described by Cullen in his original work, but Washington died on Saturday night at 11:30 P.M.[41]

The "Monday morning quarterbacks" got their licks in. It was shown that about five pints of blood had been withdrawn over thirteen hours. One author even suggested they should have drawn blood from under the tongue, near the seat of the trouble. One ounce drawn in this way was as good as a quart from the arm. However, the patient was not weakened with this technique. Other suggestions included: the tonsils should have been scarified; scarification and cupping should have been applied to the thyroid cartilage; the neck should have been rubbed with warm laudanum plus camphor followed by an application of a bag of warm salt; the patient should have been dressed in several layers of flannel; instead of calomel, he should have gotten small drafts of hot whey, laudanum, camphor, spiritus volatilis aromaticus, or spiritus nitre dulces to remove spasm.[42]

Other diagnoses were offered, including acute laryngitis, quinsy sore throat, laryngeal diphtheria, and inflammatory edema of the larynx. Later diagnoses included cardiorenal disease and Ludwig's angina. The most likely diagnosis was a streptococcus infection that spread down the submucosa to the larynx. This resulted in suffocation. A tracheotomy could have carried him through the acute process.

In his will, Washington left Dr. Craik his bureau and circular chair and "appendage of my studio." Dr. David Stuart was given his shaving and dressing table and telescope. He left land holdings in Virginia, Maryland, Pennsylvania, New York, Northwest Territory, Kentucky, and what is now Washington, D.C. He also left stock in several companies and banks as well as livestock.[43] This came to about $530,000 and did not include the slaves, which he left to his wife Martha with the proviso that they be given their freedom upon her death.

George III

BACKGROUND AND CHARACTER

George III is the British king mentioned in the Declaration of Independence:

> The history of the present King of Great Britain is a history of repeated injuries and usurpations. He has refused his assent to laws the most wholesome and necessary for the public good. He has obstructed the administration of Justice. He has erected a multitude of new offices. He has plundered our seas, ravaged our coasts, burnt our towns. He has excited domestic insurrections against us. A prince whose character is thus marked by every act which may define a tyrant is unfit to be the ruler of a free people.[44]

During the first year of the Revolution, the war was considered a fight against parliament. It was only after Jefferson's magnificent declaration that the anger of the American Patriots was directed against the king of Great Britain. The attitude of the English people was at first very favorable toward their monarch. Then, in a period of nascent imperialism, he was soundly attacked for his loss of the American prize. Gradually, with time, his position in British hearts has again been upgraded.

Before we examine his health, let us first explain how the leader of a small state in Germany became the king of the strongest nation in Europe. Sophia was the granddaughter of James I of England and Scotland. (The two were joined in his reign.) In 1658 she married Duke Ernst August. Her mother, Queen Elizabeth of Bohemia, was the sister of Charles I of Great Britain. She was strongly Protestant. While she was on the continent, Great Britain went through a series of dynastic quarrels with the civil wars and the execution of the king. After Cromwell's death, the Stuart family was brought back in the "Restoration" (Charles II). The Catholic Stuart, King James II, was deposed in the Glorious Revolution. His reign was followed by the accession of William and Mary of the House of Orange from the Netherlands. They in turn were followed by Princess Anne, a Protestant Stuart. (In 1701 the Act of Settlement was passed. This statute proclaimed that a Protestant monarch must occupy the British throne.) Queen Anne had 17 failed pregnancies. She had one weak son who died of smallpox at age eleven. She died without an heir in 1713, and the English had to search for a Protestant house. They found it in the state of Hanover where Sophia was married to the elector. She was offered the throne, but she died, and her son became George I, King of Great Britain and Hanover in 1714. He was 53 when he ascended to the British throne. He was born and brought up a prince of Germany, and he could not speak English nor understand the ways of a developing democracy. His son, George II, succeeded him in 1727. He, too, was born and raised in Germany. His first language was German, and he spoke English poorly. George II married Caroline, a Protestant princess. Their first-born was Frederick who married Augusta of Saxe-Gotha. Frederick died of pulmonary disease before he could succeed to the throne. His son, and second child, became George III after the death of his grandfather in 1760. At this time, British power was at its height in the Western World.[45]

In Hanoverian politics, the heir apparent was the center of opposition to the ruler. With his transfer to England, this political state continued. The "loyal opposition" to the king surrounded the Prince of Wales. Frederick, who detested his father, gladly became the political opponent of the king. However, Frederick was universally hated by politicians, as well as by his parents and his wife. He was described as a weak, poor, irresolute, false, lying, dishonest, and contemptible wretch. Frederick's mother, Caroline, was heard to say that she doubted her son's ability to have sex with a woman and doubted his ability to produce children. Despite this, there were nine children from his marriage. Frederick wanted his sons' education to encompass Latin, music, fencing, dancing, history, mathematics, and religion. Before he could get too far along in his plans, he died suddenly in 1751. His autopsy showed an abscess or "imposthume" in the breast that ruptured and suffocated him,[46] similar to Benjamin Franklin. His son George was twelve at the time. The king, Frederick's father, was happy his son predeceased him, but he remained on good terms with his son's widow, Augusta. (As an aside it might be mentioned that Augusta's contribution to the genetic pool was not that great. The Gotha family had their share of feeble-mindedness and possibly insanity.)[47] For four years after his father's death, George III was completely protected by his mother from outside influences, and it was believed that this stunted his intellectual growth and maturity. He supposedly grew up shy, priggish, introspective, lazy, and friendless. George preferred a secluded life in the country. He was uncomfortable with people he did not know. The future monarch was never exposed to children his own age. George had average intelligence, but he had a great curiosity. Biographers have described him as dull, apathetic, lethargic, and unteachable. He loved music and literature. His only real friend was his younger brother, Edward, who was the favorite of his parents.

Augusta's counselor-in-chief was John Stuart, the Earl of Bute. There was talk that he was her lover as well. Bute became George III's principal tutor in 1755, and he soon became the confidant and idol of the lonely boy. George depended on Bute, and he could not make a decision without consulting his "new father."[48] At an early age, George fell in love with Sarah Lennox, Lady Pembroke, but he did not pursue this quest, because his mentor felt this was a bad match. She was the sister-in-law of Fox in the British parliament who was Bute's political enemy.[49]

George II died on October 15, 1760, and the rule of George III was welcomed by the people of the country. The new king was born in England and his first language was English, although he spoke German fluently. The new monarch was the first young king to ascend the throne since 1558. He believed himself a "patriotic king," but he wished to rule as well as reign. George wanted to gain royal power, which decayed over the centuries. The king, early in his reign, resolved to stop corruption and laziness in politics. To his court he brought dignity, decency, religion, and morality. As sovereign, he showed no preference to either party in parliament. On his accession to the throne, he issued a "Proclamation for the Encouragement of Piety and Virtue." George wanted to prevent and punish vice, profanity, and immorality. He was truly pious; perhaps too much for a Great Britain with increased strength and wealth where urbanity was prized more than piety. The new king outlawed gambling and card playing at court. He ate and drank sparingly, and he took no mistresses. He failed to provide grist for the press's mill. The new ruler had normal sexual drives, and early in his reign he started searching for a Protestant princess. The search for his queen ended successfully with Charlotte of Mecklenburg-Strelitz. When she came to Great Britain, George tried to protect her from the wickedness present in the higher reaches of society. The king was a strong believer in the Established Church of England. As leader of this church, the monarch opposed Catholic emancipation, and he opposed the removal of disabilities placed upon the nonconformists under the Test and Corporation Acts. If we judged George by twentieth-century criteria, he would appear very intolerant, but he shared the religious beliefs of most of his subjects.[50]

Thackeray later was to say that George III was a dunce suited to trivia. He was "less king than cabbage." His views were as "conventional as his common subjects." The king was not a fool, nor was he easy to fool. He spoke and wrote German and French reasonably well. The monarch approved of and supported the arts and sciences. Some of his contemporaries described him as reasonably quick-witted, and he could respond to a barb quickly and appropriately. The king was devoted to his duty, and he worked hard at it. He appointed Benjamin West of Pennsylvania as court painter at 1,000 pounds per year. The ruler of America also patronized John Copley. George started a library collection, which he willed to the British Museum. It became the King's Library. He founded the Royal Academy of Science, and he paid Herschel, a famous astronomer and mathematician, to help him build his own telescope. He paid close attention to new inventions that were expanding the Industrial Revolution in England. However, his first love was agriculture, and he acquired the nickname of "Farmer George." The monarch of the most powerful nation in Europe still found time to play the flute, harpsichord, and violin.[51]

One positive biographer described the king's appearance as tall and full of "dignity and grace." His countenance was florid and good natured, his manner graceful and obliging. The king showed no warmth nor resentment toward anyone. Horace Walpole described his demeanor as "cold." The king was well built, but he tended to obesity in later years. The monarch weighed 14 stone (196 pounds). He had a high forehead and protruding eyes, a large nose, thick lips, and a dimpled chin. The royal vision was poor, and this gave him a peering look. The sovereign had a shaved head, and he wore a wig to his earlobes. Boswell felt he spoke with dignity, delicacy, and ease.[52]

George was one of nine children and he fathered 15 with one wife, two of whom died in infancy. Charlotte, like her mother-in-law, must have been of sturdy German stock, and she probably had a major prolapse of the uterus. Under British law, Protestant royalty had to marry Protestant royalty. Just as their father before them, George's sons had to turn for their wives to Germany as the only Protestant country in Europe. At this time, Germany was composed of several hundred principalities and electorates whose chief export was Protestant princesses. The English king's daughters were forced into spinsterhood, because the German princelings did not look toward England for wives. The king was a fond and doting father, but his children's upbringing, lessons, and activities were carefully regulated. The princesses grew up with deep affection for their father, but hostility developed between the king and his sons. They indulged in frivolity and vice. The Prince of Wales was notorious for frequent love affairs, drinking, and gambling; he was totally irreligious and refused to study. The boys were sent to Germany for their education and military training. The king, while born in England, remained proud of his German heritage, and he wanted to instill that pride in his sons.[53]

Politically, George III was conservative, and he believed his duty was to prevent any change in the government or the constitution. Although not a formal written document as in this country, the English constitution was a combination of the Magna Carta, the Habeas Corpus Act, the Bill of Rights, the Act of Settlement, and the Act of Union between England and Scotland. A king could not veto legislation because Great Britain at the time was a constitutional monarchy. However, he could work through his friends in Parliament to kill laws that he opposed. A king chose ministers agreeable to Parliament; the concept of a cabinet of ministers picked from Parliament developed later, during the Seven Years War (1756–1763). Although George was still the Elector of

Hanover, he did not want England entangled in European affairs. George was a pacifist at heart, and he encouraged maritime and colonial policy to increase commerce and wealth rather than war. The development of a commercial empire rather than a land empire was first propounded by Pitt the Elder.[54]

The new king ascended his throne when England seemed on the verge of vanquishing its persistent enemy, France. However, the problem of the cost of the wars of the eighteenth century worried the leaders of government. The national debt had reached 130 million pounds. In addition, Parliament needed funds to keep 10,000 British regular troops in North America to maintain their recent acquisitions against a possible resurgence of the French. The enforcement of the Sugar Act as well as the passage of the Stamp Act in 1765 were attempts to pay off the debt as well as cover current expenses. The Stamp Act was not a new tax in Great Britain. It had been used earlier in the century to help pay for the repeated British incursions on the continent. In America, the stamp tax was resented. It was believed to be the cause of George Washington's loss of any devotion to the motherland. The law was repealed before it was enforced. The anger and turbulence in the colonies produced by the Stamp Act was believed by many historians to be the first battle of the Revolution. In Great Britain, ministers followed each other in rapid succession—Grenville, Rockingham, Pitt, Fox, and Townshend. The infamous Townshend Acts of 1767 included the tea tax. Townshend was replaced by Hillsborough and he in turn by Lord North. In the colonies, the Boston Massacre of 1770 and the Boston Tea Party in 1773 led to the "Intolerable Acts." These in turn were responsible for the outbreak of hostilities. During this period of turmoil, George III remained the constitutional monarch. Inwardly, he felt the need for force to put down his rebellious subjects. The king believed he and Britain were morally right in their relations with their obstreperous colonies in America. Active warfare persisted from Lexington until Yorktown. The British defeat led to the resignation of North. Rockingham succeeded him in 1782 but died shortly thereafter. He was replaced by Shelburne. George III still refused to grant independence to his "Rebellious American Colonies," but by the fall of 1782, he was forced to accept their existence as a separate state. He was sufficiently disturbed by this to pen a letter of abdication, which he never submitted.[55]

HEALTH PROBLEMS

The monarch's health was a constant problem throughout his reign. It resulted in two national disasters: the Regency Crisis of 1788 and the Catastrophe of 1817. The first overt manifestation of his disease occurred in June of 1762. This followed a fever with cold, cough, and oppression in the breast. He was bled seven times and had three blisters applied. His physicians also prescribed a laxative and ass's milk, a recognized therapy for consumption. At this time, Charlotte was pregnant for the first time. In 1765, in the midst of parliamentary problems as well as those related to the colonies, George had his first major attack. It started with cough, fever, chest pain, rapid pulse, and fatigue. The diagnosis at the time was consumption. There was no mention of mental problems in contemporary descriptions of this attack. In fact, his mind was clear enough to urge his ministers to pass an act to provide for a regency. He believed death was imminent during this and other attacks. Part of his therapy during this spell was to apply cups in order to lower his temperature.[56] It was 50 years after this major attack, and particularly after his death, that medical writers discussed the possibility that his "indisposition" was of a mental nature. During the nineteenth century it became an accepted fact. In 1855, Dr. Isaac Ray wrote a medical treatise on the insanity of George III and argued that the attack in 1765 was of the same nature as subsequent ones. However, there was no real evidence in the medical reports of 1765 upon which to base this assumption. In 1931, Dr. Jelliffe labeled George III's illness as manic depressive psychosis.[57] Dr. Manfred Guttmacher, an eminent psychoanalyst, wrote his book, *America's Last King: An Interpretation of the Madness of George III* in 1941. Guttmacher expanded on Jeliffe's hypothesis, claiming that George III's self-blame, indecision, and frustration led to his insanity and suggesting that the king would not have developed a psychosis had he remained a country squire. Guttmacher saw the physical symptoms as subterfuges to hide the mental illness, and believed the king falsified his mental symptoms. Guttmacher felt the king had a neurotic personality as well as a hereditary taint of neuroticism. The psychiatrist argued his subject's five manic attacks were precipitated by political and domestic events that caused him to decompensate. The major attacks were caused by his impotence to act when he thwarted himself by lack of decisiveness; his minor ones followed frustration caused by the outside world. Guttmacher also blamed repressed sexual desires for Lady Pembroke, the king's first love. The eminent analyst was obviously a Freudian.

Dr. Guttmacher showed that George I's mother, Sophia, was manic depressive. His father, Ernest Augustus, had organic brain disease. George I married his cousin Sophia and had two children with her. Sophia committed adultery, and she was divorced and imprisoned. George I hated his son, George II, as well as his daughter-in-law. George II had an enormous sexual appetite, and he had many mistresses. George II and his wife Caroline hated their son Frederick. Frederick, like his father, was a womanizer. After Frederick's death, George III grew up dependent upon this mother, Augusta, who was despised by the English masses. George III transferred his dependency to Bute, who may have been his mother's lover. At the age of eighteen, George III fell in love with the Countess Pembroke who married another. This family history would have made a good soap opera. During his bouts of illness, George III constantly referred to his love for Lady Pembroke. In 1765 the new monarch had his first breakdown described by Guttmacher as an attack of manic depression, mostly depression. There was no distortion of thinking nor delusions, and he did not lose track of time or reality. This episode lasted six months. In February 1766 the monarch had a mild attack, perhaps related to the excitement over the Stamp Act. During the Revolution, there were no accounts of illness, and despite his need to grant independence to "his colonies," he still suffered no breaks. He did have an attack in 1788–89. This was the severest episode, and it started with worry and depression, according to Guttmacher's text. Worry became obsessive, and the king dwelled upon the death of his son Octavius who had died five years earlier. He was convinced he should have married Countess Pembroke rather than Charlotte. The king had auditory hallucinations in the form of Handel's oratorios. The monarch felt shame over the loss of America. The physical symptoms during the attack that started June 11, 1788, were a series of severe abdominal pains. He was sick for three days with a diagnosis of "bilious disorder" or gout. The patient took the waters at Cheltenham and recovered to a degree.

Several months later he had pains in the face, and the real attack started in the fall of that year. Dr. Baker, who cared for him early in the attack, felt his bile was not flowing properly. Baker's diagnosis was "unformed gout." The king knew it was not gout, because he could kick his foot with the other heel without pain. Gout was a frequent diagnosis at the time. There were two forms of the disease: the stationary form that settled in a joint, usually the great toe, and the unformed or diffuse or flying. Dr. Baker gave him a purge as well as laudanum for the pain. The king was told by the physician that the attack was precipitated because he did not change his wet stockings. As a result, he "caught rheumatism of his legs that flew to his stomach." Dr. Baker called Dr. Heberden, Sr., in consultation, and they both called Dr. Richard Warren. Dr. Heberden also called Dr. James Munro, head of the "Bedlam Asylum." On October 22, 1788, Dr. Baker found his patient in a delirious state declaiming against doctors and medicine. He became calm the next day, but a week later the king was hypomanic and talked continuously with a flight of ideas. This was followed by totally manic behavior. The patient ran a race with a horse, pretended to play a violin, and ate at tremendous speed. He then developed severe abdominal pain and colic. The treatment included purges and laudanum. The king developed insomnia and confusion in speech and writing. A poor night resulted in delirium the next day. The patient's vision and hearing were failing, and he continued to speak rapidly and incoherently.[58] On November 15 Dr. Francis Willis and his sons were called in on the case. Willis was a cleric who had studied medicine as a "back-up" profession. He owned a private mental asylum. On Willis's orders, the king was placed in a straitjacket repeatedly and tied to his bed as a result of violent behavior after a visit by the queen. Dr. Willis's treatment was rough and intimidating. It caused pain and irritability followed by more violence and further restraint in the straitjacket.[59]

The illness was described by the king's equerry, Robert Fulke Greville, who simply wrote down his observations. According to Greville, his king became delirious at dinner on November 15; on November 19 he talked incessantly for 19 hours without intermission; he was confused, rambling, and incoherent; on November 23 he talked indecently, which was very strange for this religious, strict individual.[60] His doctors reported that the patient lived in a world of his own. He addressed people, dead or alive, as though they were present. His speech resembled the details of a dream in its extravagant confusion. The doctors blistered his head in order to get the poisons up from his brain, and he was given large doses of the eighteenth-century panacea, bark. The queen was worn out from sleeplessness and had to remove herself from his quarters. Dr. Warren, who was the personal physician of the Prince of Wales, could not approach the king, because of his violent behavior toward the doctor. There were periods when several attendants had to sit on the king to keep him down. He was treated with Dr. James's Powders without benefit. His violent activities led to exhaustion, but the insomnia persisted despite hydrotherapy. Doctors Reynolds, Pepys, and Addington were called in consultation.[61] It was during this attack that the doctors described skin lesions and discolored urine.[62] With the further deterioration of his status, the patient was bled, cupped, and purged. The agitation was described as a "flurry of spirits." From his constant talking, of which the patient was aware, he became hoarse. His head throbbed, and his vision deteriorated further. This was accompanied by giddiness and weakening of his legs. The monarch tried to attend concerts, but his legs fidgeted constantly. His speech became garbled and repetitive, and he was more violent with an associated rapid pulse. Dr. Warren declared him insane, although there were periods of lucidity in November. During these periods, the king discussed his own bizarre behavior. These lucid periods were replaced by grandiose ideas. He saved certain vital documents from a flood, bestowed high honors on his subjects, and claimed he could see Hanover through a telescope. The patient's feet were blistered with cantharides, resulting in suppuration. This was followed by hot baths. On November 24 Dr. Addington believed the patient would recover but wanted him moved to Kew where he would exercise away from the view of the curious. The king was moved against his will, and his wife and daughters were not permitted to visit him on orders of the Prince of Wales.

Plans were started to create a regency, with the Prince of Wales as regent. The Whigs used Warren's prognosis; the Tories backed Willis. Both were called to testify. Another physician, Dr. William Battie, was also called to Parliament. In 1758 he had written a treatise on madness, dividing that illness into two parts, basically organic psychoses and functional psychoses (these were not his terms). He believed the king's problem was a functional psychosis with a hopeful prognosis. The only flaw was that the king's illnesses persisted too long, and doctors began to think of a permanent psychosis. When the king's status cleared, it was diagnosed as a form of delirium, i.e., a toxic delusional state.[63]

The Regency Act passed Commons and was sent to the House of Lords. However, by mid–February the king showed rapid improvement, and the Regency Act was dropped. By April he was practically normal, and in June he was completely recovered although he had lost three stone (42 pounds). Dr. Willis, who was in charge of his care for four months, was promised 1,500 pounds per year for 21 years. His son, John Willis, was promised 650 pounds per year for life. This attack brought the king to the brink of death, but it was followed by 11 years free of further attacks. The king suffered repeated attacks in the early nineteenth century, and he was finally declared disabled in 1811.[64]

PSYCHIATRIC DIAGNOSIS

According to Dr. Manfred Guttmacher, King George's attack was due to serious inner emotional conflicts, including his difficulties with his sons who rebelled against him as well as the activities of "his colonies." He felt his 13 living children would break away from him like the 13 colonies. (The good psychiatrist was probably a cabalist as well.) His youthful desires for Lady Pembroke versus his loyalty to his now dowdy queen caused serious emotional problems. To this was added his rigid conscience in regard to his psychosexual desires. The only way out of his impasse was to slip into a psychotic state.

The episode which began on February 13, 1801, started with a bilious attack after a heavy cold associated with hoarseness. He talked rapidly again. The Reverend John Willis, son of the earlier Reverend Willis, was called to see the patient. He declared that a state of deterioration had occurred. The king was lucid, but he slipped into a period of confusion and delirium. Reverend Willis brought his two brothers into the case to apply the same treatment started by their father. The patient became worse, and his pulse raced at 136 beats per minute. Hot vinegar and water were applied to his feet, and he was given musk and bark. A pillow filled with warm hops was used to treat his insomnia. The king was placed on a starvation diet to bring his fever down and was dosed with tartar emetic. Although he recovered from this attack more rapidly, the king showed signs of organic brain disease as well as severe debility and irritability. The fever recurred as did abdominal attacks and uncontrolled hand activity. At this time, the three Willises controlled the king and the government of Great Britain. The king hated the Willises, and they were discharged by the family, only to be called back to reinstitute their therapeutic regime. Dr. Guttmacher believed this attack was precipitated by passage of the Catholic Toleration Act of 1801, which the king opposed, as well as by the resignation of Pitt the Younger from his position as prime minister.

In February 1804, at the age of 66, the king suffered another attack with mania and hyperactivity. By mid–February his temperature was high, and he talked constantly. The Willises were not called in during this attack, because the king in his lucid periods urged his son not to use them. Dr. Samuel Simmons of St. Luke's Hospital for the Insane was called. He, too, put the king in a straitjacket. The patient developed intermittent fevers and "flurries." His behavior and judgment diminished as did his sight and hearing. This attack resulted in an overt break in the relations between the king and the queen. She refused to allow him into her bedroom. They did not eat or speak together. The king tried to "ravish" the Princess of Wales, and he grabbed his granddaughter's governess. The monarch suffered bouts of depression mixed with normal behavior. His physicians noted the development of cataracts, which partly explained his visual problems.

In 1810 his daughter Amelia died. This loss resulted in a severe psychotic break. George anguished over Amelia's illness. This was followed by denial of her illness, then the inability to deny it. Again, his only outlet was a psychotic break, according to Guttmacher.[65] When he learned of her death, he believed he could bring her back to life. The king alternated between periods of lucidity and delusion. In 1811 the Regency Act was passed, naming the Prince of Wales regent. In February 1812 the regency was made permanent after Parliament questioned many doctors, including Dr. Heberden, Jr., Monro, John Willis, Hafford, and Baillie. By 1812 George withdrew into his world of delusions completely. After 1817 he was completely deaf, and the king died on January 29, 1820, when "his body fell apart." His wife predeceased him by three years.[66]

Dr. Manfred Guttmacher was not alone in his interpretation of George's illness. Other physicians offered diagnoses of manic depressive psychoses on the basis of sexual tensions and frustrations. These frustrations caused such personality traits as obstinacy, conservatism, decorum, and strict morality which were forced upon his court. Twentieth-century historians saw him as a neurotic aware of his inability to perform the duties of his high position. This led him to take refuge in insanity. Actually, the king had no symptoms of mental illness in the attack of consumption in 1765, but the early diagnosis of insanity colored the interpretation of the monarch's conduct in political affairs. His firmness during the Revolution in his adherence to a policy that was unwise and disastrous was felt to be due to his inability to face reality. (Although his conduct relative to the colonies was supported by Parliament early in the war.) His moral qualities, which were virtues, were considered vices in the face of the diagnosis of manic depression. His perseverance in his support of Parliament's right to govern was considered obstinacy. The king's courage was interpreted as a failure to face facts. George's loyalty to his ministers was believed to be a desire to govern by corruption. His lack of mistresses implied sexual timidity. The king was not a mental giant, but he was honest, hard working, conscientious, and responsible. He was religious and supported Protestantism completely. His marriage produced 15 children, and he was faithful to his wife. He had a quick temper, and was not able to forgive slights. The king was firm and obstinate; his high moral standards he demanded of others. George grew more rigid with age, as do we all.[67]

Before a discussion of what I believe was the true cause of his problems, we should spend a little time reviewing the treatment of insanity during this period. His treatment was hideous. It was repressive, coercive, and punitive. In 1788 Willis boasted that he "broke in patients as horses in a menage," and he treated the king no differently from "one of his gardeners at Kew." For failure to obey orders, he was placed in a winding sheet or a restraining chair or straitjacket with his legs tied to the bed. The patient received medication to bring his fever down and calm his turbulent spirits. He had vomits, purges, bleedings, blisterings, cuppings, and leeches. In his last illness, he was treated by Willis's sons, Robert, Darling, and John. They kept him in solitary confinement and silence to decrease his excitement. His reaction to this terrible treatment was felt to be a form of his mania, and his hatred of the Willises was considered delusional. The Willises claimed the restraints were applied to protect him from serious injury. It was also a form of therapy, because restraining activity reduced angry passions. They isolated the patient from things with which he was acquainted. The patient was kept indoors with nothing to see or hear. He was taken away from home and familiar surroundings. They kept away people the patient knew. These were felt to stimulate associations and make the disease worse. They urged bleeding, purging, vomiting, and a "low diet" to bring down the body's natural powers.[68] These brought down the turbulent spirit and allowed reason to return. In the poor, the straitjacket could be used so that the family did not have to pay attendants, but George did not escape this treatment. Electric shocks to the head were started in 1760. In the 1780s shock for depressed patients was instituted at St. Thomas's Hospital in London. The Willises claimed that they followed the therapy laid out by William Cullen of Edinburgh in his textbook of medicine on the *Therapy of Maniacs*. Cullen urged intimidation, isolation, and restraint to make the patient afraid of his keeper. This was accomplished by physical violence in the form of whipping and striking the patient. However, Cullen urged restraint.

News of the king's problems reached America, and Benjamin Rush, the father of American psychiatry, responded. He forgave the king his injustices to the colonies, and he offered to send a restraint he had invented that was more humanitarian than those in use at that time. The monarch's doctors did not accept this offer. From what is known today, it is fairly certain that the therapy by George III's doctors probably aggravated the primary disease. Blisters led to infection and suppuration. The combination of bleeding, cupping, leeches, vomits, and purges contracted his fluid volume. The lack of protein in his "low diet" prevented him from the production of antibodies and regeneration of the depleted protein in his body.

The treatment of the insane was big business in Britain at the time. Private madhouses sprouted like mushrooms after a rain throughout eighteenth-century England. Many sane women were institutionalized for the convenience of their spouses. This allowed them to get control of their wives' fortunes as well as to dally with mistresses. A doctor could be paid to certify insanity. Many physicians opened asylums and profited from the fee of certification, as well as the "treatment" of the patient. In 1774 Parliament passed an act for "Regulating Madhouses" to protect the sane from the abuses of the system. The act called for the examination of madhouses by commissioners appointed by the College of Physicians. Records of therapy had to be kept on all patients, as well as the written certification of madness signed by a doctor, surgeon, or apothecary.[69]

MEDICAL INTERPRETATION

Doctors Ida Macalpine and Richard Hunter, who employed excellent detective work, came to a different conclusion as to the cause of the king's illness. They believed that he suffered from porphyria, a metabolic illness. They were able to trace the illness as far back as Margaret Tudor, a daughter of King Henry VII.[70]

In light of the family history, Macalpine and Hunter dissected the illnesses of George III. He had five separate attacks. The first in July 1765 at age 26, the second from October 1788 to February 1789 at age 50, the third in February and March of 1801 at age 62, the fourth from January to March 1804 at age 66, the fifth from October 10 to January 29, 1820, at age 82. There were minor attacks as well: those of May and June of 1762 at age 24, January and February of 1766, and that of June 1790, and the one in December 1795. The attacks started with a cold, cough, and malaise leading to anginoid pains (stitches in the breast). Abdominal colic, constipation, and tachycardia up to 144 beats per minute then occurred. The king then developed hoarseness, followed by painful weakness and stiffness of the arms and legs, so he could not walk, stand unaided, or hold a cup. He had cramps, paresthesia, hyperesthesia, and hypalgesia. He suffered generalized tremor and pain in the face, head, and neck. There was dysphagia along with foaming of the mouth, visual disturbances so that he could not read, nystagmus, dizziness, inability to speak, and incontinence. He suffered vasomotor disturbances like sweating, suffused face as well as oliguria and polyuria, polydipsia, pale stool, swelling of his legs and feet, and weals on his arms. There was encephalopathy as well, which caused agitation, rapid speech, sensitivity to light and sound, emotional lability, uninhibited behavior, and nocturnal confusion. The king suffered total insomnia—once he went without sleep for 72 hours. He talked constantly at one stretch for 26 hours. There was great irritability of his frame, frank delirium, inability to fix his attention, and gross errors in judgment.

George III had illusions, delusions, and hallucinations. He talked to dead people as though they were in his chamber, and he lived in his own world. He described visions of scenery around him. His conversation was confused. His excitement led to stupor, incontinence, and convulsions. As George grew older, he became more cheerful, tranquil, good humored, trifling, and silly, with alternating periods of tears and laughter. There were four references in his doctor's journals of abnormalities in his urine. It was described as bloody and left a bluish ring.[71]

Porphyria was first described by Gunther in 1912. In 1937 Waldenstrom defined acute intermittent porphyria as a chemical disorder with a chronic course and acute exacerbations, periodic in nature. It was familial and inherited as a Mendelian dominant. Original reports described a series of symptoms—abdominal pain, constipation, diarrhea, vomiting, and neurological involvement that occurred later. Mental symptoms were common and varied. Urinary porphobilinogens were elevated during attacks and may have persisted in remissions. A form called variegate porphyria occurred more commonly in South Africa. It had the same course and symptoms, but there was added fragility of the skin and intolerance to the sun. Both could occur in the same patient or in different forms in different family members. Many victims may have been free of symptoms, but they still carried the disease. Barbiturates precipitated attacks, and between attacks, feces showed large amounts of porphyrin-peptide conjugates (x-porphyrin). George III had variegate porphyria. As a young man he is said to have had acne. In the attack of 1788, he had great weals on his arms. His face had a violaceous hue during attacks, which produced the appearance of great fury. Infections and colds frequently started an attack. It could run a fulminating course, recur in attacks of varying severity, or disappear with advanced age. It started soon after puberty. The color of the patient's urine could go from deep amber to purple when passed or left standing.[72] We must conclude from this evidence that George III's problems, at least in part, were caused by an undiagnosed physical illness.

Notes

Chapter 1

1. J. Laffin, *Surgeons in the Field* (London: Dent, 1970), 7–18.
2. M. I. Roemer, "The History of the Effects of War on Medicine," *Annals of Medical History* 3d ser., no. 4, (1942): 189–99, esp. 191.
3. G. E. Ijams, and P. B. Matz, "The History of the Medical Domiciliary Care of Veterans," *The Military Surgeon* 75 (1935): 113.
4. B. A. Moxness, "Care of the War Disabled Prior to the World War" *Military Surgeon* 75 (1935): 117–121.
5. Ijams and Matz, 114.
6. E. Cutbush, *Observations on the Means of Preserving the Health of Soldiers, Sailors, and on the Duties of the Medical Department of the Army and Navy and Rewards on the Hospital and Their Internal Arrangement* (Philadelphia: Fry and Cammerer, 1809), 2–6.
7. Rush, *Medical Inquiries and Observations* (Philadelphia: Greggs and Dickinsons, 1815; reprint New York: Arno Press and New York Times, 1972), 147–48.
8. K. E. Manchester, "General Washington and the Patriot Soldiers," *Journal of the American Dietetic Association*, no. 5 (May 1776): 421–33.
9. C. K. Bolton, *The Private Soldier Under Washington* (Port Washington, NY: 1902), 81.
10. Manchester, 425.
11. H. L. Applegate, "Preventative Medicine in the American Revolutionary Army," *Military Medicine* 126 (1962): 379–82, esp. 380.
12. Cutbush, 22–29.
13. Manchester, 425, 427.
14. Applegate, 379.
15. Cutbush, 30–40.
16. L. Montross, *Rag, Tag, and Bobtail* (New York: Harper, 1952), 46–47.
17. C. H. Huzmann, "Military Sanitation in the Sixteenth, Seventeenth, and Eighteenth Century," *Annals of Medical History* 1 (1917): 281–300, esp. 296–98.
18. Cutbush, 7–13.
19. J. Jones, *Plaine, Concise, and Practical Remarks on the Treatment of Wounds and Fractures to Which Is Added an Appendix on Camps and Military Hospitals Principally Designed for the Use of Young Military and Naval Surgeons in North America* (Philadelphia, 1776), 101–14.
20. Cutbush, 14–17.
21. R. Torres-Reyes, "The 1979–80 Encampment," *A Study of Medical Services* (Washington, D.C.: U.S. Department of Interior, 1971): 22–23.

22. Cutbush, 52–57, 71.

23. G. Von Swieten, *The Diseases Incident to Armies with the Method of Cure. Also the Nature and Treatment of Gunshot Wounds by John Ranby* (Philadelphia, 1776), passim.

24. N. Mercer, "Diseases of Military Campaigns," *Military Surgeon*, 78, (1936): 130–34.

25. J. Tilton, *Economical Observations on Military Hospitals* (Wilmington, DE, 1803).

26. B. Mitchell, *The Price of Independence: A Review of the American Revolution* (New York: Oxford University Press, 1974), 143–66.

27. L. C. Duncan, *Medical Men of the American Revolution* (New York: Kelley Publishers, 1970), 13–15.

28. *Ibid.*, 15–17.

29. E. E. Hume, "The Military Sanitation of Moses in the Light of Modern Knowledge," *Military Surgeon*, 78 (1936): 39–52.

30. S. Selveyn, "Sir John Pringle: Hospital Reformer, Moral Philosopher, and Pioneer of Antisepsis," *Annals of Medical History*, 10 (1929): 266–74.

31. N. Cantlie, *History of the Army Medical Department* (Churchill Livingston Edenburgh Press, 1974), 81–84.

32. J. E. Gibson, "Captured Medical Men and Army Hospitals of the American Revolution," *Annals of Medical History* n.s. 10 (1938): 382–89.

33. Selveyn, 266–74.

34. S. Bayne-Jones, *the Evolution of Preventative Medicine in the United States Army, 1607–1939* (Washington, D.C.: Office of the Surgeon General, 1968), 10–12.

35. Tilton, 17.

36. L. Taillot, "Early American Surgeons," *Ciba Symposium* (1939–40): 334–39.

37. B. Rush, *The Letters of Benjamin Rush*, ed. L. H. Butterfield (Princeton: Princeton University Press, 1951), 140–45. The letter was originally printed in the *Pennsylvania Packet*, April 22, 1777.

38. Jones, 104–14.

39. Tilton, passim.

40. R. Block, "Military Medicine in the Eighteenth Century," *Military Surgeon*, 65 (1929): 561–76, esp. 566.

41. *Ibid.*, 571–76.

42. G. Washington, *Basic Writings of George Washington*, ed. Saxe Commins (New York: Random House, 1948), 121–27.

43. M. C. Gillett, *The Army Medical Department, 1775–1818* (Washington, D.C.: Center of Military History United States Army, 1981), 74, 84, 115.

44. P. M. Ashburn, *A History of the Medical Department of the United States Army* (Boston and New York: Houghton-Mifflin, 1929), 21–22.

45. F. Packard, *The Life and Times of Ambroise Paré, 1510–90* (New York: Paul P. Hoeber, 1921), 15–16, 27–28, 46, 114–16, 268–76.

46. A. Wooden, "The Wounds and Weapons of the Revolutionary War, 1775–83," *Delaware Medical Journal*, 44 (#3) (March 1972): 59–62.

47. Jones, 13–25.

48. J. Thacher, *Military Journal of the American Revolution 1775–83* (First published by Cottons & Barnard, Boston, 1827), 255. Dr. Thacher's book is frequently referred to by medical historians. I found it to be largely a diary of a poorly trained doctor. His references to medical aspects were minuscule in the totality of the text: pages 52 and 53 describe the treatment for rattlesnake bite to be one quart of olive oil orally, and mercury rubbed into the bite; page 112 presents his observations of the British and Hessian surgeons at

the Albany Hospital; pages 114 and 115 have his description of Captain Gregg who survived a scalping by the Indians, and page 257 describes inoculation for smallpox where an extract of the butternut tree was used to prepare the patient rather than jalap and calomel.

49. Jones, 30–100.

50. O. Wangensteen, "Some Highlights in the History of Amputation Reflecting Lessons in Wound Healing," *Bulletin of the History of Medicine*, 41 (1967): 97–98.

51. *Ibid.*, 99–106.

52. J. Phalen, "Surgeon James Mann's Observations on Battlefield Amputations," *Military Surgeon*, 87 (1940): 463–66.

53. Wangensteen, 110–12.

54. Phalen, 466.

55. W. Craig, "Neurosurgery in Military Medicine," *Military Surgeon*, 114 (1954): 21–26.

56. H. Drowne, "Dr. Salomon Drowne: A Surgeon in the Revolution," *Military Surgeon*, 86 (1940): 292–97.

57. Duncan, 120.

58. C. Jelenko, "Emergency Medicine in Colonial America," *Annals of Emergency Medicine* 11 (1) (1982): 73–77.

59. G. Marks and W. K. Beattie, *The History of Medicine in America* (New York: Scribner, 1973), 126–27.

60. Jones, 13–21.

61. C. K. Stewart and T. Miller, *Moving the Wounded*, (Fort Collins Co.: Old Army Press, 1970), 11–15.

62. Jelenko, 73–77, esp. 75.

63. G.A. Bender and J. Parascandola, eds. *American Pharmacy in the Colonial and Revolutionary Periods* (Madison, Wisc.: American Institute of the History of Pharmacy, 1977), 29–36.

64. *Ibid.*

65. H. S. Commager, *The Spirit of Seventy-Six: The Story of the American Revolution as Told by Participants* (New York: Harper and Row, 1967), 823–27.

66. F. N. L. Poynter, *Evolution of the Hospital in Britain* (London: Pitman Medical Publishing Company, 1964), 159–60.

67. Duncan, 232–233.

68. A. Shands, "James Tilton, M.D.: Delaware's Greatest Physician," *Delaware Medical Journal* (1974): 25.

69. Duncan, 217–23.

70. S. Reiser, "The Colonial Physician," *Military Medicine*, 142 (4) (1977): 47.

71. S.X. Radbill, "Francis Allison, Jr.: A Surgeon of the Revolution, 9 (*Bulletin of the History of Medicine* 9, 1941): 243–57, esp. 245.

72. C. K. Wilbur, *Revolutionary Medicine, 1700–1800* (Chester, Conn.: Globe Piquot Press, 1980), 48.

73. Poynter, 157–69.

74. R. L. Blanco, "Medicine in the Continental Army 1775–86," *New York Academy of Medicine Bulletin*, 57 (8) (October 1981): 677–701.

75. J. Black and W. Green, "A Rhode Island Chaplain in the Revolution," *Letters of Ebenezer David* (Providence: The Rhode Island Society of the Cincinnati Providence, 1949), passim.

76. Thacher, 154.

77. J. Duffy, *The Healers: A History of American Medicine* (Evanston: University of Illinois Press, 1979), 77–88.

78. Taillot, 334–38.

79. C. R. Hall, "The Beginnings of American Military Medicine," *Annals of Medical History*, 4 (1942): 122–31.

80. P. E. Kooperman, "Medical Services in the British Army, 1842–83," *Journal of the History of Medicine and Allied Sciences*, 34 (1979): 428–55.

81. W. Watson, "Four Monopolies and the Surgeons of London and Edinburgh," *Journal of the History of Medicine and Allied Sciences*, 25 (1970): 311–22.

82. W. Ball, *John Morgan* (Philadelphia: University of Pennsylvania Press, 1965), 32.

83. P. E. Kooperman, "Medical Services in the British Army, 1842–83," *Journal of the History of Medicine and Allied Sciences*, 34 (1979): 447–49.

84. Thacher, 112.

85. R. Schmitz, "Hessian Troops in the American Revolution," *Minnesota Medicine*, 7 (1976): 479–80.

86. G. Nadeau, "A German Military Surgeon in Rutland, Massachusetts, During the Revolution," *Bulletin of the History of Medicine*, 18 (1945): 243–300.

87. Block, 565–72.

88. A. Wooden, "Dr. Jean Francois Coste and the French Army in the American Revolution," *Delaware Medical Journal* 7 (1976): 397–404.

89. I. C. Selavan, "Nurses in American History: The Revolution," *American Journal of Nursing*, 4 (1975): 592–94.

90. J. Stimson, "The Forerunners of the American Army Nurses," *Military Surgeon*, 58 (1926): 133–41.

91. Bender and Parascandola, eds., 11–13, 29–35.

92. Blanco, "Medicine in the Continental Army," 687–94.

93. H. Applegate, "The Effect of the American Revolution on American Medicine," *Military Medicine*, 126 (1961): 551–53.

94. Blanco, *Medicine in the Continental Army*, 691.

Chapter 2

1. M. Ready, "Army Doctors: Four Short-Term Medical Chiefs," *Military Medicine* 132 (1967): 188–94.

2. Duffy, 80–81.

3. L. Duncan, "Beginnings of the Army Medical Service," *Military Surgeon* 20 (1932): 384–89.

4. A. French, *General Gage's Informers* (New York: Greenwood Press, 1968), passim.

5. Ready, 190.

6. French, 184–85.

7. Duncan, 389–94.

8. W.S. Middleton, "John Morgan: Father of Medical Education in North America," *Annals of Medical History* 9 (1927): 13–26.

9. V. Allen, "Medicine in the American Revolution, Part 3," *Oklahoma State Medical Association Journal* 64, no. 9 (1971): 377–81.

10. P. Ashburn, *History of the Medical Department of the United States Army* (Boston: Houghton-Mifflin, 1929), 10–12.

11. W. J. Bell, *John Morgan* (Philadelphia: University of Pennsylvania Press, 1965), 31–32.

12. Middleton, 15–16.

13. P. Olch, "The Morgan-Shippen Controversy," *Review of Surgery* 22, no. 1–2 (1965): 1–8.

14. Bell, John Morgan, 545–48.

15. Olch, 17–20.

16. C. E. Fox, and S. Berlin, "Abraham Chovet (1704–1790): The Perfect Original," *Transcriptions and Studies of the College of Physicians of Philadelphia* 38 (1970/1): 221–30.

17. W. J. Bell, *The Colonial Physician and Other Essays* (New York: Science History Publications, 1975), 221.

18. Olch, 21.

19. Allen, 378–79.

20. J. Morgan, *A Vindication of His Public Character in the Station of Director General of the Military Hospital and Physician-in-Chief of the American Army, 1776* (Boston: Powers and Willis, 1777), 1–8, 12–23.

21. Middleton, 25.

22. Bell, W. J., "The Court-Martial of William Shippen, Jr.," *Journal of the History of Medicine and Allied Sciences* 19 (1964): 218–38.

23. Bell, *John Morgan*, 202.

24. R. S. Klein, *Portrait of an Early American Family* (Philadelphia: University of Pennsylvania Press, 1975, 9–13, 47, 112–13.

25. *Ibid.*, 113–18.

26. B. C. Corner, *William Shippen, Jr.* (Philadelphia: American Philosophical Society, 1951), 11–34, 65–73, 80–91, 98–102.

27. J. B. Blake, "The Anatomical Lectures of William Shippen, 1766," *Transactions and Studies of the College of Physicians of Philadelphia* 42–43 (1974/76) 61–66.

28. W. S. Middleton, "William Shippen, Jr.," *Annals of Medical History*, n.s., 4 (1932). 441–52.

29. Bell, "The Court-Martial of William Shippen, Jr.," 218–38.

30. Corner, 115–17.

31. M. H. Saffron, *Surgeon to Washington, Dr. John Cochran* (New York: Columbia University Press, 1977), 1–25.

32. M. H. Saffron, "John Cochran, 1730–1807: Director General of the Hospital of the United States," *Transcriptions and Studies of the College of Physicians of Philadelphia* 42–43 (1974/76): 379–87.

33. Mitchell, 151.

34. Duffy, 87–88.

35. B. Rush, *The Autobiography of Benjamin Rush*, ed. B. C. Corner (Princeton: Princeton University Press, 1948), 23–74.

36. *Ibid.*, passim; and N. B. Goodman, *Benjamin Rush* (Philadelphia: University of Pennsylvania Press, 1934), 32–35.

37. D. F. Hawke, *Benjamin Rush: Revolutionary Gadfly* (Indianapolis: Bobbs-Merrill, 1971), 108; and Goodman, 32–33.

38. G. Gminder, "An Exhibit of the Life and Works of Benjamin Rush, M.D.," *Bulletin of the History of Medicine* 19 (1946): 96–112.

39. E. T. Carlson, "Benjamin Rush on Revolutionary Hygiene," *New York Academy of Medicine Bulletin* 55, no. 2, (July–August 1979): 614–35.

40. Rush, *Letters,* 124–31.

41. Goodman, 48.

42. Allen, 379–380.

43. Rush, 130–35.

44. *Ibid.,* 137.

45. Rush, 158–71, 182–84.
46. Rush, *Autobiography*, 136.
47. Carlson, 616–18.
48. B. Rush, *Medical Inquiries*, 147–150.
49. *Ibid.*, 37–115, 151–225.
50. J. I. Waring, "The Influence of Benjamin Rush on the Practice of Bleeding in South Carolina," *Bulletin of Medical History* 35 (1961): 230–37.
51. Rush, *Autobiography*, 87, 93, 159.
52. J. E. Gibson, "Benjamin Rush's Apprentice Students," *Transactions and Studies of the College of Physicians of Philadelphia* 14, 4th ser. (1946) 127–32.
53. M. P. Rucker, "Benjamin Rush, Obstetrician," *Annals of Medical History*, 3rd ser. (1941): 487–500.

Chapter 3

1. R. Ketchum, ed. *American Heritage Book of the Revolution* (New York: American Heritage Publishing, 1958), 22–24, 46, 50, 55–68.
2. J. Phalen, "Doctors at Arms: Joseph Warren, Minute Man," *Military Surgeon*, 92 (1943): 658–61, esp. 659.
3. Ketchum, ed., 69.
4. Stanley, G. F. G., *Canada Invaded* (Toronto: Hakkert Publishers, 1973), 3–6, 16.
5. Ketchum, 69–72, 99.
6. Commager, 105–7, 112–13.
7. Ketchum, 100–102.
8. Duncan, 35–37.
9. Phalen, 660.
10. Ketchum, 107–112.
11. H. Thursfield, "Smallpox in the American War of Independence," *Annals of Medical History* 2, 2nd. ser. (1940): 312–18.
12. J. Duffy, "Smallpox and the Indians in the American Colonies," *Bulletin of the History of Medicine* 25 (1957): 324–41.
13. D. R. Hopkins, *Princes and Peasants: Smallpox in History* (Chicago: University of Chicago Press, 1983), 260.
14. W. B. Blanton, *Medicine in Virginia in the Eighteenth Century* (Richmond, Va.: Garrett and Massie, 1931), 64.
15. D. Van Swenenberg, "The Suttons and the Business of Inoculation," *Medical History* 22 (1978): 71–82.
16. J. B. Blake, "The Medical Profession and Public Health in Colonial Boston," *Bulletin of the History of Medicine* 26 (1952): 218–30.
17. Ketchum, 172.
18. Commager, 277.
19. R. Truax, *The Brothers Warren of Boston: The First Family of Surgery*, (Boston: Houghton Mifflin, 1968), 36.
20. E. A. Maclay, *History of the U.S. Navy, 1775–1893* (New York: Appleton, 1849), 9.
21. J. J. Henry, *Arnold's Campaign Against Canada* (Albany: Joel Munsell, 1877), 2–3.
22. Stanley, 28–64.

23. Henry, 3–4.
24. I. Senter, *The Journal of Isaac Senter* (Philadelphia: Historical Society of Pennsylvania, 1946), 6–10.
25. J. A. McSherry, "Reiter's Syndrome and the American Revolutionary War," *Practitioner* 26, no. 1366 (April 1982): 794–95.
26. Senter, 2–28.
27. Stanley, 84.
28. Senter, 32.
29. Stanley, 98–103.
30. Henry, 134–39, 169.
31. Montross, 78–80.
32. D. B. David, "Medicine in the Canadian Campaign of the Revolutionary War," *Bulletin of the History of Medicine* 44 (1970): 461–73.
33. Stanley, 115.
34. Senter, 38.
35. R. Blanco, *Jonathan Potts: American Revolutionary Physician* (Gailand: STPM Press, 1974), 91–92.
36. L. Roberts, *Memoirs of Captain Lemuel Roberts* (Bennington, Vt., 1808), 28–41.
37. Blanco, "Medicine in the Continental Army," 683–84.
38. Stanley, 133, 138–42.
39. Mitchell, 16–17.
40. Blanco, *Dr. Jonathan Potts*, 94.
41. J. E. Gibson, *Bodo Otto and the Medical Background of the American Revolution*, (Springfield, Ill., and Baltimore, Md.: Charles C. Thomas, 1937), 98–101.
42. Commager, 539–90.
43. Thacher, 257–58.
44. Ketchum, 254.
45. Thacher, 259.
46. W. Owen, *Medical Department of the United States Army During the Revolution* (New York: Paul B. Hoeber, 1920).
47. Hopkins, 13–20.
48. R. Parkhurst, "The History and Traditional Treatment of Smallpox in Ethiopia," *Medical History* (1975): 343–53.
49. Hopkins, 200.
50. A. G. Carmichael, and A. M. Silverstein, "Smallpox in Europe Before the Seventeenth Century," *Journal of the History of Medicine and Allied Sciences* 42 (1984): 147–68.
51. G. Miller, *The Adoption of Inoculation for Smallpox in England and France* (Philadelphia: University of Pennsylvania Press, 1957), 27–28, 242–56.
52. Hopkins, 117–18, 140.
53. Miller, 40–42.
54. K. Dewhurst, *Dr. Thomas Sydenham* (Berkeley: University of California Press, (1966), 106.
55. Hopkins, 295–99.
56. *Ibid.*, 37–59.
57. D. Bernoulli, (Translated from French by Bradley, L.) *Smallpox Inoculation: An Eighteenth Century Controversy*, trans. L. Bradley Paris, 1767, 14–15.
58. Hopkins, 14–15, 37–41, 107, 111.
59. Miller, 48–49.
60. *Ibid.*, 50–64.

61. *Ibid,*. 68–130.

62. J. I. Waring, "James Killpatrick and Smallpox Inoculation in Charleston," *Annals of Medical History* 10 (1938): 301–8.

63. L. Clarkson, *Disease, Death, and Famine in Pre-Industrial England* (Dubbin: Gill and McMillin, 1975), 99.

64. Miller, 109–150.

65. *Ibid.*, 123–95, 219–25.

66. *Ibid.*, 42–44.

67. Parkhurst, 47–48.

68. Miller, 41.

69. Van Swenenberg, 71–74.

70. *Ibid.*, 75–81.

71. Miller, 163.

72. J. Simmons, "Influence of Epidemic Disease on the Early History of the Western Hemisphere," *Military Surgeon* 71 (1932): 133–43.

73. Hopkins, 207–36.

74. Truax, 17–18.

75. M. C. Lerkund, "Colonial Epidemic Disease," *Ciba Symposium* 1 (1939-40): 376.

76. J. T. Barnett, "The Inoculation Controversy in Puritan New England," *Bulletin of the History of Medicine* 12 (1942): 169–90.

77. R. Shyrock, *Eighteenth-Century Medicine in America* (Worcester, Md.: American Antiquary Society, 1950), 15.

78. Winslow, *A Destroying Angel* (Boston: Houghton Mifflin, 1874), 32–33, 44–49, 56, 86.

79. Blake, "Smallpox Inoculation in Colonial Boston," 287.

80. Colman *Some Observations on the New Method of Receiving the Smallpox by Ingrafting and Inoculation* (Boston: Green 1721), 6–14.

81. Hopkins, 255.

82. Blake, "Smallpox Inoculation in Colonial Boston," 287–91.

83. J. B. Blake, "The Medical Profession and Public Health In Colonial Boston," *Bulletin of the History of Medicine* 26 (1952): 218–30.

84. J. Cary, *Joseph Warren: Physician, Politician, Patriot* (Evanston: University of Illinois Press, 1964), 20–22.

85. C. Heaton, "Medicine in New York During the English Colonial Period," *Bulletin of the History of Medicine* 17 (1945): 9–37.

86. Hopkins, 243–54.

87. Waring, 301–04.

88. Winslow, 94–101.

Chapter 4

1. G. Rosen, "Occupational Diseases of English Seamen During the Seventeenth and Eighteenth Centuries," *Bulletin of Medical History* 7 (1939): 751–8, esp. 754.

2. L. H. Roddis, "A Short History of Nautical Medical Care," *Annals of Medical History* 3 (1941): 203–47, esp. 204–6.

3. A. Chaplin, *Medicine in England During the Reign of George III* (New York: AMS Press, 1917), 100–101.

4. Roddis, 222–29.

5. W. Watson, "Two British Surgeons in the French Wars," *Medical History* 13 (1969): 213–25.

6. C. Lloyd, and Coulter, *Medicine and the Navy*, vol. 3 (Livingston, 1961), 10–18.

7. Cutbush, 224–46.

8. A. E. A. Hudson and A. Herbert, "James Lind: His Contributions to Shipboard Sanitation," *Journal of the History of Medicine and Allied Sciences* 11 (1956): 1–3.

9. Watson, 215–20.

10. Lloyd and Coulter, 38, 67.

11. L. H. Roddis, *A Short History of Nautical Medicine* (New York and London: Paul B. Hoeber Publishers, 1941), 252–58.

12. Cutbush, 79–82.

13. Rosen, 752.

14. Roddis, *A Short History of Nautical Medicine*, 236–40.

15. Cutbush, 109–19.

16. Roddis, *A Short History of Nautical Medicine*, 223–41.

17. Cutbush, 77–79.

18. V. E. Levine, "Scurvy: The Soldier's Calamity," *Military Surgeon* 89 (1941): 140–54.

19. T. Devlin, ed., *Textbook of Biochemistry* (New York: Wiley Medical Publications, 1982), 946–48, 1225–27.

20. J. M. Kissane, ed., *Anderson's Pathology*, 8th ed. (Mosby, 1985), 509–10; 569; 1742–43.

21. Hudson and Herbert, 1–13.

22. C. Lloyd, *The Health of Seamen* (London and Colchester: Naval Records Society, Spottswood Ballantyne, 1965), 12–23.

23. Von Swieten, 89–93.

24. W. Buchan, *Domestic Medicine of the Family Physician* (Philadelphia: Printer Joseph Cruikshank, Philadelphia, 1774), 276–80.

25. W. Northcote, *Extracts from the Marine Practice of Physic and Surgery Including the Nature and Treatment of Gunshot Wounds* (Philadelphia: John Ranby, 1776), 138–50.

26. W. Mann, Jr., "Health and Physical Efficiency, Naval Warfare," *Military Surgeon* 94 (1944): 4–8.

27. E. H. Ackerknecht, *History and Geography of Most Important Diseases*, (New York and London: Hefner Publishing, 1965), 146.

28. Jones and Hughes, "Copper Boilers and the Occurrence of Scurvy," *Medical History* 20 (1976): 80–81.

29. R. E. Hughes, "James Lind and the Cure of Scurvy: An Experimental Approach," *Medical History* 19 (1975): 342–51.

30. Lloyd, 88–95.

31. Roddis, "Short History of Nautical Medicine," 210–11.

32. Clarkson, 146.

33. L. G. Wilson, "The Clinical Definition of Scurvy and the Discovery of Vitamin C," *Journal of the History of Medicine and Allied Sciences* 30 (1975): 40–60.

34. R. L. Blanco, "The Soldier's Friend Sir Jeremiah Fitzpatrick, Inspector of Health for Land Forces," *Medical History* (1976): 402–21.

35. Maclay, 3.

36. W. A. Fowler, *Rebels Under Sail* (New York: Scribner's, 1976), 14–20.

37. E. Dupuy and G. Hammerman, *The American Revolution: A Global War* (New York: David McKay, 1977), 285–88.

38. Maclay, 4–12.
39. Fowler, 20–29.
40. W. B. Clark, *George Washington's Navy* (Baton Rouge: Louisiana State University Press, 1960); 3–4, 8–12, 20–26, 49, 185.
41. Fowler, 49–52.
42. Maclay, 34–36.
43. Fowler, 60.
44. Maclay, 36–42.
45. Fowler, 65–118.
46. E. S. Maclay, *History of American Privateers* (New York: Burt Franklin Publishers, 1899), 4–8, 69–78, 208.
47. C. K. Wilbur, *Picture Book of the Revolution's Privateers* (Harrisburg, Penn.: Stackpole, 1973), 91–92.
48. Maclay, *History of American Privateers*, 8–9, 17–18, 79, 103, 131.
49. Fowler, 89–90, 225.
50. Commager, 912, 926–27.
51. Maclay, *History of the U.S. Navy*, 51–59.
52. Fowler, 101–10, 120–27.
53. S. E. Morrison, *John Paul Jones* (Boston: Northeastern University Press, 1959), 39, 59–64.
54. *Ibid.*, 103–10, 143–48, 156–63.
55. C. H. Preble, ed., *The Diary of Ezra Green, M.D., Surgeon on Board the Continental Ship of War Ranger* (Boston, 1875), 21–25.
56. Morrison, 71.
57. Dupuy and Hammerman, 212–14.
58. Morrison, 186–90, 226–40.
59. J. Barnes, ed., *Fanning's Narrative* (New York: New York Times and Arno Press, 1968), 38, 58–59.
60. Morrison, 315, 326, 333, 360.
61. W. G. Eckert, "Identification of the Remains of John Paul Jones," *American Journal of Forensic Medical Pathology* 2 (June 3, 1982): 143–52.
62. Ketchum, 265, 285–86.
63. M. B. Gordon, *Naval and Maritime Medicine During the American Revolution* (New Jersey: Ventnor, 1978).
64. J. Ranby, *Nature and Treatment of Gunshot Wounds* (Philadelphia, 1776), 115–28.
65. Cutbush, 125–33, 212–46.
66. Jones, 15–29, 90–100.
67. Gordon, 16–84 and passim.
68. Roddis, *A Short History of Nautical Medicine*, 260–62.

Chapter 5

1. Ketchum, 178–79.
2. Duncan, 112–15.
3. Saffron, 108–116.
4. Ketchum, 180–88.
5. C. C. Dennie, *A History of Syphilis* (Springfield, Ill.: Charles C. Thomas, 1962), 3–9.

6. *Ibid.*, 12–18.

7. T. Rosebury, *Microbes and Morals* (New York: Viking Press, 1971), 5–13.

8. Ackerknecht, 18–19.

9. F. Swediaur, *Symptoms, Effects, and Therapy of Syphilis* (Philadelphia: Thomas Dobson, 1815), 270–386, 395–509. Originally published in London in 1784, this book of 509 pages is entirely devoted to the disease. It represents the thoughts about the disease in the eighteenth century. The first 269 pages describe the disease and its complications. The author, like most physicians of the time, felt gonorrhea and syphilis were different manifestations of the same disease.

10. W. Buchan, *Domestic Medicine or the Family Physician* (Philadelphia: Joseph Cruikshank, 1774), reprinted as *Domestic Medicine; or, A Treatise on the Prevention and Cure of Diseases by Regimen and Simple Medicine* [Boston, 1809]), ch. 47.

11. Von Swieten, pp. 94 ff. and passim.

Chapter 6

1. R. C. Heflebower, "Prisoners of War," *Military Surgeon* 63 (1928): 625–42.

2. Packard, 219–20, 235–39.

3. Heflebower, 631.

4. J. E. Gibson, "Captured Medical Men and Army Hospitals of the American Revolution," *Annals of Medical History* 10 (1938): 382–89.

5. D. Dandridge, *American Prisoners of the Revolution* (Baltimore, Md.: Genealogical Publishing House, 1967), 25.

6. Fowler, 257, 260.

7. Nadeau, 249–99.

8. C. Hawkins, *The Adventures of Christopher Hawkins* (New York: Charles J. Bushwell, 1864), 223.

9. Barnes, 165.

10. Gibson, 383–88.

11. Hawke, 205–209.

12. Gibson, 385.

13. Mitchell, 168–73.

14. Dandridge, 25–60, 91–138.

15. Hawkins, 65–74, 206–74.

16. Duncan, 318–20.

17. Barnes, 1–8.

18. I. R. Potter, *Life and Remarkable Adventures of Israel Potter* (New York: Counth Books, 1962), 16–21.

19. C. Herbert, *A Relic of the Revolution* (Boston: Charles H. Pierce, 1847, reprinted New York: The New York Times and Arno Press, (1968), passim.

20. S. Lutnick, *The American Revolution and the British Press 1775–1763*, (Columbia, Missouri: University of Missouri Press, 1967), 1–8, 10–20, 45–47, 81–83, 147–48.

21. Simmons, 133–43.

22. Hawke, 204–05.

23. E. Beardsley, "History of a Dysentery in the Twenty-Second Regiment of the Late Continental Army Occasioned by Barracks Being Overcrowded and Not Properly Ventilated," in H. S. Commager *The Spirit of Seventy-Six*, 835–36.

24. Hawkins,

25. Buchan, 220–26.

26. Duffy, 220–21.

27. Hawke, 396.

28. Mardell, Douglas, Bennett, *Principles and Practices of Infectious Disease* (New York: Wiley Medical Publications, 1979), 1751–59.

Chapter 7

1. H. Zinsser, *Rats, Lice, and History* (Boston: Atlantic Monthly Press, 1934), 66.

2. *Ibid.*, 117–45.

3. *Ibid.*, 195–259.

4. Ketchum, 178.

5. Saffron, 106–13.

6. Duncan, 117–40.

7. Mitchell, 148.

8. Duncan, 170–71.

9. Mitchell, 149–57.

10. Rush, 358–60.

11. *Ibid.*

12. W. D. Tiggert, "A 1759 Spotted Fever Epidemic in North Carolina," *Journal of the History of Medicine and Allied* Sciences 41 (July 1987): 296–304.

13. Mitchell, 155–57.

14. Buchan, 146–52.

15. Von Swieten, 82–88.

16. Roddes, 212–13.

17. Ackerknecht, 32–35.

18. Clarkson, 43.

19. *Ibid.*, 44–47.

20. C. Heaton, "Medicine in New York During the English Colonial Period," *Bulletin of the History of Medicine* 6–7 (1975–6): 49–54.

21. J. Duffy, *Epidemics in Colonial America* (Baton Rouge: Louisiana State University Press, 1953), 230.

Chapter 8

1. Ketchum, 210–16.

2. J. B. B. Trussel, Jr., *Birthplace of an Army: A Study of Valley Forge* (Harrisburg: Pennsylvania History and Museum Commission, 1979), 1–35.

3. *Ibid.*, 39–40.

4. *Ibid.*, 41–44.

5. *Ibid.*, 62–74.

6. *Ibid.*, 77–116.

7. Ketchum, 221–24.

8. Duncan, 227–43.

9. Commager, 639–41.

10. W. S. Middleton, "Medicine at Valley Forge," *Annals of Medical History* 3, 3rd ser. (1941): 461–86.

11. Thacher, 148–49.

12. R. Friedman, *The Story of Scabies* (New York: Froben Press, 1947), 104.

13. Middleton, 476.

14. Von Swieten, 94–98.

15. Buchan, 286–88.

16. Friedman, *Story of Scabies,* passim.

17. Orkin et al, *Scabies and Pediculosis* (Philadelphia: Lippincott, 1977), 1.

18. Friedman, *Story of Scabies,* 368–69.

19. B. B. Beeson, "Scabies," *Archives of Dermatology and Syphilology* 16 (1927): 294–307.

20. Friedman, *Story of Scabies,* 4.

21. Orkin et al., 4.

22. Friedman, *Story of Scabies,* 6, 16–17, 20, 28, 30, 35, 57–59.

23. R. Friedman, "Scabies in Colonial America," *Annals of Medical History* 2 (1940): 402.

24. Friedman, *Story of Scabies*, 79–80,378.

25. G. Cumston, "Some Remarks on the History of the Discovery of the Acarus," *British Journal of Dermatology* 36 no. 13 (1924): 13–19.

26. Friedman, *Story of Scabies*, 82–85, 211.

27. Beeson, 301.

28. W. Libmann, "Complications of Scabies," *Military Surgeon* 99 (1946): 116–26.

Chapter 9

1. P. F. Russell, *Man's Mastery of Malaria* (London: Oxford University Press, 1955), 2.

2. M. A. Barber, *A Malariologist in Many Lands* (Lawrence: University of Kansas Press, 1946), 4–5.

3. W. B. Blanton, *Medicine in Virginia in the Eighteenth Century* (Richmond, Va.: Garrett and Massie, 1931), 66.

4. J. Duffy, *Epidemics in Colonial America*, 207–14.

5. Wooden, 394–404.

6. D. G. Carlson, *African Fever* (Canton, Mass.: Science History Publications, 1984), 28–30.

7. Ketchum, 334.

8. *Ibid.*, 264–67.

9. Commager, 704–705.

10. *Ibid.*, 1062–63.

11. *Ibid.*, 107.

12. Ketchum, 311–32.

13. Commager, 1160.

14. Ketchum, 334–58.

15. Duncan, 352–53.

16. Wooden, 401–404.

17. Duncan, 352–54.

18. Ketchum, 364, 375.

19. R. Jackson, *A Treatise on the Fevers of Jamaica with Some Observations on the Intermitting Fever of America*, (Philadelphia: Robert Campbell bookseller, 1795), 192–214.

20. Russell, 3–6.

21. W. H. S. Jones, *Malaria: A Neglected Factor in the History of Greece and Rome* (Cambridge and London: Bowes and Bowes, 1907), 7–48.

22. Jones, 19–28.

23. Russell, 9.

24. Jones, 64–68.

25. A. Celli, *The History of Malaria in the Roman Campagna* (London: John Bale and Danielson, 1933), 26–28. *See also* R. A. Major, *Disease and Destiny* (New York: Appleton Century, 1936), 165–68.

26. Russell, 9.

27. L. J. Bruce-Chwatt, *The Rise and Fall of Malaria in Europe* (London: Oxford University Press, 1980), 107.

28. Russell, 22, 182.

29. Clarkson, 50.

30. S. Jarcho, "A Cartographic and Literary Study of the Word Malaria," *Journal of the History of Medicine and Allied Sciences* 25 (1970): 31–39.

31. Bruce-Chwatt, 131.

32. Russell, 78–91.

33. Goodman and Gilman, *The Pharmacological Basis of Therapeutics* 5th ed. (New York: MacMillan, 1975), 1062–65, esp. 1063.

34. Major, 174–75.

35. Russell, 90.

36. *Ibid.*, 94–101. Major, 176–177.

37. Major, 178–80.

38. Russell, 103, 132–133.

39. Russell, 96–102.

40. Goodman and Gilman, 1063–65.

41. Jackson, 186–212.

Epilogue

1. Washington, *Basic Writings*, 39.

2. Ketchum, 191.

3. J. T. Flexner, *The Forge of Experience, 1732–1775*, (Boston: Little Brown, 1965), 23–24.

4. Tobey, "Preventable Disease in the Washington Family," *Hygeia* 13 (1935): 118–21.

5. F. A. Williams, and T. E. Reys, "The Medical History of George Washington"—*Proceedings of the Staff Meetings of the Mayo Clinic*, 17 (1941): 92–96.

6. Flexner, 19, 39, 163–70.

7. Williams, and Keys, 93.

8. J. W. Estes, "George Washington and the Doctors," *Medical Heritage* 1 no. 1 (January–February 1985): 44–58.

9. G. Washington, *The Diaries of George Washington*, ed. D. Jackson (Charlottesville: University Press of Virginia, 1976), 30–34.

10. M. Knox, "The Medical History of George Washington, His Physician, Friends, and Advisers," *Bulletin of the History of Medicine* 1, (1933): 174–91.

11. S. L. Liston, "Traumatic Amputation of the External Ear, the War of Jenkin's Ear, and George Washington," *American Journal of Surgery* 148 no. 5 (1984): 599–601.

12. Flexner, 52–113.

13. Washington, *Basic Writings*, 39.

14. Flexner, 121–25.

15. P. M. Dale, *Medical Biographies* (Norman: University of Oklahoma Press, 1952), 102–11.

16. Flexner, 127–31.

17. Washington, *Basic Writings*, 41–55.

18. Flexner, 184.

19. *Ibid.*, 184–92.

20. *Ibid.*, 193–223.

21. Washington, 122–211.

22. Washington, *Basic Writings*, 84.

23. Washington, *Diaries*, vols. 2 and 3.

24. *Ibid.*, vol. 1.

25. W. B. Blanton, "Washington's Medical Knowledge and Its Sources," *Annals of Medical History* 5 (1933): 52–61.

26. Washington, *Diaries*, 2:128, 226, 246–47.

27. J. Hay, "George Washington Conquest of Physical Handicaps," *Hygeia* 9 (1931): 736–39.

28. Washington, *Diaries,* 2:113, 3:275–80.

29. Hay, 737.

30. Estes, 44–58.

31. *Ibid.*, 57.

32. Washington, 4:16, 5:152.

33. Washington, *Basic Writings*, 517–18.

34. Marx, *The Health of Presidents* (New York: Putnam, 1960), 17–89.

35. Washington, *Diaries*, 6:76–77, 222.

36. Estes, 49–53.

37. *Ibid.*, 52.

38. Washington, *Diaries*, 6:263.

39. F. O. Lewis, "Washington's Last Illness," *Annals of Medical History* 4 n.s., (1932): 245–48.

40. S. Friedberg, "Laryngology and Otology in Colonial Times," *Annals of Medical History* 1 (1917): 86–101.

41. Lewis, 247–48.

42. J. Burchell, "Observations on the Medical Treatment of General Washington in His Illness," *Transactions of the College of Physicians of Philadelphia*, 25, 3rd ser. (1903): 90–94. *See also* Friedberg, 89.

43. Washington, *Basic Writings*, 663–73.

44. From the Declaration of Independence.

45. J. Brooke, *King George III* (New York: McGraw Hill, 1972), 2–9.

46. G. S. Ayling, *George the Third* (New York: Knopf, 1972), 16–31.

47. M. S. Guttmacher, *America's Last King: An Interpretation of the Madness of George III*, (New York: Scribner, 1941), 10–17.

48. Ayling, 37–41.

49. Brooke, 71.

50. Ayling, passim.

51. *Ibid.*, 176–208.

52. Brooke, 288.

53. Ayling, 210–24.

54. Brooke, 307–08.

55. *Ibid.*, 125–26, 170–72, 221.

56. Ayling, 124–26.

57. I. Macalpine, and R. Hunter, *George III and the Mad Business* (London: Penguin Press, 1960), 186, 354.

58. Guttmacher, 75–259.

59. Ayling, 334–44.

60. *Ibid.*, 334.

61. Guttmacher, 200, 333.

62. Macalpine and Hunter, 15.

63. I. Macalpine and R. Hunter, "The Insanity of George III: A Classic Case of Porphyria," *British Medical Journal* 1 (1966): 65–67.

64. Ayling, 346, 450.

65. Guttmacher, 281–363.

66. Ayling, 453–56.

67. J. Brooke, "Historical Implications of Porphyria," *British Medical Journal* 1 (1968): 109–11.

68. Macalpine and Hunter, "The Insanity of George III," 69.

69. Macalpine and Hunter, *George III and the Mad Business*, 277–325.

70. I. Macalpine and R. Hunter, "Porphyria in the Royal Houses of Stuart, Hanover, and Prussia," *British Medical Journal*, 1 (1968): 7–18.

71. Macalpine and Hunter, "The Insanity of George III," 68–70.

72. Macalpine and Hunter, "Porphyria in the Royal Houses of Stuart, Hanover, and Prussia," 8–9.

Bibliography

Ackerknecht, E. H. *History and Geography of the Most Important Diseases.* New York: Hefner Publishers, 1965.

Allen, V. "Medicine in the American Revolution, Part 3." *Oklahoma State Medical Association Journal.* 64 (9/71): 377–81.

Allison, F. "A Surgeon of the Revolution, Samuel X. Radbull." *Bulletin of the History of Medicine* 9 (1941): 243–57.

Applegate, H. "The Effect of the American Revolution on American Medicine." *Military Medicine* 126 (1961): 551–53.

Applegate, H. "Preventive Medicine in the American Revolutionary Army." *Military Medicine* (126) (1962): 379–82.

Ashburn, P. *History of the Medical Department of the U. S. Army.* Boston: Houghton-Mifflin, 1929.

Ayling, G. *George III* New York: Knopf, 1972.

Barber, M. A. *A Malariologist in Many Lands.* Lawrence: University of Kansas Press, 1946.

Barnes, J., ed. *Fanning's Narrative* New York: New York Times and Arno Press, 1968.

Barnett, J. T. "The Inoculation Controversy in Puritan New England." *Bulletin of the History of Medicine* 121 (1942): 169–90.

Bayne-Jones, S. *The Evolution of Preventive Medicine in the United States Army, 1607–1939* Washington, D.C. Office of the Surgeon General, 1968.

Beardsley, E. "History of a Dysentery in the Twenty-Second Regiment of the Late Continental Army Occasioned by Barracks Being Overcrowded and Not Properly Ventilated." In H. S. Commager, *The Spirit of Seventy-Six: The Story of the American Revolution* as Told by Participants. New York: Harper and Row, 1967. Originally read before a medical meeting January 2, 1788.

Bell, W. J. *The Colonial Physician and Other Essays.* New York: Science History Publications, 1975.

Bell, W. J. *John Morgan.* Philadelphia: University of Pennsylvania Press, 1965.

Beeson, B. B. "Scabies." *Archives of Dermatology and Syphilalogy* 16 (1927): 294–307.

Bell, W. J. "The Court Martial of William Shippen, Jr." *Journal of the History of Medicine and Allied Sciences* 19 (1964): 218–38.

Bender, G.A. and J. Parascandola eds. *American Pharmacy in the Colonial and Revolutionary Periods.* Madison, Wisc.: American Institute of the History of Pharmacy, 1977.

Bernouilli, D. *Smallpox Inoculation: An Eighteenth-Century Controversy.* Trans. L. Bradley. Paris 1767.

Black, J. and W. Green. "A Rhode Island Chaplain in the Revolution." *Letters of Ebenezer David.* Providence: The Rhode Island Society of the Cincinnati, 1949.

Blake, J. B. "The Anatomical Lectures of William Shippen 1766." *Transactions and Studies of the College of Physicians of Philadelphia* 42–43 (1974/76): 61–66.

Blake, J. B. "The Medical Profession and Public Health in Colonial Boston." *Bulletin of the History of Medicine* 26 (1952): 218–30.

Blake, J. B. "Smallpox Inoculation in Colonial Boston." *Journal of the History of Medicine and Allied Sciences* 8 (1953): 284–300.

Blanco, R. L. "The Soldier's Friend: Sir Jeremiah Fitzpatrick, Inspector of Health for Land Forces." *Medical History* (1976): 402–21.

Blanco, R. *Jonathan Potts: American Revolutionary Physician.* Gailand: STPM Press, 1974.

Blanco, R. "Medicine in the Continental Army," 1775–81. *Bulletin of the New York Academy of Medicine* 57, no. 8 (1981): 677–701.

Blanton, W. B. *Medicine in Virginia in the Eighteenth Century* Richmond, Va.: Garrett and Massie, 1931.

Blanton, W. B. "Washington's Medical Knowledge and Its Sources." *Annals of Medical History*, n.s., 5 (1933): 52–61.

Block, F. "Military Medicine in the Eighteenth Century." *Military Surgeon* 65 (1929): 561–76.

Bolton, C. K. *The Private Soldier Under Washington.* Port Washington, N.Y.: Kennebet Press, 1902.

Brooke, J. "Historical Implications of Porphyria." *British Medical Journal* 1 (1968): 109–11.

Brooke, J. *King George III.* New York: McGraw Hill, 1972.

Bruce-Chewatt, L. J. *The Rise and Fall of Malaria in Europe.* London: Oxford University Press, 1980.

Buchan, W. *Domestic Medicine of the Family Physician.* Philadelphia: Joseph Criekshank, Printer, 1774; reprinted 1804.

Burchell, J. "Observations on the Medical Treatment of George Washington in His Illness." *Transactions and Studies of the College of Physicians of Philadelphia*, 3rd. ser., 25 (1903): 90–94.

Cantlie, N. *History of the Army Medical Department.* Edinburgh: Churchill Livingston Press, 1974.

Cantlie, N. Inspector-General of Hospitals "Robert Jackson" (1750–1827) *Proceedings of the Royal Society of Medicine*, 1972, December 65(12).

Carlson, D. G. *African Fever.* Canton, Mass.: Science History Publications, 1984.

Carlson, E. T. "Benjamin Rush on Revolutionary Hygiene," *New York Academy of Medicine Bulletin* 55, no. 2 (July–August, 1979): 614–35.

Carmichael, A. G. and A. M. Silverstein, "Smallpox in Europe Before the Seventeenth Century." *Journal of the History of Medicine and Allied Sciences* 42 (1984) 147–68.

Cary, J. *Joseph Warren: Physician, Politician, Patriot.* Evanston: University of Illinois Press, 1964.

Cascini, A. M. "War and Typhus." *Military Surgeon* 50 (1922): 403–18.

Celli, A. *History of Malaria in the Roman Campagna.* London: John Bale Sons and Danielson, 1963.

Chaplin, A. *Medicine in England During the Reign of George III.* New York: AMS Press, New York, 1917.

Clark, W. B. *George Washington's Navy.* Baton Rouge: Louisiana State University Press, 1960.

Clarkson, L. *Disease, Death, and Famine in Pre-Industrial England.* Dublin: Gill and McMillan, 1975.

Clendenning, P. H. "Dr. Thomas Dimsdale and Smallpox Inoculation in Russia." *Journal of the History of Medicine and Allied Sciences.* 8 (1973): 109–27.

Colman, M. *Some Observations on the New Method of Receiving the Smallpox by Ingrafting and Inoculation.* Boston: B. Green Publishers, 1721.

Commager, H. S. *The Spirit of Seventy-Six: The Story of the American Revolution as Told by Participants.* New York: Harper and Row, 1967.

Corner, B. C. *William Shippen, Jr.* Philadelphia: American Philosophical Society, 1951.

Cray, W. "Neurosurgery in Military Medicine." *Military Surgeon* 114 (1954): 21–26.

Cumston, G. "Some Remarks on the History of the Discovery of the Acarus." *British Journal of Dermatology* 36, no. 13 (1924): 13–19.

Cutbush, E. *Observations on the Means of Preserving Health of Soldiers and Sailors, and on the Duties of the Medical Department of the Army and Navy and Remarks on the Hospital and Their Internal Arrangement.* Philadelphia: Fry and Cammerer, 1809.

Dale, P. M. *Medical Biographies.* Norman: University of Oklahoma Press, 1952.

Dandridge, D. *American Prisoners of the Revolution.* Charlottesville, Va., 1911; reprinted Baltimore, Md.: Genealogical Publishing House, 1967.

David, D. B. "Medicine in the Canadian Campaign of the Revolutionary War." *Bulletin of the History of Medicine* 44 (1970): 461–73.

Dennie, C. C. *A History of Syphilis.* Springfield, Ill.: Charles C. Thomas Publishers, 1962.

Devlin, T. ed. *Textbook of Biochemistry.* New York: Wiley Medical Publications, 1982.

Dewhurst, K. *Dr. Thomas Sydenham.* San Francisco: University of California at Berkeley, 1966.

Drowne, H. "Dr. Salomon Drowne: A Surgeon in the Revolution." *Military Surgeon* 86 (1940): 292–97.

Duffy, J. *Epidemics in Colonial America.* Baton Rouge: Louisiana State University Press, 1953.

Duffy, J. *The Healers: A History of American Medicine.* Evanston: University of Illinois Press, 1979.

Duffy, J. "Smallpox and the Indians in the American Colonies." *Bulletin of the History of Medicine.* 25 (1957): 324–41.

Duncan, L. C. "Beginnings of the Army Medical Service." *Military Surgeon.* 20 (1932): 384–89.

Duncan, L. C. *Medical Men of the Revolution.* New York: Augustus M. Kelley Publishers, 1970.

Dupuy, E. and G. Hammerman. *The American Revolution: A Global War.* New York: David McKay, 1977.

Eckert, W. "Identification of the Remains of John Paul Jones." *American Journal of Forensic Medical Pathology* 3, no. 2 (June 1982): 143–52.

Edward, L. "The Edge of Utility: Slaves and Smallpox in the Early Eighteenth Century." *Medical History* 29 (1985): 511–70.

Estes, J. W. "George Washington and the Doctors." *Medical Heritage*, no. 1, 1 (January–February 1985): 44–58.

Fitz, R. "The Treatment of Inoculated Smallpox in 1764 and How it Felt." *Annals of Medical History.* 4 (1942): 110–113.

Flexner, J. T. *George Washington: The Forge of Experience, 1732–1775*, Boston: Little Brown, 1965.

Fowler, W. M. *Rebels Under Sail.* New York: Scribner, 1976.

Fox, C. E. and S. Berlin, "Abraham Chovet (1704–1790): The Perfect Original." *Transactions and Studies of the College of Physicians of Philadelphia* 38 (1970): 221–30.

Fracastor, G. *Syphilis or the French Disease.* Trans. H. Wynne-Finch. London: Heineman Medical Books, 1935.

French, A. *General Gage's Informers.* New York: Greenwood Press, 1968.

Friedberg, S. "Laryngology and Otology in Colonial Times." *Annals of Medical History*, no. 1, 1 (1917): 86–101.

Friedman, R. "Scabies in Colonial America." *Annals of the History of Medicine* 2 (1940): 401–03.

Friedman, R. *The Story of Scabies*. New York: Froben Press, 1947.

Gibson, J. E. "Benjamin Rush's Apprentice Students." *Transactions and Studies of the College of Physicians of Philadelphia*, 4th ser., 14 (1946): 127–32.

Gibson, J. E. *Bodo Otto and the Medical Background of the American Revolution.* Springfield, Ill., and Baltimore, Md.: Charles C. Thomas, 1937.

Gibson, J. E. "Captured Medical Men and Army Hospitals of the American Revolution." *Annals of Medical History*, n.s., 10 (1938): 382–89.

Gibson, J. E. "John Howard and the Gaol Fever." *History of Medicine*. 6/7 (1975–76): 49–54.

Gillett, M. C. *The Army Medical Department, 1775–1818.* Center of Military History, U. S. Army, 1981.

Gminder, G. "An Exhibit of the Life and Works of Benjamin Rush, M.D. " *Bulletin of the History of Medicine* 19 (1946): 96–112.

Goodman, N. B. *Benjamin Rush.* Philadelphia: University of Pennsylvania Press, 1934.

Goodman, L. S. and A. Gilman, *The Pharmacological Basis of Therapeutics.* 5th ed., New York: Macmillan, 1975; reprinted 1985.

Gordon, M. B. *Naval and Maritime Medicine During the American Revolution.* Ventnor, New Jersey: Ventnor Publishers, 1978.

Greene, A. *Recollections of the Jersey Prison Ship, Captain Dring Thomas.* New York: Counth Books, 1829.

Guttmacher, M. S. *America's Last King: An Interpretation of the Madness of George III.* New York: Scribner, 1941.

Hall, C. R. "The Beginnings of American Military Medicine." *Annals of the History of Medicine* 4 (1942): 122–31.

Hawke, D. F. *Benjamin Rush: Revolutionary Gadfly.* Indianapolis: Bobbs Merrill, 1971.

Hawkins, C. *The Adventures of Christopher Hawkins.* New York: Charles I. Bushwell, 1964.

Hay, J. "George Washington, Conquest of Physical Handicaps." *Hygeia* 9 (1931): 736–39.

Heaton, C. "Medicine in New York During the English Colonial Period." *Bulletin of the History of Medicine* 17 (1945): 9–37.

Heflebow, R. C. "Prisoners of War." *Military Surgeon* 63 (1928): 625–42.

Henry, J. J. *Arnold's Campaign Against Canada.* Albany, N.Y.: Joel Munsell, 1877.

Herbert, C. *A Relic of the Revolution.* Boston: Charles A. Pierce, 1847; reprinted New York: The New York Times and Arno Press, 1968.

Hopkins, D. R. *Princes and Peasants: Smallpox in History.* Chicago: University of Chicago Press 1983.

Hudson, A. E. A and A. Herbert. "James Lind: Historical Contributions to Shipbound Sanitation." *Journal of the History of Medicine and Allied Sciences* 11 (1956): 1–13.

Hughes, R. E. "James Lind and the Cure of Scurvy." An Experimental Approach. *Medical History* 19 (1975): 342–51.

Jackson, R. *A Treatise on the Fevers of Jamaica with Some Observations on the Intermitting Fever of America.* Philadelphia: Robert Campbell, Book Seller, 1795.

Jarcho, S. "A Cartographic and Literary Study of the Word Malaria." *Journal of the History of Medicine and Allied Sciences* 25 (1970): 31–39.

Jelenko, C. "Emergency Medicine in Colonial America, Revolutionary War Casualties." *Annals of Emergency Medicine*, 11, no. 1 (1982): 73–76.

Jones, Goether, Watson. *Handbook of Nautical Medicine.* New York: Springer Verlag,

Jones, E. and R. E. Hughes. "Copper Boilers and the Occurrence of Scurvy." *Medical History* 20 (1976): 80–81.

Jones, J. *Plain, Concise, and Practical Remarks on the Treatment of Wounds and Fractures to Which Is Added an Appendix on Camps and Military Hospitals Principally Designed for the Use of Young Military and Naval Surgeons in North America.* Philadelphia, 1776.

Jones, W. H. S. *Malaria: A Neglected Factor in the History of Greece and Rome.* Cambridge and London: Bowes and Bowes, 1907.

Ketchum, R. E., ed. *American Heritage Book of the Revolution.* New York: American Heritage Publishing, 1958.

Kissane, J. M., ed. *Anderson's Pathology.* 8th ed. St. Louis: Mosby, 1985.

Klein, R. S. *Portrait of an Early American Family.* Philadelphia: University of Pennsylvania Press, 1975.

Knox, M. "The Medical History of George Washington, His Physicians, Friends, and Advisers." *Bulletin of the History of Medicine* 1 (1933): 174–91.

Kooperman, P. E. "Medical Services in the British Army 1742–1783." *Journal of the History of Medicine and Allied Sciences* 34 (1979): 428–455.

Laffin, J. *Surgeons in the Field.* J. M. London: Dent, 1970.

Lee, H. *Memoirs of the War in the Southern Department of the United States.* New York: New York Times and Arno Press, 1969.

Lerkund, M. C. "Colonial Epidemic Disease." *Ciba Symposium* 1 (1939–40).

Levine, V. E. "Scurvy: The Soldier's Calamity." *Military Surgeon* 89 (1941): 140–54.

Lewis, F. O. "Washington's Last Illness." *Annals of Medical History*, n.s., 4 (1932): 245–48.

Libmann, W. M. "Complications of Scabies." *Military Surgeon* 99 (1946): 116–26.

Liston, S. L. "Traumatic Amputation of the External Ear, the War of Jenkin's Ear, and George Washington." *American Journal of Surgery* 148, no. 5 (1984): 599–601.

Lloyd, C., ed. *Health of Seamen.* London and Colchester: Navy Records Society, Spottswood Ballantyne, 1965.

Lloyd, C. and J. L. S. Coulter. *Medicine and the Navy.* Vol. 3. E&S Livingston 1961.

Lutnick, S. *The American Revolution and the British Press, 1775–83.* Columbia: University of Missouri Press, 1967.

Macalpine, I. and R. Hunter. *George III and the Mad Business.* London: Penguin Press, 1969.

Macalpine, I. and R. Hunter. "The Insanity of George III: A Classic Case of Porphyria." *British Medical Journal* 1 (1966): 65–67.

Macalpine, I. and R. Hunter. "Porphyria in the Royal House of Stuart, Hanover, and Prussia." *British Medical Journal* 1 (1968): 7–18.

Maclay, E. S. *A History of American Privateers.* New York: B. Franklin Publishers, 1899.

Maclay, E. S. *A History of the U. S. Navy, 1775–1893.* New York: Appleton, 1894.

Major, J. H. *Disease and Destiny.* New York: Appleton Century, 1936.

Manchester, K. E. "General Washington and the Patriot Soldiers." *Journal of the American Dietetic Association* 68, no. 5 (May 1976): 421–33.

Mandell, C. and R. G. Douglas, J. E. Bennett. *Principles and Practices of Infectious Disease.* NY, Edinburgh, London, Melbourne: Wiley Medical Publisher, 1979.

Mann, W. J. "Health and Physical Efficiency, Naval Warfare." *Military Surgeon* 94 (1944): 4–8.

Marks, G. and W. K. Beathe. *The History of Medicine in America.* New York: Scribner, 1973.

Marx. R. *The Health of Presidents.* New York: Putnam, 1960.

McSherry, J. A. "Reiter's Syndrome and the American Revolutionary War" *Practitioner* 226, no. 1366 (April 1982): 94–95.

Middleton, W. S. "John Morgan: Father of Medical Education in North America." *Annals of Medical History* 9 (1927): 13–26.

Middleton, W. S. "Medicine at Valley Forge." *Annals of the History of Medicine,* 3rd ser., 3, no. 6 (1941): 461–86.

Middleton, W. S. "William Shippen, Jr." *Annals of Medical History,* n. s., 4 (1922): 441–52.

Miller, G. *The Adoption of Inoculation for Smallpox in England and France.* Philadelphia: University of Pennsylvania Press, 1957.

Mitchell, B. *The Price of Independence: A Review of the American Revolution.* New York: Oxford University Press, 1974.

Montross, L. *Rag, Tag, and Bobtail The Story of the Continental Army, 1775–1783.* New York: Harper and Brothers, 1952.

Morgan, J. *A Vindication of His Public Character in the Station of Director of the Military Hospital and Physician-in-Chief of the American Army, 1776.* Boston: Powers and Willis, 1777.

Morrison, S. E. *John Paul Jones.* Boston: Northeastern University Press, 1959.

Moxness, B. A. "Care of the War Disabled Prior to the World War." *Military Surgeon* 75 (1935): 113–32.

Nadeau, G. "A German Military Surgeon in Rutland, Massachusetts, During the Revolution." *Bulletin of the History of Medicine* 18 (1945): 243–300.

Northcote, W. *Extracts from the Marine Practice of Physic and Surgery, Including Nature and Treatment of Gunshot Wounds by John Ranby.* Philadelphia 1776.

Olch, P. "The Morgan-Shippen Controversy." *Review of Surgery* 22, nos. 1–2, (1965): 1–8.

Orkin, M., Parish, Schwartzman. *Scabies and Pediculosis.* Philadelphia: Lippincott, 1977.

Owen, W. *Medical Department of the United States Army During the Revolution.* New York: Paul B. Hoeber, 1920.

Packard, F. *The Life and Times of Ambroise Paré, 1510–90.* New York: Paul B. Hoeber, 1921.

Parkhurst, R. "The History and Traditional Treatment of Smallpox in Ethiopia." *Medical History* 9 (1975): 343–53.

Phalen, J. "Doctors at Arms: Joseph Warren, Minute Man." *Military Surgeon* 92 (1943): 658–61.

Phalen, J. "Surgeon James Mann's Observations on Battlefield Amputations." *Military Surgeon* 87 (1940): 463–66.

Potter, I. R. *Life and Remarkable Adventures of Israel R. Potter.* New York: Counth Books, 1962.

Poynter, P. *Evolution of the Hospital in Britain.* London: Medical Publishing, 1964.

Preble, C. H. ed. *The Diary of Ezra Green, M. D. , Surgeon on Board the Continental Ship of War, Ranger,* Boston, 1875.

Pringle, J. *Observations on the Diseases of the Army.* 1752.

Radbill, S. X. "Francis Allison, Jr.: A Surgeon of the Revolution." *Bulletin of the History of Medicine,* 9 (1941): 243–57.

Ranby, J. *Nature and Treatment of Gunshot Wounds.* Philadelphia, 1776.

Ready, M. "Army Doctors, Four Short-Term Medical Chiefs." *Military Medicine* 132 (1967): 188–94.

Reiser, S. "The Colonial Physician." *Military Medicine* 142, no. 4, ( ) 306–07.

Roberts, L. *Memoirs of Captain Lemuel Roberts.* Bennington, Vt., 1808.

Roddes, L. H. "A Short History of Nautical Medicine," *Annals of Medical History* 3 (1941): 203–47.

Roddes, L. H. *A Short History of Nautical Medicine.* New York and London: Paul B. Hoeber, 1941.

Roemer, M. I. "The History of the Effects of War on Medicine." *Annals of Medical History* 3rd ser., 4 (1942): 189–99.

Rosebury, T. *Microbes and Morals.* New York: Viking Press, 1971.

Rosen, G. "Occupational Diseases of English Seamen During the Seventeenth and Eighteenth Centuries." *Bulletin of Medical History* 7 (1939): 251–58.

Rucker, M. P. "Benjamin Rush Obstetrician." *Annals of Medical History,* 3rd ser., 3 (1941): 487–500.

Rush, B. *The Autobiography of Benjamin Rush.* Ed. B. C. Corner. Princeton: Princeton University Press, 1948.

Rush, B. *The Letters of Benjamin Rush.* Ed. L. H. Butterfield. Princeton: Princeton University Press, 1951.

Rush, B. *Medical Inquiries and Observations.* Philadelphia: Greggs and Dickinsons, 1815, Philadelphia: Thomas Dobson, 1794–1798.

Russell, P. F. *Man's Mastery of Malaria.* London: Oxford University Press, 1955.

Saffron, M. "Rebels and Disease, The New York Campaign 1776." *Academy of Medicine New York Bulletin* 13 (June 1967): 104–18.

Saffron, M. "John Cochran, 1730–1807: Director General of the Hospital of the United States." *Transcriptions and Studies of the College of Physicians of Philadelphia* 42–3 (1974/76): 379–87.

Saffron, M. *Surgeon to Washington, Dr. John Cochran.* New York: Columbia University Press, 1977.

Schmitz, R. "Hessian Troops in the American Revolution." *Minnesota Medicine* 7 (1976).

Selavan, I. C. "Nurses in American History: The Revolution." *American Journal of Nursing.* 4 (1975): 592–94.

Selveyn, S. "Sir John Pringle: Hospital Reformer, Moral Philosopher, and Pioneer of the Antisepsis." *Medical History* 10: 266–74.

Senter, I. *The Journal of Isaac Senter.* Philadelphia: Historical Society of Pennsylvania, 1946.

Shands, A. "James Tilton, M. D.: Delaware's Greatest Physician." *Delaware Medical Journal* (January 1974).

Shyrock, R. *Eighteenth-Century Medicine in America.* Worcester, Md.: American Antiquarian Society, 1950.

Simmons, J. "Influence of Epidemic Disease on the Early History of the Western Hemisphere." *Military Surgeon* 71 (1932): 133–43.

Stanley, G. F. G. *Canada Invaded.* Toronto: Hakkert Publishers, 1973.

Stein, J. H. *Internal Medicine.* 2nd ed. Boston: Little Brown, 1987.

Stewart, C. K. and T. Miller. *Moving the Wounded.* Fort Collins, CO: Old Army Press, 1979.

Stimson, J. "The Forerunners of the American Army Nurses." *Military Surgeon* 58 (1926): 133–41.

Swediaur, F. *Symptoms, Effects, and Therapy of Syphilis.* Philadelphia: Thomas Dobson Publishers, 1815, originally published in London, 1784.

Taillot, L. "Early Army Surgeons," *Ciba Symposium* (1939–40).

Thacher, James. *Military Journal of the American Revolution, 1775–83.* Boston: Coltons and Barnard, 1827.

Thoms, H. "Albigence Waldo, Surgeon." *Annals of Medical History* 10 (1928): 486–97.
Thursfield, H. "Smallpox in the American War of Independence." *Annals of Medical History*, 3rd ser. of 2 (1940): 312–18.
Tiggert, W. D. "A 1759 Spotted Fever Epidemic in North Carolina," *Journal of the History of Medicine and Allied Sciences*. 42, no. 7, (1987): 296–304.
Tilton, J. *Economical Observations on Military Hospitals*. Wilmington, Del. 1803.
Tobey, I. A. "Preventable Disease in the Washington Family." *Hygeria* 13 (1935): 118–21.
Torres-Reyes, R. "The 1779–80 Encampment." *A Study of Medical Services*. Washington, D.C.: U.S. Department of Interior, 1971.
Truax, R. *The Brothers Warren of Boston: First Family of Surgery*. Boston: Houghton-Mifflin, 1968.
Trussel, J. B. B. *Birthplace of an Army: A Study of Valley Forge*. Harrisburg: Pennsylvania History and Museum Commission, 1976.
Van Swenenberg, D. "The Suttons and the Business of Inoculation." *Medical History* 22 (1978): 71–82.
Von Swieten, G. *The Diseases Incident to Armies with the Method of Cure. Also the Nature and Treatment of Gunshot Wounds by John Ranby*. Philadelphia 1776.
Wangensteen, O. et al. "Some Highlights in the History of Amputation, Reflecting Lessons in Wound Healing." *Bulletin of the History of Medicine* 41 (1967): 97–131.
Waring, J. I. "James Killpatrick and Smallpox Inoculation in Charleston." *Annals of Medical History* 10 (1938): 301–18.
Waring, J. I.—"The Influence of Benjamin Rush on Bleeding in South Carolina." *Bulletin of Medical History*. 35 (1961): 230–7.
Washington, G. *Basic Writings of George Washington*. Ed. S. Commins. New York: Random House, 1948.
Washington, G. *The Diaries of George Washington*. Ed D. Jackson. Vols. 1–6. Charlottesville: University of Virginia Press, 1976.
Watson, W. "Two British Naval Surgeons of the French Wars." *Medical History* 13 (1969): 213–25.
Wilbur, C. K. *Revolutionary Medicine, 1700–1800*. Chester, Conn.: Globe Pequot Press, 1980.
Williams, F. A. and T. F. Keys. "The Medical History of George Washington." *Proceedings of the Staff Meetings of the Mayo Clinic* 17 (February, 1942): 92–112.
Wilbur, C. K. *Picture Book of the Revolution's Privateers*. Harrisburg, Pa.: Stackpole, 1973.
Wilson, L. "The Clinical Definition of Scurvy and the Discovery of Vitamin C." *Journal of the History of Medicine and Allied Sciences* 30 (1975): 40–60.
Winslow. *A Destroying Angel*. Boston: Houghton-Mifflin, 1874.
Wooden, A. C. "Dr. Jean Francois Coste and the French Army in the American Revolution." *Delaware Medical Journal* 48, no. 7 (1976): 397–402.
Wooden, A. C. "The Wounds and Weapons of the Revolutionary War, 1775–1783." *Delaware Medical Journal* 44, no. 3 (March 1972).
Zinsser, H. *Rats, Lice, and History*. Boston: Atlantic Monthly Press, 1934.

Index